The
ACNES

The
ACNES

SECOND EDITION

Editor
Jayakar Thomas
MD DD MNAMS FRCP FRCPCH PhD DSc
Emeritus Professor
Department of Dermatology
Chettinad Academy of Research and Education
Chennai, Tamil Nadu, India

Co-editor
Parimalam Kumar
MD DD MNAMS FRCP iFAAD FIAD
Former Head of Dermatology
Madras Medical College
Chennai, Tamil Nadu, India

Foreword
D Prabhavathy

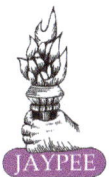

JAYPEE BROTHERS MEDICAL PUBLISHERS
The Health Sciences Publisher
New Delhi | London

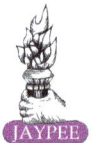 **Jaypee Brothers Medical Publishers (P) Ltd**

Headquarters
EMCA House
23/23-B, Ansari Road, Daryaganj
New Delhi 110 002, India
Landline: +91-11-23272143, +91-11-23272703
+91-11-23282021, +91-11-23245672
E-mail: jaypee@jaypeebrothers.com

Corporate Office
Jaypee Brothers Medical Publishers (P) Ltd.
4838/24, Ansari Road, Daryaganj
New Delhi 110 002, India
Phone: +91-11-43574357
Fax: +91-11-43574314
E-mail: jaypee@jaypeebrothers.com

Overseas Office
JP Medical Ltd.
83, Victoria Street, London
SW1H 0HW (UK)
Phone: +44-20 3170 8910
Fax: +44(0)20 3008 6180
E-mail: info@jpmedpub.com

Website: www.jaypeebrothers.com
Website: www.jaypeedigital.com

© 2024, Jaypee Brothers Medical Publishers

The views and opinions expressed in this book are solely those of the original contributor(s)/author(s) and do not necessarily represent those of editor(s) or publisher of the book.

All rights reserved. No part of this publication may be reproduced, stored or transmitted in any form or by any means, electronic, mechanical, photocopying, recording or otherwise, without the prior permission in writing of the publishers.

All brand names and product names used in this book are trade names, service marks, trademarks or registered trademarks of their respective owners. The publisher is not associated with any product or vendor mentioned in this book.

Medical knowledge and practice change constantly. This book is designed to provide accurate, authoritative information about the subject matter in question. However, readers are advised to check the most current information available on procedures included and check information from the manufacturer of each product to be administered, to verify the recommended dose, formula, method and duration of administration, adverse effects and contraindications. It is the responsibility of the practitioner to take all appropriate safety precautions. Neither the publisher nor the author(s)/editor(s) assume any liability for any injury and/or damage to persons or property arising from or related to use of material in this book.

This book is sold on the understanding that the publisher is not engaged in providing professional medical services. If such advice or services are required, the services of a competent medical professional should be sought.

Every effort has been made where necessary to contact holders of copyright to obtain permission to reproduce copyright material. If any have been inadvertently overlooked, the publisher will be pleased to make the necessary arrangements at the first opportunity.

Inquiries for bulk sales may be solicited at: jaypee@jaypeebrothers.com

The Acnes / Jayakar Thomas

First Edition: 2019

Second Edition: **2024**

ISBN: 978-93-5696-275-0

Dedicated to

The many dermatologists who provide care to their patients with acne, to my committed teachers of dermatology, and, most of all, to my beloved spouse for her care, love, and affection without which this humble piece of work would not have been a reality.

Foreword

It is a privilege to write the foreword for the book by Professor Jayakar Thomas. I have listened to numerous orations and talks delivered by him as well as gone through a lot of his books, chapters in books, and articles.

In medicine, it is important to diagnose and treat common conditions more effectively rather than concentrating on rare disorders since the bulk of our patients fall into the former category. Acne is one of the most common conditions encountered in clinical practice and it is also one of the most psychologically crippling disorders. The social and psychological aspects of acne are very important notably because it affects individuals during adolescence when personality development takes place.

When acne is very severe or not properly treated, it leads to scars which persist for life and cannot be cured completely leading to decrease in self-esteem in some individuals. Moreover, the treatment for scars is considerably more painful and also expensive compared to the treatment of acne. Therefore, it is important to hit acne early and hit it hard. It is also important to rule out various conditions associated with acne.

The Acnes covers every aspect of acne and should be read by every dermatologist since the bulk of patients coming to a dermatologist have acne. The boxes and tables are especially informative and help in easy understanding.

D Prabhavathy MD DD
Former Professor and Head
Department of Dermatology
Madras Medical College
Chennai, Tamil Nadu, India

Preface to the Second Edition

Acne is among the most common skin conditions worldwide. Despite this fact, accurate information about acne is scarce.

Myths about acne are as common as the skin problem. It is essential that all medical practitioners know about acne.

This second edition of *The Acnes* is aimed to serve both general practitioners and dermatologists—mainly for the latter.

We hope this book is a helpful tool, not only for the student who needs an expert source of basic knowledge in the different forms of acne, but also for the pressured practitioner who needs a clear, concise, and balanced distillation of the best information on which to base daily clinical decisions.

At times, the science presented might seem overwhelming. But one can start reading from any chapter, based on one's interests, tastes, and preferences. A chapter on **What is New in Acne Vulgaris—from Recent Literature** has been included.

Jayakar Thomas
Parimalam Kumar

Preface to the First Edition

Acne is among the most common skin condition worldwide. Despite this fact, accurate information about acne is scarce.

Myths about acne are as common as the skin problem. It is essential that all medical practitioners know about acne.

This book, *The Acnes*, is aimed to serve both general practitioners and dermatologists—mainly for the latter.

We hope this book is a helpful tool, not only for the student who needs an expert source of basic knowledge in the different forms of acne, but also for the pressured practitioner who needs a clear, concise, and balanced distillation of the best information on which to base daily clinical decisions.

At times, the science presented might seem overwhelming. But one can start reading from any chapter, based on one's interests, tastes, and preferences.

Jayakar Thomas
Parimalam Kumar
Deepthi Ravi

Contents

CHAPTER 1: Introduction — 1

CHAPTER 2: Etiopathogenesis — 3

CHAPTER 3: Clinical Features — 26

CHAPTER 4: Types and Variants of Acne — 39

CHAPTER 5: Course and Complications — 87

CHAPTER 6: Assessment and Investigation — 99

CHAPTER 7: Treatment — 106

CHAPTER 8: What is New in Acne Vulgaris—from Recent Literature — 143

Suggested Readings — 165

Index — 171

CHAPTER 1

Introduction

Acne vulgaris (*acme* meaning prime of life and *vulgus* meaning common) is a common inflammatory disorder of the pilosebaceous unit seen primarily in adolescents. It is one of the most common skin diseases affecting the youth. Nevertheless, acne is seen worldwide in all age groups from newborn to old age. It affects all ethnicities and races. The clinical manifestations of varying extents and severities pose a challenge to the treating physician. Although the course of acne may be self-limiting even without treatment in some of the affected individuals, the sequela like scars persist lifelong in many. Despite best of treatment, not infrequently in disease results in significant psychosocial morbidity leading to tremendous stress in the affected individual. With proper understanding of the etiopathogenesis, astute knowledge about the various clinical presentations, and updated data on the therapeutic armamentarium currently available to treat the disease, every person with acne can be assured of the best medicosurgical assistance and better outcome to give the best cosmetic result possible.

EPIDEMIOLOGY

Acne is a disorder seen worldwide. It is a disorder primarily of the teenagers but can be seen even in newborn children and old adults. Apart from genetics, various factors play a role in the onset, course, severity, and response to treatment in an acne patient.

Age and Gender

Acne is, by and large, a disease of the teenagers. However, the age of acne can be from as early as newborn till as old as even sixth decade. The age of onset of acne varies considerably. Acne vulgaris can have its onset even in the prepubertal age and may start as early as 6–8 years of age. In some persons, the onset can be delayed to as late as 20 years of age or even later. It is not uncommon to see acne in the neonate and as a disturbing ailment in adults as late as in their sixth decade. Acne often heralds the onset of puberty and is not until such time is considered as a significant problem. Though >85% of adolescents develop acne, not all seek medical attention at an earlier date, may be because of the self-limiting nature of the disease in some, if not all. Earlier onset of puberty, obesity, diet, and other lifestyle factors play significant role in earlier onset of the disease in addition to the positive family history. Awareness and recognition of the problem contribute to increased hospital attendance.

Acne most commonly presents between 10 and 13 years of age. There is no major gender difference in the onset and clinical manifestation. However, girls have an earlier onset which can be easily attributed to the earlier onset of puberty in girls than in boys.

No ethnic group is exempt from the development of acne and a higher prevalence was observed between 15 and 20 years of age. As the age of menarche in girls advances, so does the age of onset of acne in the female gender. However, the disease severity is more in boys during the late adolescence. Persistence of acne through the third decade is not uncommon. Both persistent and late or onset acne are seen more frequently in females. Women with XYY genotype are more prone for such severe forms of acne. A more severe form of acne variant, acne fulminans, is more common in males as against females, which affects males between 13 and 22 years of age.

Based on the age of onset, acne is classified as given in **Table 1**.

TABLE 1: Acne classification based on the age of onset.

Age of onset	Classification of acne
Birth to 6 weeks	Neonatal acne
6 weeks to 1 year	Infantile acne
1–7 years	Mid-childhood acne
7–12 years	Preadolescent or prepubertal acne
12–19 years or after menarche in girls	Adolescent acne

CHAPTER 2

Etiopathogenesis

Etiopathogenesis of acne (**Figs. 1 to 40**) is multifactorial and is influenced by the hormonal and immune functioning of a genetically prone individual. As quoted by Shelly, acne is regularly diagnosed by public, but the physicians need to make observations of the cause without which effective management with no or minimum disfigurement is difficult to be accomplished. There are four important key elements interrelated in the development of acne. These fundamental components of etiological causes of acne include follicular hyperkeratinization, seborrhea, inflammation, and infection by *Cutibacterium acnes*. The four major pathologic factors in the ethology of acne are given in **Box 1**.

In recent days, there is enough evidence to prove the role played by the innate immunity in the pathogenesis of acne. The influence of genetics, diet, and environmental factors in the precipitation or perpetuation of acne are also discussed.

BOX 1	Major pathogenic factors in acne.
• Follicular epidermal hyperproliferation • Increased sebum production • Inflammation • *Cutibacterium acnes*	

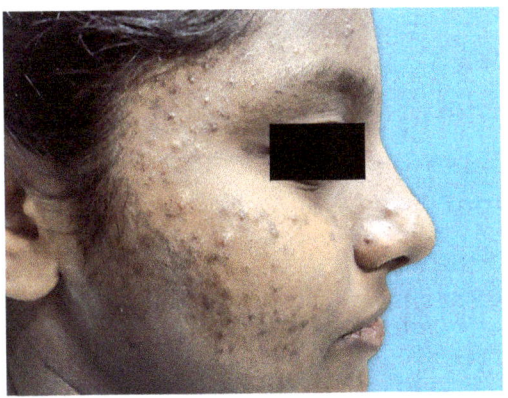

FIG. 1: Ductal hypercornification is an important feature in the etiology of acne which can be seen histologically as microcomedones and clinically as macrocomedones.

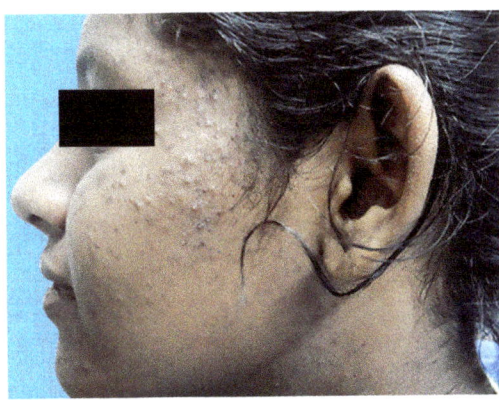

FIG. 2: Same patient as in Figure 1.

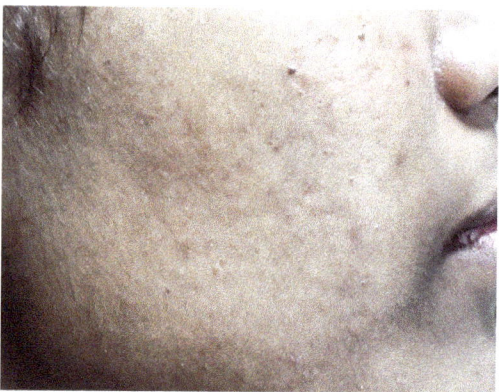

FIG. 3: Presence of microcomedones is a measure of comedogenesis.

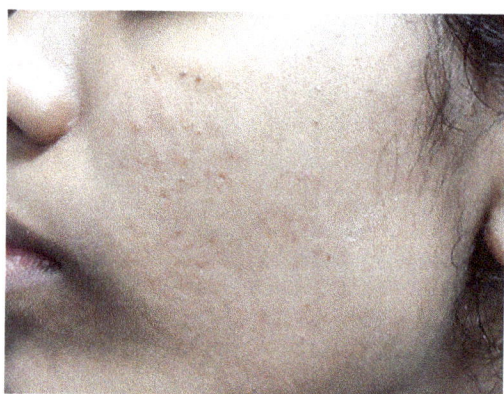

FIG. 4: Severity of acne correlates well with the number and size of microcomedones.

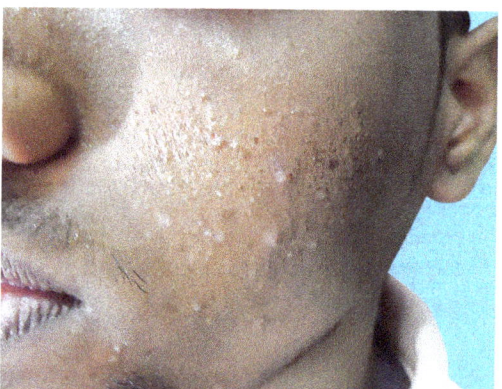

FIG. 5: A boy with comedones resulting from abnormalities in the proliferation and differentiation of ductal keratinocytes.

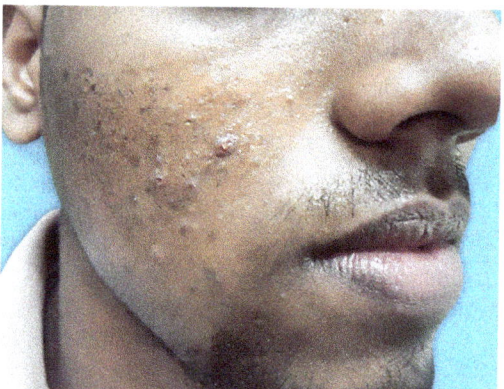

FIG. 6: Same patient as in Figure 5.

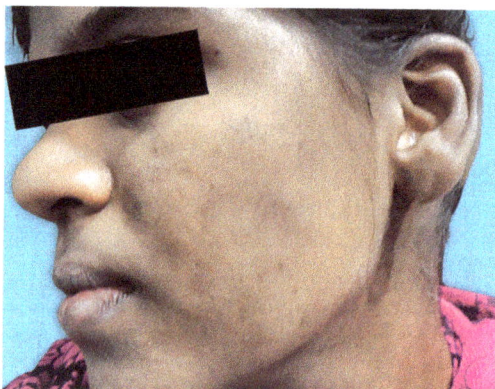

FIG. 7: Teenager showing few papules along with comedones representing the retention of keratinocytes in the duct.

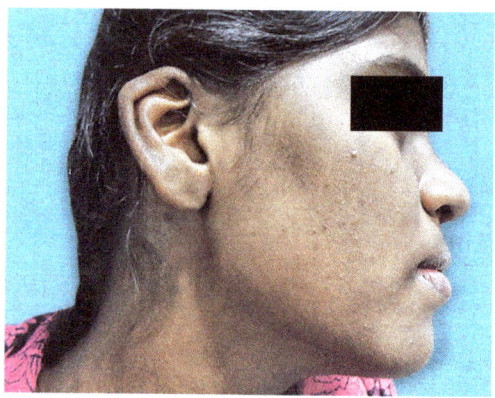

FIG. 8: Same patient as in Figure 7.

CHAPTER 2: Etiopathogenesis

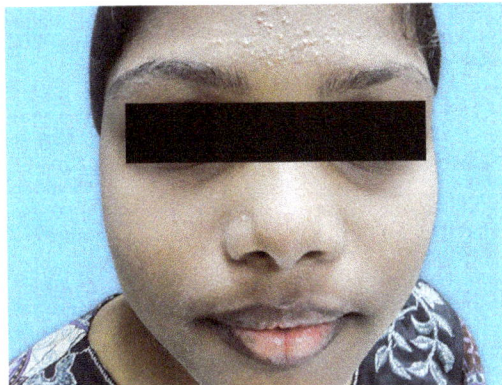

FIG. 9: A young girl with acne where microcomedones are found even in clinically normal looking adjacent skin.

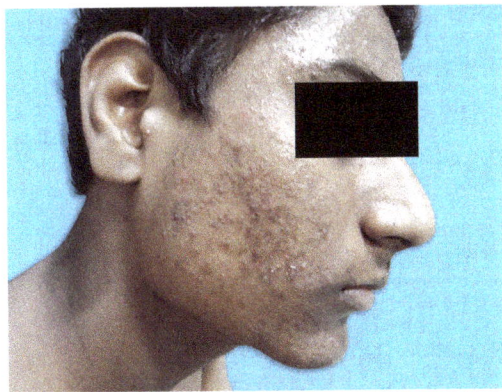

FIG. 10: Comedones are temporary structures which either evolve to more severe form of acne or resolve.

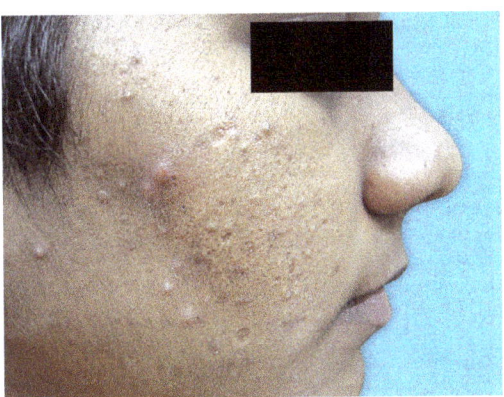

FIG. 11: A woman with premenstrual flare probably due to increased skin hydration temporarily blocking the pilosebaceous orifice.

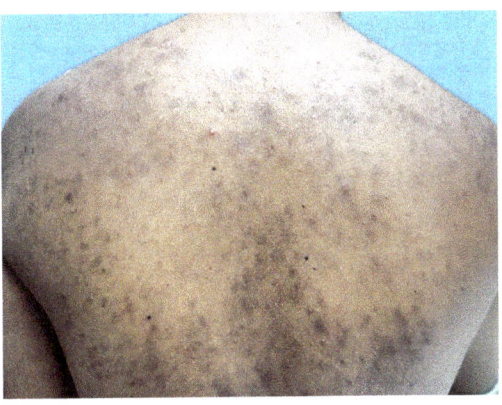

FIG. 12: Acne over a male's back skin shows higher numbers of microorganisms in the upper part of the follicles.

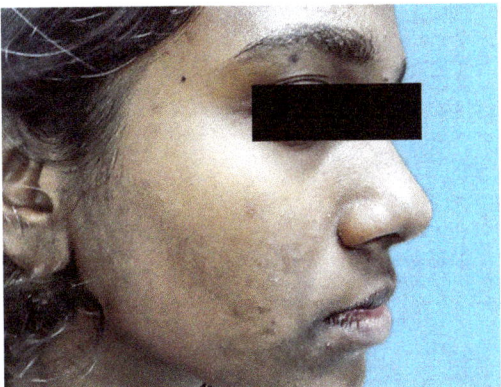

FIG. 13: Female facial skin with acne shows higher numbers of microorganisms in the upper part of the follicles.

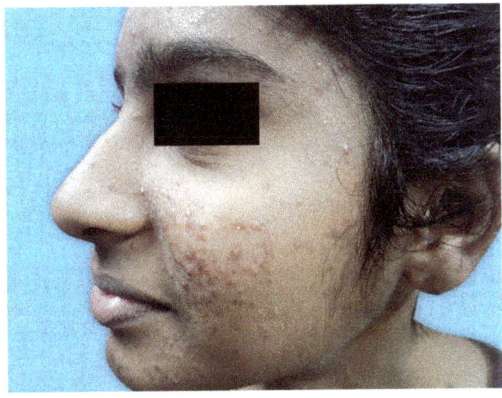

FIG. 14: Acne in a patient who regularly used creams where comedogenesis is induced by isopropyl myristate.

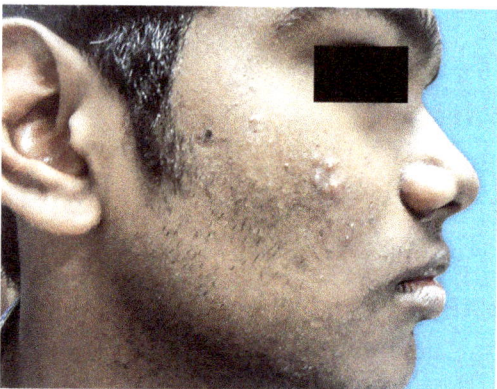

FIG. 15: Ingredients of some cosmetics such as propylene glycol, and D and C red dyes inducing comedone formation in this boy.

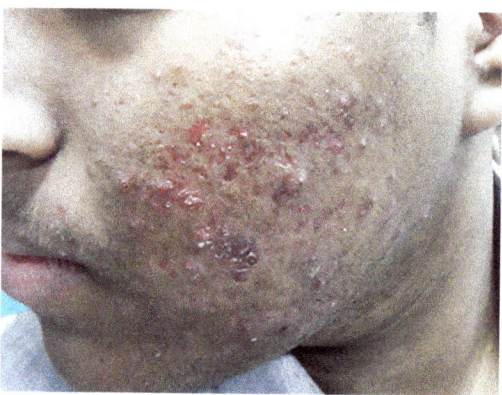

FIG. 16: Rupture of the sebolamellar sheath leading to discharge of excretion of products which may contribute to comedogenesis.

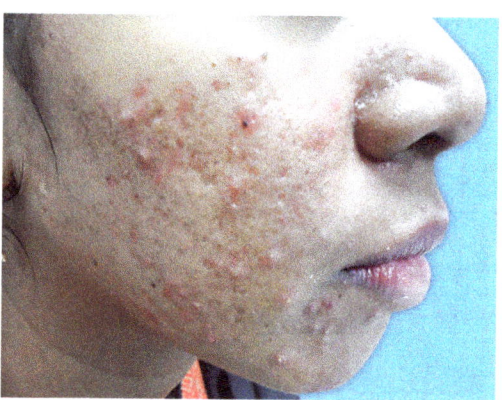

FIG. 17: Acne is primarily a noninfective disease.

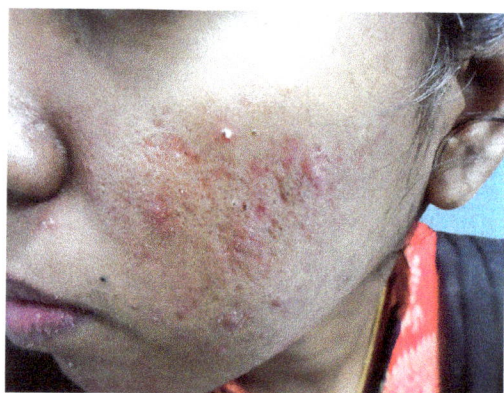

FIG. 18: Same patient as in Figure 17.

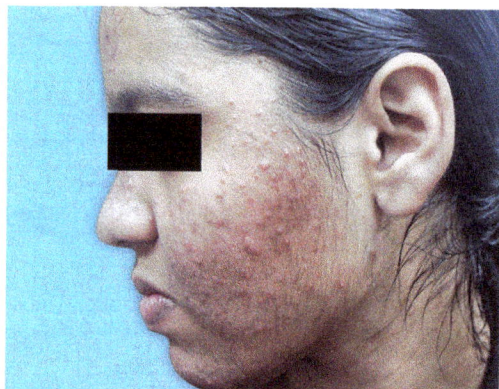

FIG. 19: Inflammatory acne can be viewed as an infection of the blocked pilosebaceous ducts with cutibacteria trapped by cornified plugs within the follicular ducts.

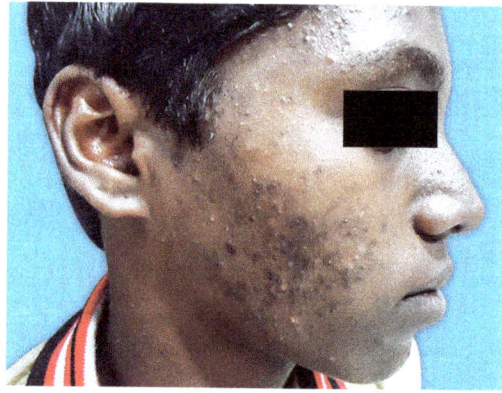

FIG. 20: Seborrhea in an adolescent which is associated with significant increase in *Cutibacterium acnes* numbers.

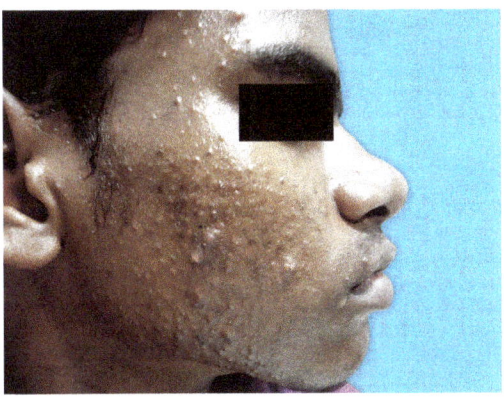

FIG. 21: Grade III acne with seborrhea; however, there is little or no relationship between the number of bacteria on the skin surface and the severity of acne.

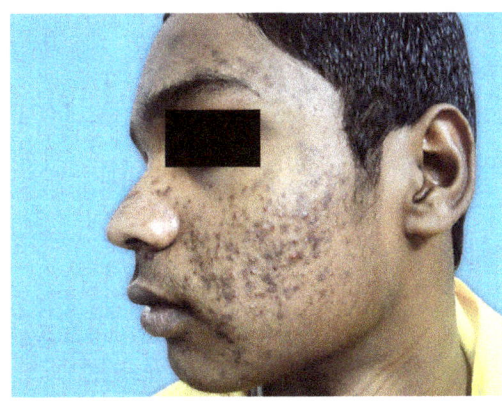

FIG. 22: A boy with severe acne; there seems to be a direct relationship between the number of follicular organisms and severity of the disease

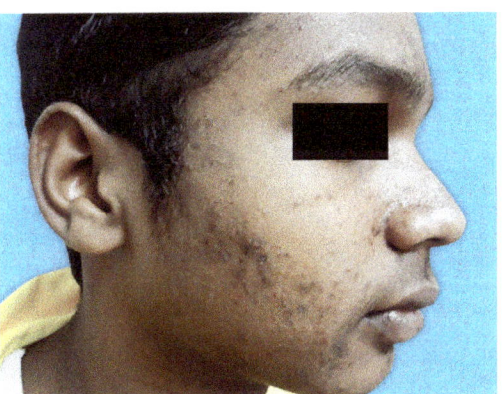

FIG. 23: Same patient as in Figure 22.

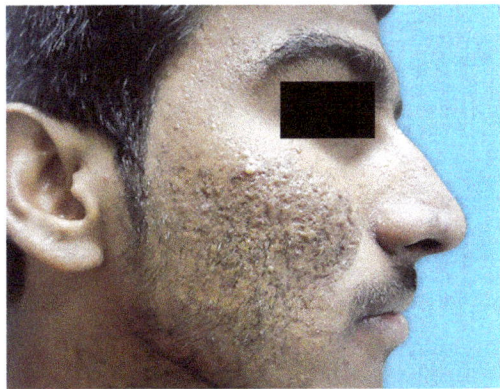

FIG. 24: Damage to basement membrane, leakage of comedonal contents in dermis triggers adaptive immune response to ductal antigens leading to inflammation as in this boy with severe acne.

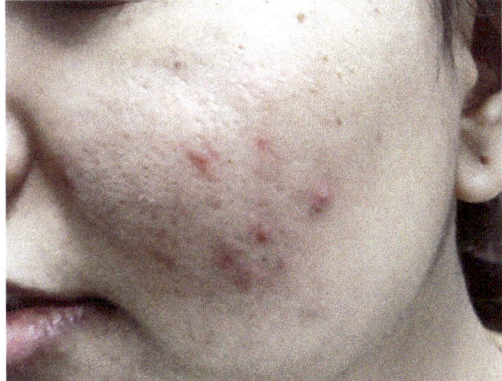

FIG. 25: Infiltrate around early inflamed lesions is predominantly comprised of CD4+ T cells and macrophages.

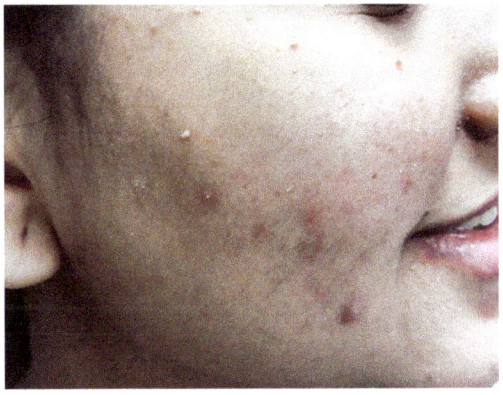

FIG. 26: Right lateral view of Figure 25.

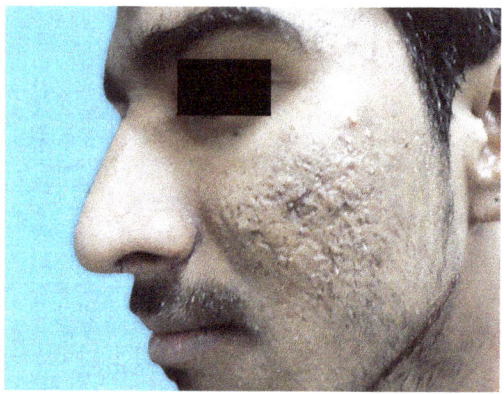

FIG. 27: Inflammatory acne with pustules and scars; it has been documented that inflammation in acne occurs prior to hyperproliferation of the follicular wall.

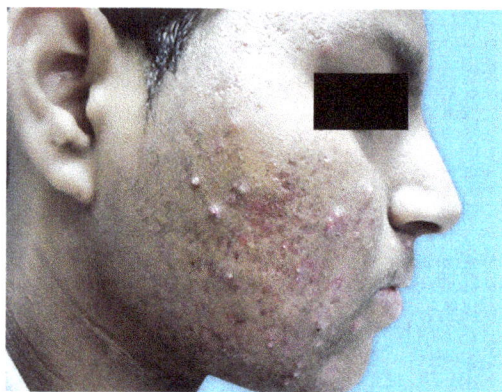

FIG. 28: A boy showing comedones and pustules; individual sensitivity and tolerance to potential causal antigens determine the clinical manifestations.

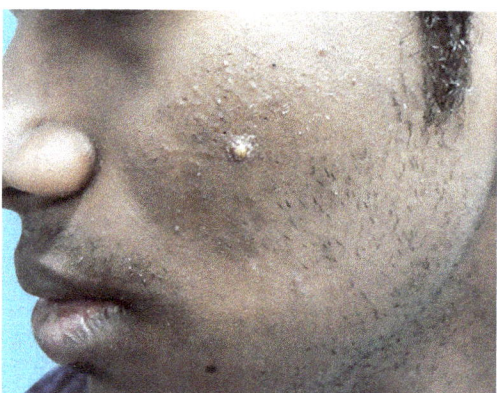

FIG. 29: A boy with comedonal acne; the integrity of the skin and ductal barrier function influence the type of acne lesion.

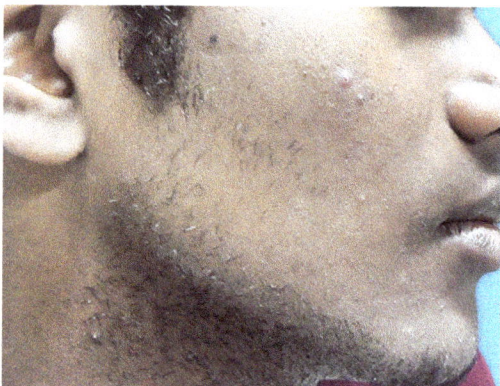

FIG. 30: Same patient as in Figure 29.

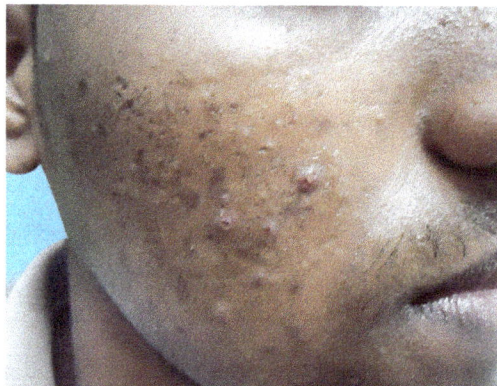

FIG. 31: Acne in a boy consuming junk food which is a cause or an aggravator of acne.

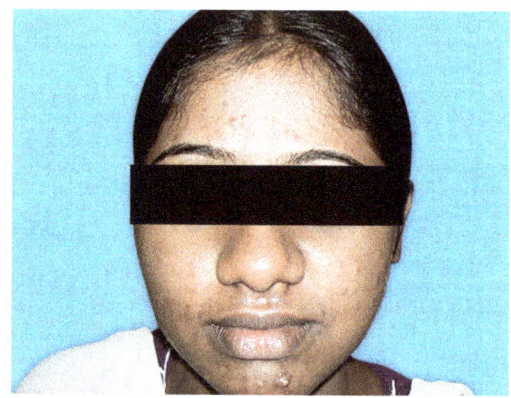

FIG. 32: Premenstrual seborrhea in a girl, a frequent and distressing feature in acne patients.

CHAPTER 2: Etiopathogenesis

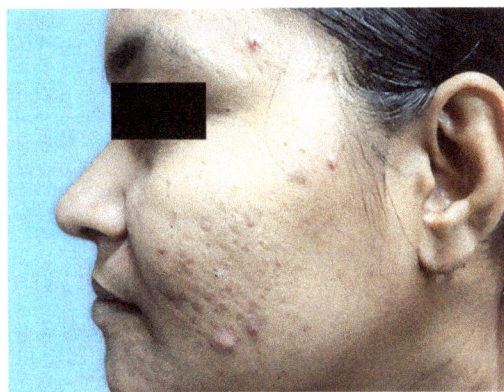

FIG. 33: Grade II acne in a cook—sweating and ductal hydration may be the responsible factors.

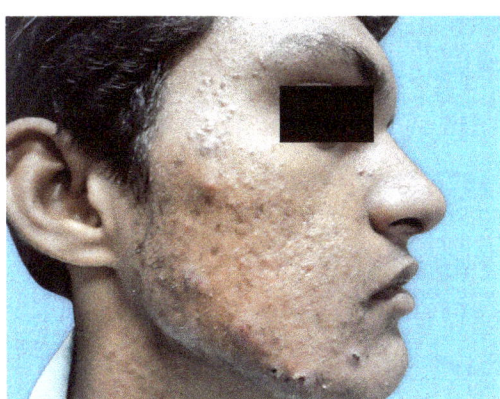

FIG. 34: Severe acne in a smoker.

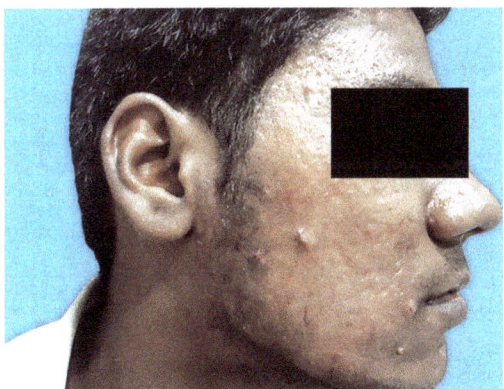

FIG. 35: Stress can aggravate and define chronicity of acne.

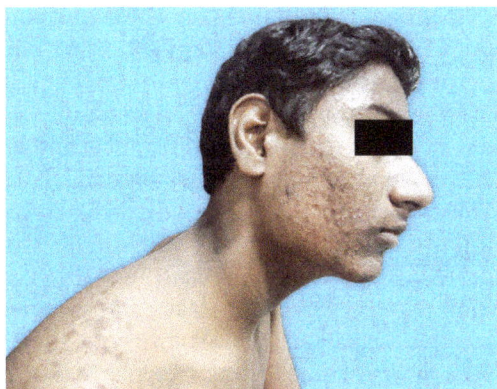

FIG. 36: Acne in a boy with strong family history indicates a chronic course.

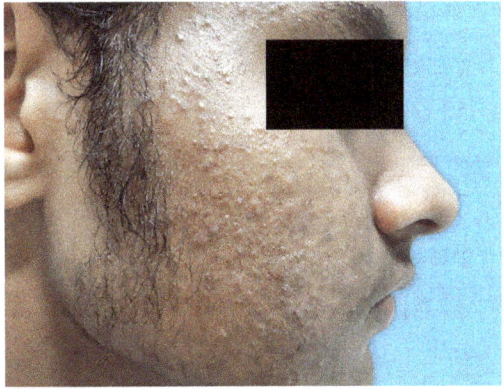

FIG. 37: Acute outbreak after a period of remission, a forerunner for chronic course of the disease.

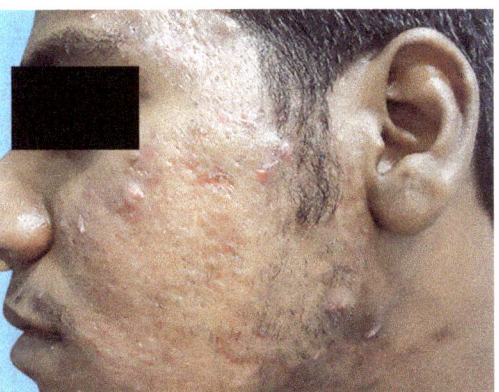

FIG. 38: Prolonged course despite proper adherence to therapy designates a chronic course.

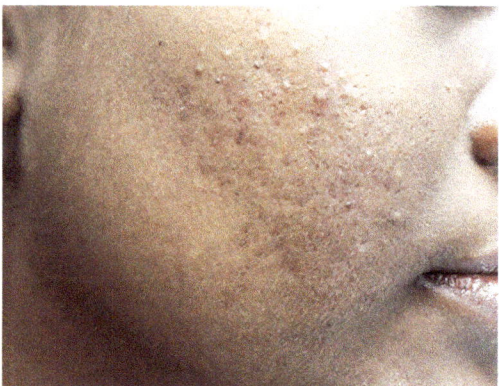

FIG. 39: Premenstrual lesions in a girl with acne; note the ice pick scars.

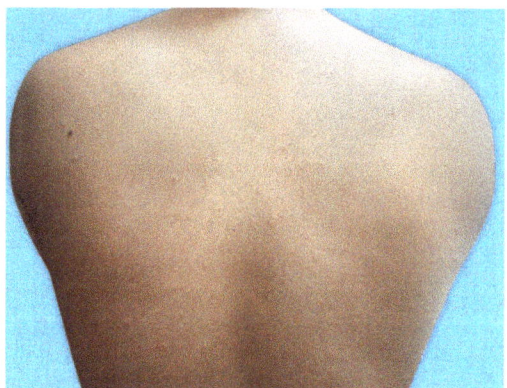

FIG. 40: Few scattered papules of acne in a boy with regular oil application.

Numerous predisposing factors attribute to the development, manifestation, and perpetuation of acne. These are mostly metabolic disturbances involving androgenic steroids, a state of insulin resistance, and an enhanced growth factor receptor-2 signaling. There is always an increased tendency for inflammation in those individuals who develop severe acne and scarring. However, underlying endocrinological abnormalities could not be detected in majority of patients with severe grades of acne. This makes it important that the term "endocrine acne" should be reserved only to those individuals exhibiting clear symptoms and signs of endocrine disturbance supported by laboratory evidence.

Polycystic ovarian syndrome (PCOS) and insulin resistance are common conditions predisposing a person to acne.

Box 2 gives the list of predisposing/associated conditions in acne.

PATHOGENESIS

Acne is a dynamic disorder with several contributing factors and causal pathways.

However, the essential pathognomonic features are follicular epidermal hyperproliferation and an increased amount of sebum production leading to adherence of the dead cells in the follicle leading to clogging

BOX 2	Predisposing or associated conditions in acne.

- Premature adrenarche
- Premature puberty
- Polycystic ovarian syndrome
- Insulin resistance
- Hyperinsulinemia
- Nonclassical congenital adrenal hyperplasia
- Apert's syndrome
- Anorexia nervosa
- Turner syndrome
- Laron syndrome
- Mayer–Rokitansky–Küster–Hauser syndrome
- Cushing's syndrome
- Ectopic ACTH syndrome
- SAHA syndrome
- APAAN syndrome
- PAPA syndrome
- PASH syndrome
- PASS syndrome
- SAPHO syndrome
- HAIR-AN syndrome
- Adrenal and ovarian tumors
- Male pseudohermaphroditism
- Complete androgen insensitivity syndrome
- Exaggerated adrenarche

(ACTH: adrenocorticotropic hormone; APAAN: acne, patterned alopecia, acanthosis nigricans; HAIR-AN: hyperandrogenism, insulin resistance, and acanthosis nigricans; PAPA: pyogenic arthritis, pyoderma gangrenosum, and acne; PASH: pyoderma gangrenosum, acne, and suppurative hidradenitis; PASS: pyoderma gangrenosum, acne, suppurative hidradenitis, ankylosing spondylitis; SAHA: seborrhea, acne, hirsutism, alopecia; SAPHO: synovitis, acne, pustulosis, hyperostosis, and osteitis)

CHAPTER 2: Etiopathogenesis

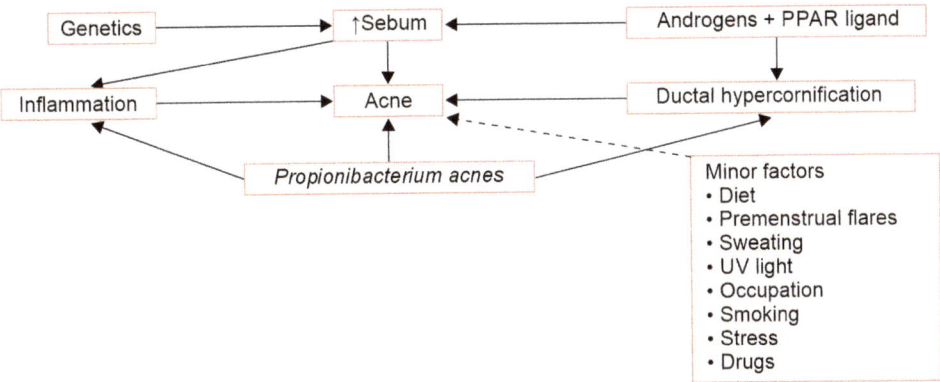

FLOWCHART 1: Schematic representation of contributing factors in the development of acne.
(PPAR: peroxisome proliferator-activated receptor; UV: ultraviolet)

of the follicle which may herald the onset of development of acne, subsequently developing microcomedones and papulopustules. Role of *C. acnes* and release of cytokines will further add on to the evolution of disease. **Flowchart 1** will schematically represent the contributing factors in the development of acne.

The etiopathogenesis of acne involves a variety of factors which sometimes may precipitate acne and acneiform eruptions in a person already having acne or *de novo*. The key factors are always complemented by other coexisting factors in the manifestation of the disease, its severity and therapeutic outcome including the sequelae. **Box 3** gives the list of internal as well as external factors involved in the entire course of the disease.

Genetics

For any disease to manifest, genetic predisposition plays an important role as a major contributing factor. Various aspects of acne influenced by genetics are given in **Box 4**.

The influence of genetic factors in the development of acne is more with monozygotic than dizygotic twins. Similarly, the risk of developing acne is more in first-degree relative of someone with history of acne is up to five times higher than in relatives without a history of acne. It was also documented that genetic susceptibility to adolescent acne is more strongly linked to maternal than paternal lineage. The risk is proportionately increased with the number of family members being affected. It has also been noted that there are many genetic loci identified for sebaceous gland size and lipogenesis. Genetic studies

> **BOX 3** Factors involved in etiopathogenesis of acne.
>
> - *General factors involved in etiopathogenesis of acne:*
>   - Genetics
> - *Environmental factors:*
>   - Diet
>   - Birth weight and body mass index
>   - Smoking and alcohol
>   - Stress and sleep deprivation
>   - Menstrual cycle and pregnancy
>   - Cosmetics
>   - Occupation
>   - Seasonal variation and ultraviolet radiation
>   - Drugs and hormones
>   - Miscellaneous
> - *Key etiopathogenic factors:*
>   - Follicular epidermal hyperproliferation
>   - Increased sebum production
>   - Inflammation
>   - *Cutibacterium acnes*

> **BOX 4** | **Role of genetics in acne.**
>
> *Genetic influence in acne*:
> - Severity
> - Distribution
> - Course
> - Scarring
> - Response to treatment
> - Psychological impact

have predicted the role of candidate genes involved in the innate as well as the acquired immunity in acne patients and their families.

Studies have confirmed that acne presents earlier in persons with a positive family history. This has also got a bearing on the clinical manifestation and response to treatment. Studies have shown greater concordance between sebum excretion rates in monozygotic than dizygotic twins. There is a dysregulation of transforming growth factor-beta (TGF-β)-mediated signaling in acne patients. This is supported by the identification of 11q13.1, 5q11.2, and 1q41 loci that contain genes linked to TGF-β cell signaling pathway. In acne fulminans, human leukocyte antigen (*HLA*)-*Cw6* gene and genetically determined change in neutrophil activity have been proposed.

Familial cases have been reported in hidradenitis suppurativa with linkage to chromosome 15q24-26 in the region of interleukin (IL)-16 and *CRABPI* genes.

A single nucleotide polymorphism between *HLA-DR* and *BTNL-2* and three alleles coding for major histocompatibility complex (MHC) class II proteins were identified in a genome-wide study to be significantly associated with rosacea.

Syndromes associated with acne have genetic influence. The Apert's syndrome; synovitis, acne, pustulosis, hyperostosis, and osteitis (SAPHO); and pyogenic arthritis, pyoderma gangrenosum, and acne (PAPA) syndromes have an autosomal dominant inheritance.

- *Apert's syndrome*: The Apert's syndrome has an autosomal dominant inheritance and is said to result from mutation in the gene encoding fibroblast growth factor receptor 2 (FGFR-2) and amino acid substitution of exon 7 of chromosome 10.
- *SAPHO syndrome*: The HLA association of SAPHO has been much debated. The association with HLA-B27 is controversial because of the overlap of spondyloarthropathies (condition with a known association with HLA-B27) with SAPHO syndrome. Some authors have shown a positive association between SAPHO syndrome and HLA-39 and 61. It has also been observed that genes responsible for SAPHO syndrome are located in chromosome 18.
- *PAPA syndrome*: Ongoing research in PAPA syndrome has picked up the gene responsible to be located on chromosome 15q24-q25. Though the mutations were detected in CD2-binding protein, the exact role played by this mutation in causing the disease is not yet clearly documented.

Environmental Factors

Acne is influenced by various environmental factors. Environmental factors involved in the etiopathogenesis are given in **Box 5**.

> **BOX 5** | **Environmental factors influencing acne.**
>
> - Lifestyle
> - Diet
> - Birth weight and body mass index
> - Smoking and alcohol
> - Stress and sleep deprivation
> - Menstrual cycle and pregnancy
> - Cosmetics
> - Occupation
> - Seasonal variation and ultraviolet radiation
> - Drugs and hormones
> - Miscellaneous

Among environmental factors studied, diet, smoking, drugs, seasonal variation, and role of anabolic and androgenic steroids seem to have moderate-to-high index of evidence in influencing development of acne. Whereas the evidence is not so high for factors such as body mass index (BMI), alcohol consumption, psychological stress, cosmetics, sunlight, and insomnia.

Lifestyle: Sedentary lifestyle has a negative effect and predisposes a person to develop acne.

Diet: There are different schools of thought regarding the influence of diet on acne, the results of various studies showing contradicting reports. Higher glycemic index and increased consumption of dairy products are thought to bring an upsurge in the insulin-like growth factor-1 (IGF-1). Increased IGF increases androgen activity and has a possible proacne effect. Studies have defined the role of obesity and insulin resistance in the development of acne.

According to some authors, milk and milk products can worsen acne. However, the results have not been consistent documenting the role of milk in the pathogenesis of acne. Similarly, the link between dairy products and worsening of acne has not been proven beyond doubt. While high calorie diet and dairy products are connected to worsening of acne, some authors believe that the anti-inflammatory effects of diet are protective in acne mediated via the effects of dietary components on the gut microbiota. Similarly, diet rich in polyunsaturated fatty acids and probiotics can reduce acne severity. This has also been proven by demonstrating reduction in the perilesional IL-8 in those consuming diet rich in omega-3 fatty acid and probiotics. Results on the link between diet with high glycemic load and acne are controversial. Some studies show worsening of acne while others do not.

Birth weight and BMI: While in adults obesity is linked with severe acne, it was found that acne was more common among those with low birth weight. The possible explanation offered is that the positive link between low birth weight and insulin resistance. In girls, in addition to insulin resistance, low birth weight is regarded as a risk factor for PCOS, which, in turn, is a well-established association of acne.

There are enough research studies proving the relationship between acne and BMI. In women, obesity and acne are frequent observations in patients with PCOS. Numerous studies have examined the relationship between acne and BMI, especially in adult women as acne and obesity coexist as symptoms of PCOS. Studies to date suggest the risk of having acne and the severity appear to increase with age-adjusted BMI in adolescents. Paradoxically, acne may be less prevalent in overweight women with PCOS.

Alcohol: There is no consistent categorically documented evidence that alcohol consumption is a risk factor for acne at any age. Some studies suggest the positive correlation of alcohol consumption and acne and some no correlation at all.

Smoking: Based on the available evidence, smoking does not play a major role in the development of acne. The weight of evidence suggests smoking has very little effect on severity of acne. However, it was observed that mature women who are persistent smokers are susceptible to noninflammatory acne and women with comedonal acne were, on average, older in comparison to adult women with papulopustular acne and reported notably higher rates of smoking than their counterparts with papulopustular acne. It was postulated that in heavy smokers there seems to be a protective effect by the nicotine against inflammation, and hence, these are seen as noninflammatory lesions. Smoking by mothers has been found to be associated with earlier onset of acne in children.

***Stress*:** Psychological stress was identified as one of the factors which can worsen acne. Changes in stress scores correlated with changes in acne severity in both genders. The values were more statistically significant in males when compared to that of females. Many studies have documented stress to be a risk as well as an aggravating factor for severe acne. Enough data are available linking acne and stress. There is strong evidence on the role of hypothalamic–pituitary–adrenal axis on sebaceous gland function which explains the positive link between stress and acne.

***Insomnia*:** It has been observed that sleep deprivation can aggravate acne in adolescent and postadolescent acne. However, the evidence is not strong enough to classify insomnia as a definite precipitating factor.

***Menstruation and pregnancy*:** Premenstrual flare of acne is a common complaint in women. According to some, there is no evidence to directly link premenstrual flare of acne and sebum production as there is no documented increase in sebum production in the luteal phase of menstrual cycle. Nevertheless, fluctuations in androgen levels during menstrual cycle account for premenstrual flare observed by many documented by clinical research.

According to a study conducted in females in the age group of 12–52 years, 44% reported premenstrual flares which were much higher in women older than 33 years when compared to younger women. This study clearly ruled out the possibility of oral contraceptive pills to be the cause for the premenstrual flare. In another study, nearly two-thirds of the study population showed a premenstrual flare showing up to 25% increase in the lesion count. The authors explain this cyclical flare to be due to the increased testosterone–estrogen ratio during the late luteal phase of menstrual cycle.

***Pregnancy*:** In pregnant women, acne can be really troublesome due to the unpredictable course and the challenges involved in choice of drug to be prescribed. The main reason for exacerbation of acne during pregnancy is the change in the hormonal pattern. Acne is said to improve during first trimester but during the last trimester, due to an increase in the maternal androgen leading to increased sebum production, there is an exacerbation of acne lesions. It has also been suggested that gestation associated immunologic factors may also contribute to worsening of the disease during pregnancy.

***Cosmetics*:** Chronic use of cosmetics is known to induce acne or acneiform eruptions due to comedogenic substances present in them like lanolin, petrolatum, certain vege box oils, butyl stearate, lauryl alcohol, and oleic acid. Topical corticosteroids present in skin lightening creams are a major cause for concern in the development or exacerbation of acne.

Pomades are greasy preparations commonly used in hair treatment that can cause noninflammatory acne.

Frequent washing with alkaline soaps and soaps containing acnegenic compounds, like hexachlorophene, may trigger inflammatory lesions.

***Occupation*:** Those working in the industry exposed to compounds like coal tar derivatives chlorinated hydrocarbons and cutting oil, are prone to develop acne and acneiform eruptions. Oil acne, tar acne, chloracne, and acne mechanica are some of the occupational acnes.

Toxic halogenated aromatic hydrocarbons occur as trace contaminants during synthesis of many industrial chemicals. Chloracne results from exposure to these halogenated aromatic hydrocarbons by any one of the routes, namely percutaneous, inhalation, or ingestion. The most potent of all the halogenated aromatic hydrocarbons is tetrachlorodibenzo-p-dioxin (TCDD). Other

| BOX 6 | Chemicals inducing chloracne. |

- Polyhalogenated biphenyls
- Polyhalogenated naphthalenes
- Polychlorinated dibenzofurans
- Polybrominated dibenzofurans
- Polychlorophenols

chloracnegenic chemicals include other halogenated dioxins, naphthalenes, biphenyls.

The important chemicals inducing chloracne are listed in **Box 6**.

Triazoloquinoxalines are several times more chloracnegenic than dioxins on a weight-to-weight basis. Both TCDD and polychlorinated biphenyls (PCBs) cause follicular hyperkeratosis. The TCDD, in addition, can cause impairment of differentiation of keratinocytes while PCB can cause mucocutaneous and nail pigmentation, nail dystrophy, and dental anomaly as well. It was also observed that TCDD can interfere with androgen receptors and impede the action of androgen. According to recent studies, it has been postulated that dioxins can activate skin stem cells there by shifting the differentiation commitment of their progeny. Activation of aryl hydrocarbon (AH) or dioxin receptor and subsequent gene expression play a critical role in the cornification and differentiation of human epidermal cells. It has to be remembered that dioxins have long half-life in fat tissue as they are lipophilic and low turnover rate in the human system.

Seasonal variation: The observation in acne patients on seasonal variation yielded different opinions. Western countries show winter exacerbation while temperate zones recorded summer aggravation, which could be attributed to humidity and increased sweating.

Sunlight and radiation: Both ultraviolet radiation (UVR) and ionizing radiation can induce acneiform eruptions. It has been hypothesized that sunlight is beneficial to acne and improvement during summer months has been observed in many countries. However, the beneficial effect of UVR is questionable as the summer improvement is not observed globally, though many studies show seasonal variation with lesser number of patients seeking medical help during summer months for their acne. It was also observed that the beneficial effect of sunlight can be countered by humidity. Acne aestivalis is the name given to acne that develops on exposure to sunlight in a hot humid environment. Histologically, the follicles show focal destruction and neutrophil infiltration. Based on the scientific data, it can be clearly stated that UVR can exacerbate or induce acne over unprotected sun-exposed skin.

Ionizing radiation induces follicular epithelial metaplasia leading to adherent keratotic plug within the follicle which is resistant to extraction and treatment.

Drugs and hormones: It has been proved beyond doubt that many drugs can induce acne-like eruptions. The single most important clinical finding that helps differentiate drug-induced acneiform eruption from acne vulgaris is the absence of comedones and monomorphic nature of lesions in the former. Another important finding is the lack of preference to seborrheic areas. Drugs inducing acneiform eruption are listed in **Box 7**. It is of interest to note that drug-induced acneiform eruption constitutes up to 1% of all drug reactions. Hence, it becomes important to be aware of such entities, the clinical details and the list of drugs that can cause them. Thus, elicitation of drug history is mandatory in every patient with acne. It has been identified that elevated levels of testosterone and anabolic androgenic steroids act as trigger factor for acne fulminans.

The following drugs have been documented in the etiology of rosacea fulminans:
- High-dose vitamin B6 and B12
- Oral contraceptive pills
- Interferon alfa-2b
- Ribavirin

BOX 7: Drugs inducing acneiform eruptions.

- *Hormones:*
  - Corticosteroid in all forms such as oral, parenteral, topical, and inhaled
  - Adrenocorticotropic hormone (ACTH)/synthetic ACTH
  - Anabolic steroid/synthetic androgen
    - Danazol
    - Nandrolone
    - Stanozolol
    - Medroxyprogesterone
- *Anticonvulsant:*
  - Carbamazepine
  - Phenytoin
  - Phenobarbitone
  - Troxidone
  - Gabapentin
  - Topiramate
- *Antidepressant:*
  - Amineptine
  - Lithium
  - Sertraline
- *Neuroleptic/Antipsychotic:*
  - Pimozide
  - Risperidone
- *Antitubercular:*
  - Isoniazid
  - Pyrazinamide
- *Antineoplastic:*
  - Actinomycin D
  - Cetuximab
  - Cisplatin
  - Epidermal growth factor receptor antagonists
    - Cetuximab
    - Panitumumab
  - Tyrosine kinase inhibitor:
    - Erlotinib
    - Gefitinib
    - Lapatinib
  - Mitogen-activated protein kinase inhibitors:
    - Trametinib
    - Selumetinib
  - Fluorouracil
  - Pentostatin
- *Antiviral:*
  - Ritonavir
  - Ganciclovir
- *Calcium antagonist:*
  - Nilvadipine
  - Nimodipine
- *Halogen:*
  - Sodium fluoride
  - Potassium iodine
- *Antimalarial:*
  - Quinine
- *Immunosuppressives:*
  - Cyclosporine
  - Sirolimus
  - Tacrolimus
  - Methotrexate
  - Cyclophosphamide
- Genetically engineered human growth hormone
- Vitamin B12
- *Miscellaneous:*
  - Buserelin
  - Cabergoline
  - Clofazimine
  - Dantrolene
  - Disulfiram
  - Famotidine
  - Follitropin alfa
  - Isosorbide mononitrate
  - Mesalazine
  - Ramipril
  - Sulfur
  - Thiouracil
  - Thiourea

Miscellaneous: Cosmetic preparations are known to cause acne-like lesions. Acnegenic cosmetics are capable of inducing comedones as well as papulopustular eruptions, whereas comedogenic cosmetics are capable of inducing only follicular keratin impaction. It is important to know that while using acnegenic preparations, papulopustules develop in a few days much earlier than comedones that are quite different from the regular evolution of acne vulgaris. Sebum secretion along with other lipids and biophysical parameters, including skin surface pH, UV-induced fluorescence, and the patencies of pores determine the clinical manifestation in a given patient.

PATHOGENESIS

The major pathogenic mechanisms involved in acne under the influence of genetic background and increased androgen production are schematically represented in **Figure 41**.

The major pathogenic factors are as follows:
- Follicular epidermal hyperproliferation
- Increased sebum production
- Inflammation
- *C. acnes*

Follicular Epidermal Hyperproliferation

Follicular epidermal hypercornification seems to be the most important key pathogenic factor which heralds the onset of acne and clinically manifests as microcomedones that can be easily missed unlike the macrocomedones. Androgen stimulation, decreased linoleic acid, increased IL-1 effects of *C. acnes* all seem to play important role in the formation of follicular plug. As the follicular plug expands, leading to follicular wall distension, ultimately it results in rupture of the follicular which is followed by inflammatory response.

Increased Sebum Production

Excess sebum production seems to play the second most important key factor in the pathogenesis of acne. There are enough evidences demonstrating excess sebum production in acne patients when compared to persons without acne in both genders. Soon after birth, the sebaceous gland activity is high and it has been documented that sebum excretion rates in newborn are transiently elevated in the perinatal period. As the effect of maternal hormones ceases in the newborn, there is a decline in the level of sebum production. There is an age-related change in the sebaceous gland activity showing low level of activity during childhood until just before puberty. With puberty, the sebaceous glands become active, the activity of which rises during the mid-to-late teens, continues to remain high, and declines during the seventh decade, which correlates well with the fall in the endogenous androgen production.

Factors like diet and stress seem to influence sebum production apart from the genetic makeup of a person. The importance of genetic predisposition in sebum production is evident from the fact that identical twins

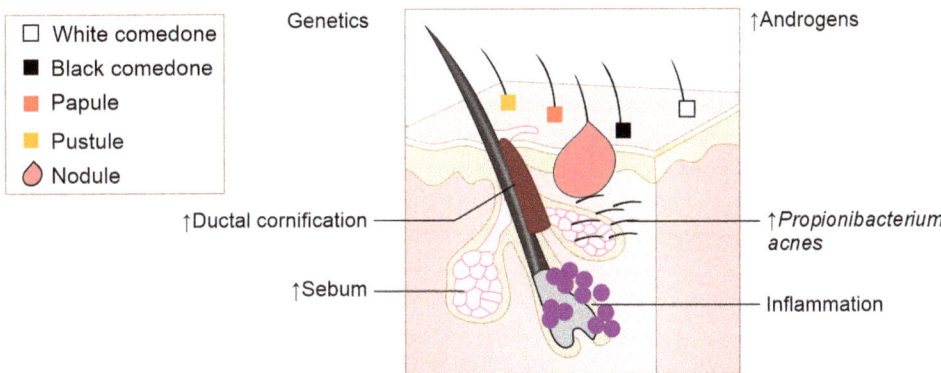

FIG. 41: Diagrammatic depiction of acne pathogenesis.

exhibit essentially the same sebum excretion rate with significantly divergent acne severity, whereas in nonidentical twins, both sebum excretion rate and acne severity were different.

Peroxisome proliferator-activated receptors (PPARs) are ligand-activated transcription factors involved in the genetic regulation of lipid metabolism and play an important role in inflammation. Lipid peroxidation, a "starter gun" in acne pathogenesis, is a well-known concept. Cytokines produced by lipid peroxidase activate the PPAR pathway promoting increased sebum production. Androgenic hormones influence sebum production and male pattern hair in females while estrogen suppresses sebum production.

The effect of androgen in sebum production is depicted in **Figure 42**.

Though the concept is not very well proved, it is suggested that estrogen can suppress sebum production by one of the following two mechanisms:
1. Directly opposing the effects of androgens within the sebaceous gland
2. Inhibiting the production of androgen by gonadal tissue via a negative feedback loop on pituitary gonadotropin release

Stress-induced seborrhea is best explained by the demonstration of upregulation of corticotropin-releasing hormone receptors present on sebocytes.

Cutibacterium acnes

Cutibacterium acnes is a gram-positive anaerobic and microaerobic bacterium, resident as a normal flora of the pilosebaceous unit. *C. acnes* breaks the triglycerides present in the sebum into free fatty acids. This further promotes colonization of *C. acnes* provoking inflammation. It has been scientifically proved that *C. acnes* induces inflammation. The inflammation induced by *C. acnes* involves one or more of the following pathways:
- *Antibody-mediated inflammation*: The anti-*C. acnes* antibody enhances the inflammatory response by complement activation further initiating a cascade of proinflammatory events.

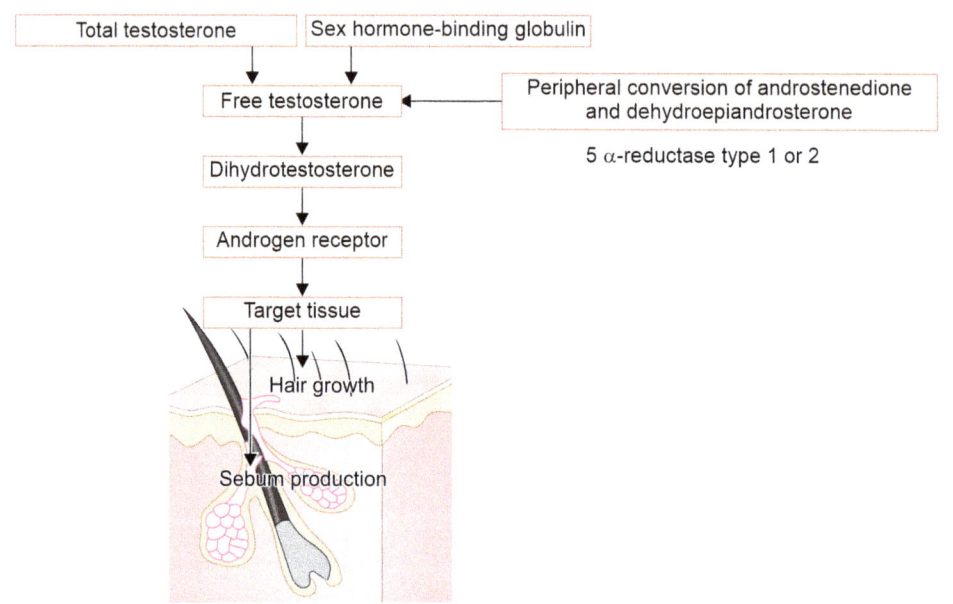

FIG. 42: Effect of androgen in sebum production.

- C. acnes stimulates toll-like receptor (TLR) expression on the keratinocytes, monocytes, and polymorphonuclear cells surrounding the sebaceous follicle which may play an essential role in inducing inflammation. After binding to TLR, proinflammatory cytokines like IL-1, IL-8, IL-12, and tumor necrosis factor (TNF) are released, thus enhancing inflammation
- It has been observed that individuals who show hypersensitivity to C. acnes may develop severe inflammatory acne when compared to those who do not. C. acnes also facilitates inflammation by eliciting delayed hypersensitivity response and by producing many inflammatory mediators such as lipase, proteases, and hyaluronidase as well as chemotactic factors.

The earlier concepts explained the role of inflammation in acne to be a result of combination of follicular epidermal hyperproliferation, increased sebum production, role of C. acnes, and the activation of adaptive immune system. However, there has been a lot of development in the research throwing more light on the inflammatory cascade in acne. The pathophysiology of inflammation in acne has taken a new dimension with the growing research in this field.

Intradermal extrusion of sebum and keratin following rupture of the expanding follicular wall initiates a brisk inflammatory response. Presence of C. acnes and various cellular components plays a major role in the initiation and promotion of inflammation. The role of *Pseudomonas* has also been studied in the exacerbation of acne.

Pathophysiology of Inflammation

The pathophysiology of inflammation, a multifactorial process in acne, has been studied in depth by many researchers. In genetically prone individuals, many factors such as the role of androgen, diet, proinflammatory lipids, and neuroendocrine regulatory mechanism, all contribute to the final outcome of the disease.

Earlier it was thought that inflammation follows follicular hyperkeratinization. However, recent data have shown that the influx of inflammatory cells precede the hyperkeratinization of the follicular duct. The CD4+ lymphocytes which are predominantly seen around the pilosebaceous units and CD8+ cells around the blood vessels play a major role in the ensuing inflammatory cascade. Studies have documented that there is a strong indication to prove that dermal inflammation precedes comedone formation. This is well supported by demonstrating the presence of microscopic inflammation in the clinically normal skin in an acne patient. These observations emphasize the fact that there is interplay between all of the pathogenic factors not to forget that clinically normal looking skin may well be throwing inflammation in a patient with acne. This hypothesis of inflammation preceding ductal hypercornification conceptualized following perifollicular demonstration of increased IL-1 activity in the uninvolved pilosebaceous units of acne patients. The perifollicular inflammation triggers the activation of keratinocytes leading to follicular hypercornification. In acne patients with inflammatory lesions, upregulated genes such as matrix metalloproteinases, human beta-defensin 4, IL-8, and granulysin are found to be involved in inflammatory process. Similarly, proinflammatory cytokine genes are also activated in acne lesions. There is also a significant upregulation of TNF-α, IL-1, IL-8, and IL-10 in involved skin of acne patients compared to the uninvolved adjacent skin. These chemokines attract inflammatory cells to the site leading to a cascade of events observed in acne patients. It was also observed that there is a noticeable increase in the number of neutrophils and lymphocytes. Markedly raised inflammatory infiltrates were demonstrated in the acne lesions when compared to that of the uninvolved skin of normal controls. In addition to the above, it was also shown that there is activation of T-helper (Th) 17-related cytokines in acne lesions indicating that the Th17 pathway is also triggered playing a pivotal role in the inflammatory response in acne. Active inflammatory mediators, such as prostaglandins and leukotrienes, are also involved in the pathophysiology of acne.

The above was supported by the selective expression and upregulation of cyclooxygenase-2 (COX)-2 expression in involved sebaceous units of acne patients. Studies have documented that COX-2-mediated prostaglandin E2 (PGE2) synthesis and an increased PGE2 levels can cause sebaceous gland hyperplasia.

Both 5-lipoxygenase and leukotriene A4 hydrolase show strong expression in acne lesions further adding evidence to the presence of inflammation as a major component in acne pathophysiology. Macrophages and *C. acnes* lead to release of considerable amounts of IL-1 beta and further exacerbate the inflammation. All the research and the results prove beyond doubt that it is the uncontrolled inflammation that leads to disease manifestation and its sequelae.

Neurophysiology of Inflammation in Acne

It has been shown that sebaceous glands express receptors for many neuropeptides such as corticotropin-releasing hormone, melanocortin, beta-endorphin, and calcitonin gene-related peptides. These receptors are known to modulate the production of inflammatory cytokines, and proliferation, differentiation, and androgen metabolism of sebocytes. The role of substance P in the acne lesions becomes significant by the fact that it can promote proliferation and differentiation of sebaceous glands by promoting development of cytoplasmic organelles, increasing the number of sebum vacuoles, and stimulating germinative cells, thereby significantly increasing the sebaceous gland area.

It is of interest to know that in patients with acne, facial skin is richly innervated, the increased number of substance P containing nerves and mast cells attributing to local substance P activity. Ectopeptidases involved in the degradation of substance P have been found to be expressed in sebocytes and can modulate certain sebocytes function indicating a significant role in the pathophysiology of inflammation involved in acne.

Causative Organisms

Different strains of *C. acnes* modulate expression of immune markers differently. The strain type III shows the highest proinflammatory potential. This, according to the researchers, is through an upregulation of expression of TNF-α and other proinflammatory cytokines. *C. acnes* induces IL-17 expression, promotes a mixed Th17/Th1 response, and triggers monocyte macrophage and sebocytes activation. The main role of *C. acnes* in the causation of acne is given in **Box 8**.

Cutibacterium acnes activates keratinocytes and sebocytes via TLRs, CD14, and CD1 molecules provoking the release of IL-1 alpha. Certain strains of *C. acnes* upregulate the expression of psoriasin, human β-defensins and cathelicidin. Certain strains of *C. acnes* worsen acne lesion by inducing opportunistic infections. It has been studied and documented that neonatal acne/neonatal cephalic pustulosis (NCP) seen in newborn is due to the colonization of hair follicles by *Malassezia sympodialis* and *Malassezia globosa*.

BOX 8	Role of *Cutibacterium acnes* in the causation of acne.

- Enzyme production
- Complement activation
- Recognition by toll receptors
- Prostaglandin production

Innate Immunity

In addition to the abovementioned inflammatory and immune responses, there seems to be a strong role played by the innate immunity in the pathogenesis of acne.

There is an upregulation of expression of antimicrobial peptides such as psoriasin and human β-defensins and cathelicidin in pilosebaceous units in acne patients. Histone H4 and cathelicidin—the antimicrobial proteins secreted locally in response to *C. acnes* play an important role in the regulation of immune protection. While histone H4 exerts direct microbial killing, cathelicidin interacts with components of innate immune system. This apart, the peripheral conversion of blood monocytes to CD209 macrophage and CD1b dendritic cells in response to *C. acnes* indicate the role of innate immunity in the pathogenesis of acne. **Figure 43** gives the clinicopathological correlation of different stages of acne. Thorough knowledge about the entire etiopathogenesis and the transformation of the microscopic finding to the clinical events will go a long way in the better understanding of pathophysiology of different spectra of acne. This will enhance the potential of physician to effectively manage patients with reference to both investigation and treatment, which may range from simple noninterference to vigorous systemic therapy including hormones. Newer concepts in the pathophysiology of acne are summarized in Box 9.

Special Situations

The pathogenesis of special and severe forms of acne is discussed below:
- Pediatric acne
- Adult-onset acne
- Acne fulminans
- Acne rosacea
- Pathogenesis of scar formation

BOX 9: Newer concepts in the pathophysiology of acne.

- Inflammation precedes follicular hyperkeratinization
- Clinically normal looking skin histologically shows signs of inflammation
- *Cutibacterium acnes* contributes to inflammation via toll-like receptors
- Sebaceous glands act as neuroendocrine element to induce local response to stress
- Peroxisome proliferator-activated receptors regulate sebum production
- Matrix metalloproteinases play an important role in inflammatory acne

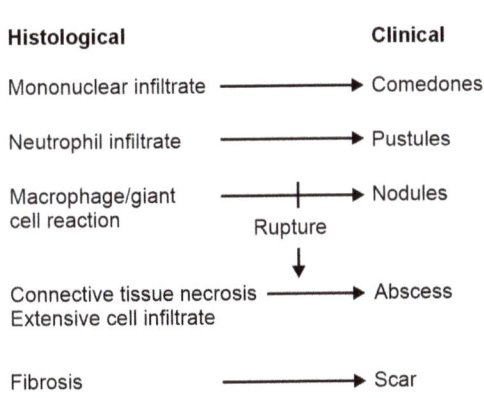
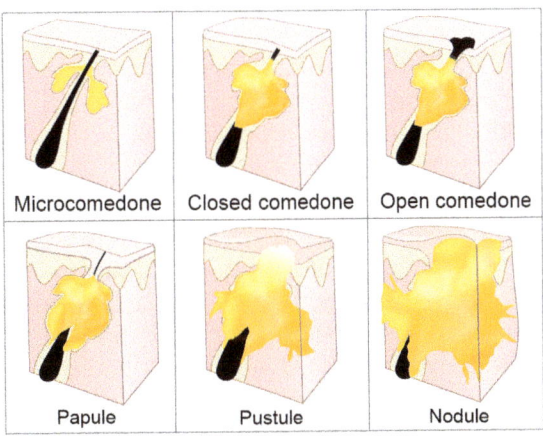

FIG. 43: Histoclinical correlation of acne.

Pediatric Acne

Acne in children is not uncommon. Whatever be the age, it is known that the hormonal influence is the cause for development of acne even in children. The real pathogenic factor for neonatal acne is not clearly understood. However, the resultant clinical picture is due to increased androgen secreted by the testes in case of boys and adrenals in both boys and girls leading to hyperactivity of the sebaceous glands. Transplacental transfer of maternal androgens along with the androgen produced by the hyperactive adrenals result in an increase in the production of dehydroepiandrosterone (DHEA) and its sulfated form. In boys from birth till 1 year of age, the luteinizing hormone (LH) is as high as to match the pubertal level. This leads to production of testosterone in excess explaining the neonatal and infantile acne in boys. Similar to neonatal acne, infantile acne is associated with increased levels of androgen produced by the adrenals and testes. Up to 1 year of age, the elevated levels of DHEA can cause increased sebum production which however, starts dropping from 6 months and is completed by 1 year. Maternal ingestion of drugs like phenytoin has been implicated in the etiology of neonatal and infantile acne. Mid-childhood acne denotes acne between the age 1 and 7 years. Acne during this age should raise the possibility of virilization as gonadal secretion of androgen is very low between 1 and 7 years of age by when the DHEA levels have also dropped down.

Prepubertal Acne

During adrenarche, there is an increase in the secretion of DHEA and dehydroepiandrosterone sulfate (DHEAS) by the adrenal glands in both boys and girls leading to androgen-mediated sebum production. It was also observed that DHEAS levels are significantly higher in prepubertal girls with acne than their counterparts without acne. However, gonadal secretion of androgen is very low at this stage. The role of *C. acnes* and *Malassezia furfur* has been well documented in the pathogenesis of childhood acne as in acne vulgaris.

Pathogenesis of Adult Female Acne

Adult-onset acne, especially in women, has a complex pathogenesis. In addition to the pathogenic factors common for acne vulgaris, adult-onset acne involves the role of androgen to a greater extent in women. The role of cosmetics in the causation of adult-onset acne has been long debated. However, use of cosmetics has not been proven to play an important role in the causation and severity of adult-onset acne.

Coming to the role of androgen, it has been proved by many researchers that androgen excess plays a major role in the onset and severity of the disease. The supporting research has demonstrated that in androgen-insensitive individuals, adult-onset acne is not reported. This is probably because of reduced sebum production in such individuals with poor response to androgen. The ovaries and adrenal glands are the major sources of androgen in women supplemented by the increased peripheral conversion. Androstenedione and testosterone are secreted by the ovaries while DHEAS, androstenedione, and testosterone are adrenal-derived. In women, testosterone is generated in excess by the peripheral conversion of androstenedione and DHEA.

As it is known that androgen-stimulated sebum secretion is a main factor in the pathophysiology of adult-onset acne, it is the androgen receptors located in the sebaceous gland and outer root sheath of hair follicle that play an important role in the pathophysiology of late-onset acne. Sebocytes proliferation and activity is stimulated by 5 alpha-dihydrotestosterone by peripheral conversion of DHEA. Apart from androgen, other hormones such as estrogen, growth hormone, insulin, IGF-1, glucocorticoids, adrenocorticotropic hormone, and melanocortin also are involved in the regulation of sebum production.

Thus, the multihormonal influence of acne in adult females has to be understood better and managed accordingly.

Acne Fulminans

The exact pathogenesis of acne fulminans remains unclear. As in acne vulgaris, genetic predisposition, infection, inflammation, and immunological factors including autoimmunity have been included in the pathogenesis of acne fulminans. Rapid response to steroid is a supportive evidence for its autoimmune etiology. Increased levels of gamma globulin and fall in complement levels have also been documented. In patients with musculoskeletal abnormalities, immune complexes have been demonstrated. The association of acne fulminans with other autoinflammatory disorders has led to the concept that abnormal innate immunity like IL-1 pathway is involved. The role of testosterone in inducing acne fulminans is supported by the presence of elevated blood levels of testosterone in young males with acne fulminans. All these observations further explain the role of inflammation and immunity in the disease manifestation.

Similarly, anabolic steroids also play as an important trigger factor. Anabolic steroids, being derivatives of testosterone, lead to sebaceous gland hypertrophy and increased sebum production, which further increases the density of *C. acnes*. Isotretinoin drug commonly used in severe forms of acne can precipitate acne fulminans. In such patients, the evolution of lesions will be rapid than usual with demonstrable circulating immune complexes. It has been hypothesized that isotretinoin induced fragility of the pilosebaceous duct epithelium leads to exposure of *C. acnes* antigens and *C. acnes* chemoattractants to the immune system. Following factors that support abnormal immune response in the etiology of acne fulminans:
- Microscopic hematuria
- Increased response to *C. acnes* antigen on skin tests showing extensive immediate and delayed reaction revealing types II and IV hypersensitivity reaction
- Depressed response to intradermal tests with purified protein derivatives

Acne Rosacea

Acne rosacea is a chronic inflammatory dermatosis sometimes cosmetically disabling having multifactorial pathomechanisms. In addition to the pathogenic factors involved in acne vulgaris, rosacea encompasses vasoactive and neurocutaneous mechanisms to a greater extent.

Causes: The definite cause of rosacea is unknown. However, there are evidences to prove that it is due to combination of hereditary and environmental factors. **Box 10** gives the list of factors aggravating rosacea.

Pathogenesis: The etiology of rosacea is unknown. However, **Boxes 11 and 12** give some of the risk factors and probable etiological factors attributed to its cause.

Both innate and adaptive immune dysfunctions are major events leading to the disease. More and more of research into this field have helped evolve newer therapeutic approach to rosacea. There is increased keratinocyte transcription of procathelicidin and serine protease leading to secretion of inflammatory and angiogenic peptides. In rosacea, mast cells are an important source of pivotal inflammatory mediators leading to vasodilatation and IL-37 generation. It has

BOX 10	Factors aggravating rosacea.
- Hot foods or beverages
- Spicy foods
- Alcohol
- Temperature extremes
- Sunlight
- Stress, anger, or embarrassment
- Strenuous exercise
- Hot baths
- Corticosteroids
- Drugs	

BOX 11	**Risk factors in rosacea.**

- Fair skin, light hair, and eye color
- Age group of 30 and 60 years, especially perimenopausal age group
- History of frequent flushing or blushing
- Positive family history of rosacea

BOX 12	**Probable etiological factors involved rosacea.**

- Vasculature
- Climatic exposures
- Dermal matrix degeneration
- Chemicals and ingested agents
- Pilosebaceous unit abnormalities
- Microbial organisms
- Ferritin expression
- Reactive oxygen species
- Increased neoangiogenesis and vascular endothelial growth factor
- Dysfunction of antimicrobial peptides

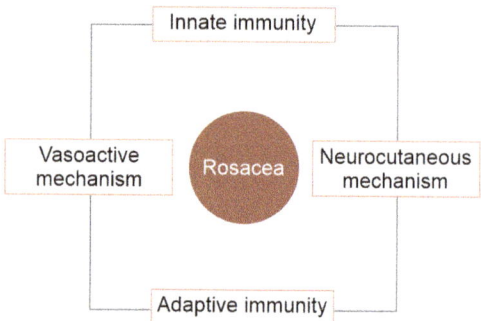

FIG. 44: Major etiological factors in rosacea.

also been observed that there is colocalization of mast cells with unmyelinated sensory nerves, vasculature, and myofibroblasts. The major etiological factors in rosacea are given in **Figure 44**.

The distinct subtype of rosacea depends much on the patient's unique sensitivity and response to these triggers.

Vasculature: Vasodilatation is pronounced or exaggerated in those individuals with rosacea. Face being richly supplied by blood vessels, adds to the cause.

Climatic exposures: Exposure to solar irradiation can worsen the disease manifestation though not in all cases.

Dermal matrix degeneration: Damage to the endothelium and degeneration of the dermal matrix are also found to be major factors in the causation of the disease.

Chemicals and ingested agents: Spicy foods, alcohol, and hot beverages trigger flushing and worsen rosacea. However, most evidence does not support dietary factors playing a central role in the pathogenesis. Certain drugs such as amiodarone, topical/intranasal steroids, and high doses of vitamins B6 and B12, may cause flare-up of lesions in patients with rosacea.

Pilosebaceous unit abnormalities: Perivascular and/or a perifollicular inflammation may attribute to the clinical inflammatory findings and symptoms in many patients.

Microbial organisms: Demodex species (mites that normally inhabit human hair follicles) may play a role in the pathogenesis of rosacea. However, the results are conflicting, as not all individuals with large colonization with the mite develop rosacea. More studies need to be performed to determine whether *Demodex folliculorum* truly is pathogenic agent in the evolution and or causation of the disease.

There seems to be a positive association between *Helicobacter pylori* and acne rosacea. However, many of the studies which documented the above, have not controlled for confounding variables that influence *H. pylori* prevalence, such as sex, age, socioeconomic status, and medications. Furthermore, these studies were not statistically powered to account for the ubiquitous nature of *H. pylori* infection.

Ferritin expression: Increased release of free iron from proteolysis of ferritin can result in oxidative damage to the skin, which may contribute to the pathogenesis of rosacea.

Reactive oxygen species (ROS): Early in the inflammatory process, ROS are released by neutrophils, which are postulated to have a central role in the inflammation associated with rosacea. Free radicals, in addition to other reactive molecules, lead to oxidative tissue damage. ROS thus released are found in greater amounts in the facial skin of affected individuals and result in inflammation.

Neoangiogenesis and vascular endothelial growth factor (VEGF) overexpression: There is increased neoangiogenesis, blood vessel enlargement and increased VEGF expression in vascular endothelium in lesional versus nonlesional skin of rosacea patients.

Antimicrobial peptides: Antimicrobial peptides (AMPs) are small molecular weight proteins that are a part of the innate immune response. They are rapidly released upon injury and/or infection of the skin, and they have been implicated in the pathogenesis of many inflammatory skin diseases. Cathelicidin, a well-known type of AMPs, is expressed in abnormally high levels in patients with rosacea.

Pathogenesis of Scar Formation

Scar is a telltale evidence of acne even after resolution of the clinical lesions of the disease. The process of scar formation begins with the rupture of the affected hair follicle. The resultant perifollicular abscess under normal circumstances is repaired by the body in 7–10 days' time without formation of a scar. This can happen when the cells grow to surround the inflammatory zone to form an encapsulation. The normal course of events of acne healing in a person not prone for scar formation will be as follows:
- The course—typical of a type IV delayed hypersensitivity response
- There is demonstration of significant angiogenesis
- Pronounced vascular cell adhesion molecule (VCAM) expression
- Large influx of activated CD4+ T cells, macrophages, and LH cells
- Cell recruitment peaking at 48 hours
- Followed by reduction in leukocytes, cellular activation
- Resumption of normal levels of blood vessels and VCAM

If the encapsulation is incomplete, further rupture happens leading to enhanced inflammatory reaction which ultimately results in development of fistulous tracts. Histologically, this is characterized by reticulate tunnels lined by hyperplastic epithelium. If the inflammatory process extends deeper, into the subcutis, there is destruction of subcutaneous fat and deep scars ensue. The different stages of healing include inflammation, granulation tissue formation, neovascularization, wound contracture, and tissue remodeling. In the process of healing, enzymatic activity and inflammatory mediators also destroy surrounding deeper structures. In acne, atrophic scars are more common than hypertrophic scars and the severity of scar is determined by the depth and extent of inflammation. **Table 1** gives the depth of inflammation and the outcome.

It is emphasized that in majority of patients, proper, appropriate, and adequate treatment will prevent scar formation. Even in genetically prone patients, a complete anti-acne treatment started early with adequate follow-up will reduce the severity of scarring.

TABLE 1: Depth of inflammation and the clinical presentation.

Pathology of depth of inflammation	Clinical outcome
Epidermis–superficial dermis	Erythematous or pigmented macule
Mid-dermis	Superficial scar
Deep dermis (localized)	Ice pick scars
Extensive dermal damage	Rolling or box scars
Perifollicular elastolysis	Atrophic perifollicular macules
Thick parallelly oriented type III collagen and numerous myofibroblasts	Hypertrophic scars
Disorganized type I collagen and few myofibroblasts	Keloidal scars

CHAPTER 3

Clinical Features

It is important to elicit proper history to gather information regarding onset, evolution symptoms such as itching, burning, and photosensitivity, details about menstrual history, associations like diabetes, and drug history in all patients with acne. Detailed history of treatments pertaining to intake of drugs for acne including specifics of contraceptive pills and procedures undergone, if any, should also be recorded. Daily routine, diet habits, and cleansers used should be noted, as well. Family history of acne will give a clue to the course of the disease and, therefore, will help assess the patient well. Complete and thorough examination is mandatory, which includes both dermatological and systemic examination wherever applicable. Assessment of quality of life (QOL) will certainly help manage the patients better and more effectively. Most patients, both males and females, report gradual onset of lesions around puberty. However, acne can manifest from newborn period to adulthood as late as sixth decade.

CLINICAL MANIFESTATIONS (FIGS. 1 TO 50)

Onset and Evolution

By and large, adolescent acne vulgaris is usually gradual in onset. Hence, history of an abrupt onset should give a clue to suspecting an underlying cause. Similarly, in females with severe acne even if the onset is gradual, hyperandrogenism should be considered and evaluated. More so, if acne is resistant to treatment. This should be taken more seriously toward endocrine workup if there is an associated menstrual irregularity and hirsutism.

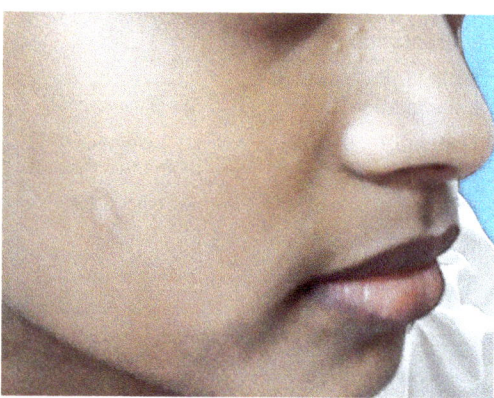

FIG. 1: Oily skin, the first clinical presentation and complaint from the preadolescent.

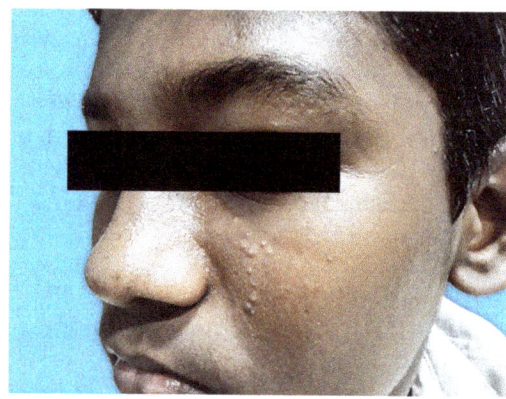

FIG. 2: Oily skin of 6 months' duration; increased sebum production starts manifesting well before the clinical onset of acne.

CHAPTER 3: Clinical Features

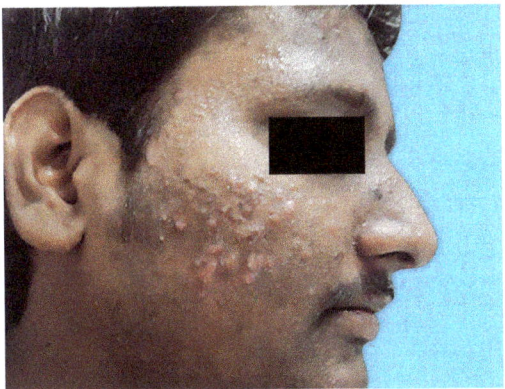

FIG. 3: Comedone papule pustule; all primary lesions of acne seen in this man.

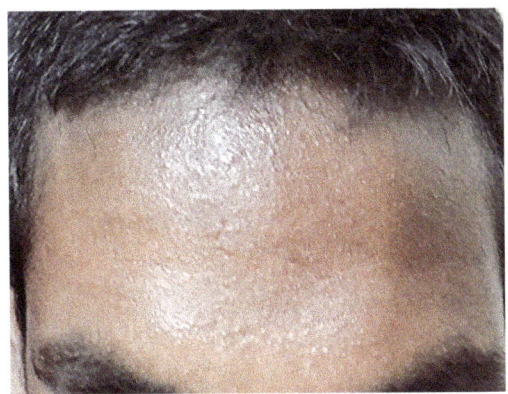

FIG. 4: Sandpaper comedones consist of multiple closed comedones predominantly distributed over the forehead with androgenetic alopecia.

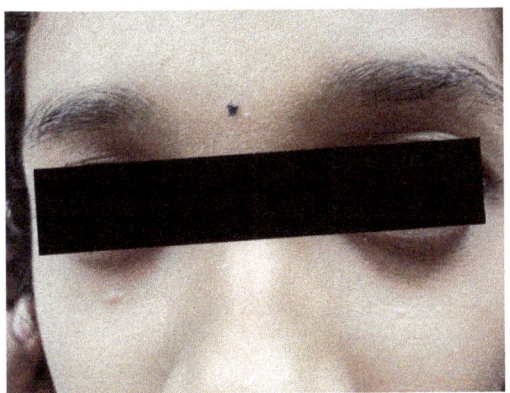

FIG. 5: White heads or closed comedones are often inconspicuous requiring adequate lighting and stretching of skin as in this girl.

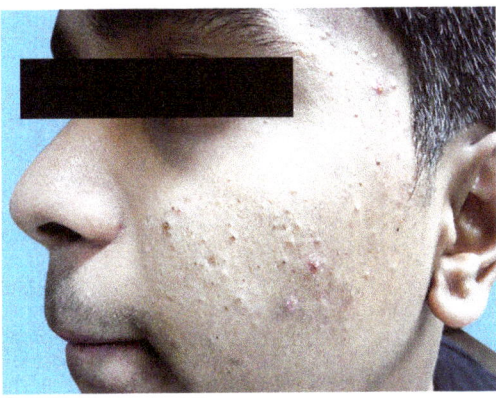

FIG. 6: A boy with open comedones; the black color is thought to be due to melanin, deposited within the cellular debris.

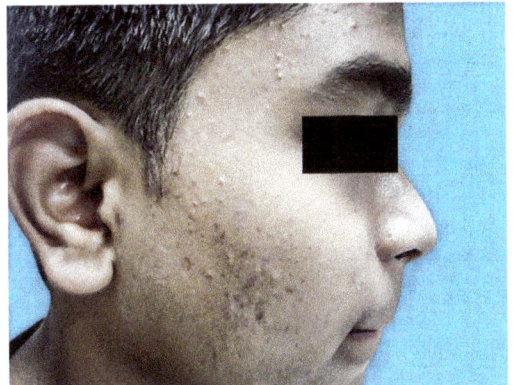

FIG. 7: Same patient as in Figure 6 with white heads which have no visible follicular opening.

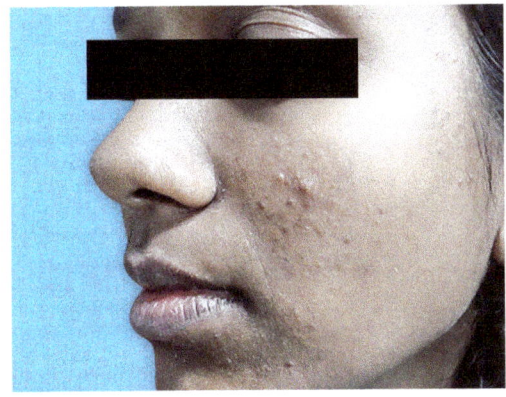

FIG. 8: Comedones starting in the T-zone; note the V-zone is not involved.

CHAPTER 3: Clinical Features

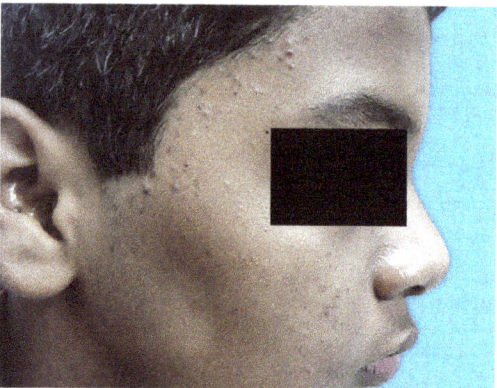

FIG. 9: Noninflamed lesions, the earliest lesions developing in younger patients embrace both white and black comedones.

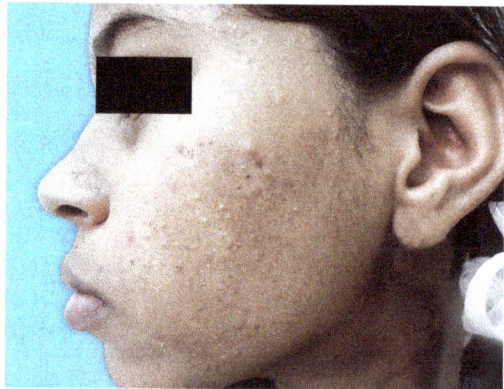

FIG. 10: Submarine comedones are greater than 0.5 cm residing deeply which are the common cause for recurrent inflammation.

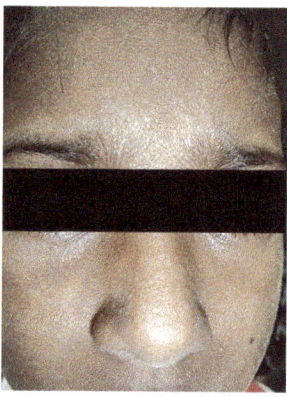

FIG. 11: Sandpaper comedones in a child consisting of multiple, very small whiteheads over the forehead.

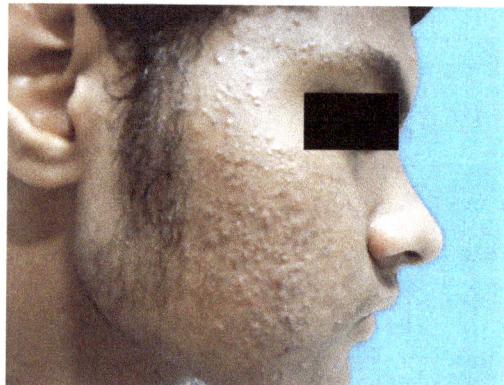

FIG. 12: Face is the most common site of involvement in acne.

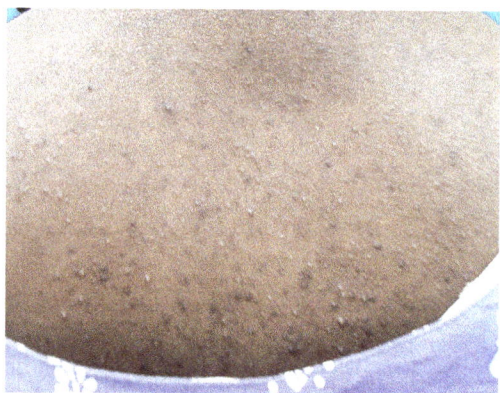

FIG. 13: A girl showing truncal involvement.

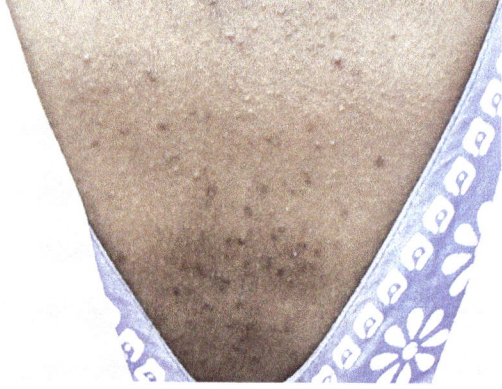

FIG. 14: A girl showing truncal involvement; same patient as in Figure 13.

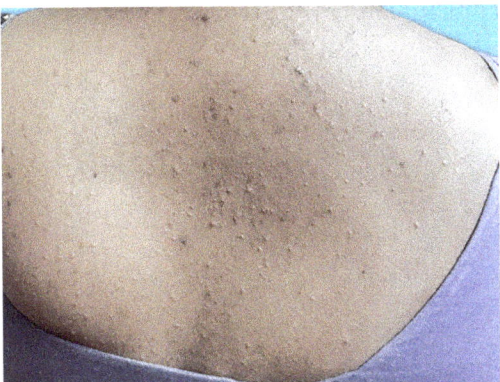

FIG. 15: Truncal acne in an older woman.

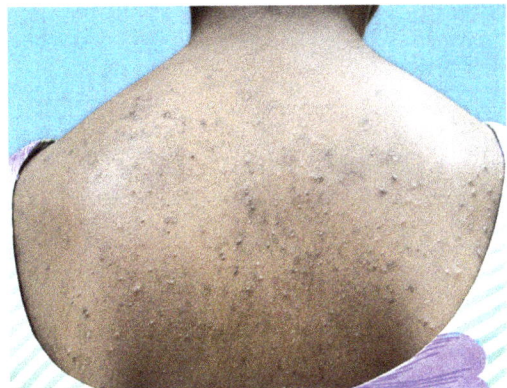

FIG. 16: A girl with truncal acne whose face was spared.

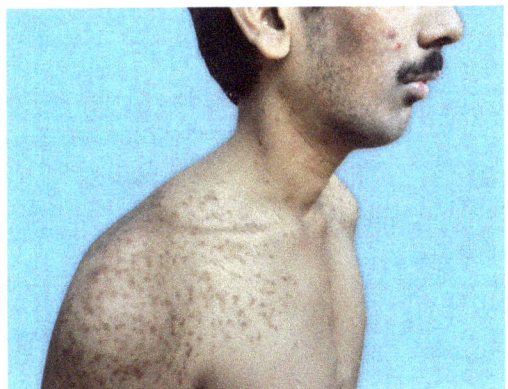

FIG. 17: Truncal involvement lesions predominately seen over the shoulder.

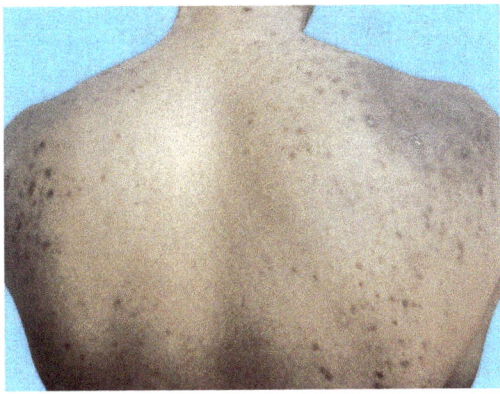

FIG. 18: Comedones over the back; note the pigmentation over shoulder following topical application.

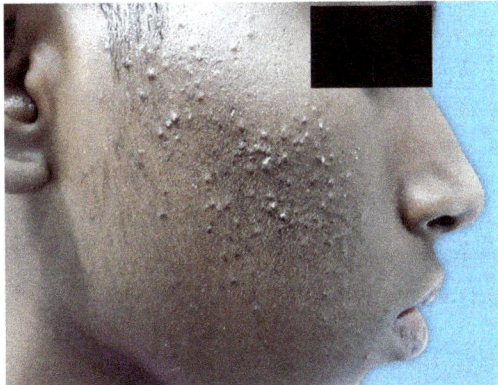

FIG. 19: A boy showing comedones and few papules; the picture can vary from mild to aggressive form with or without systemic features.

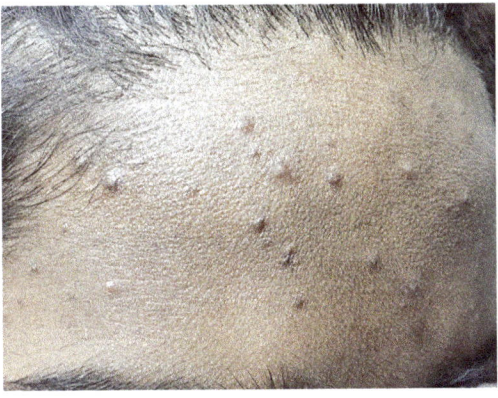

FIG. 20: Noninflammatory papules; note the receding hair line.

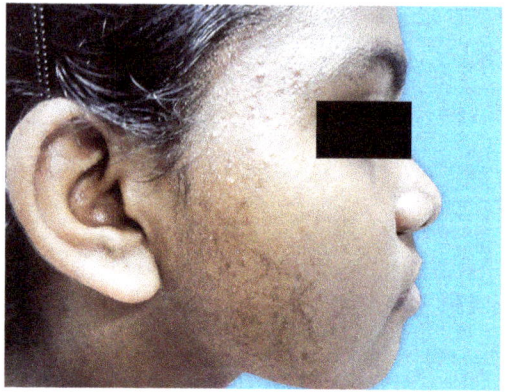

FIG. 21: Noninflamed lesions in a preadolescent; note the temporal involvement.

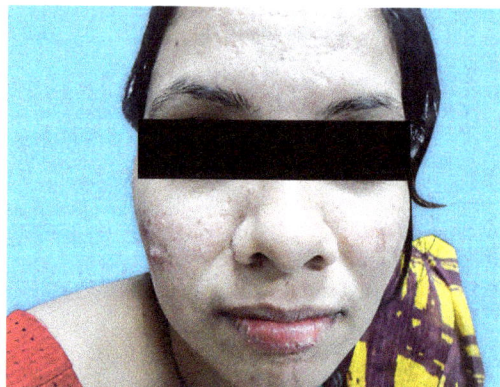

FIG. 22: Acne polymorphic inflammatory disease of the skin occurring most commonly on the face.

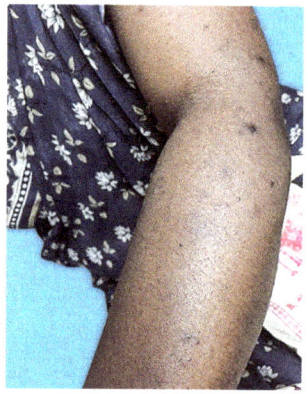

FIG. 23: Keratotic papules seen over the arm.

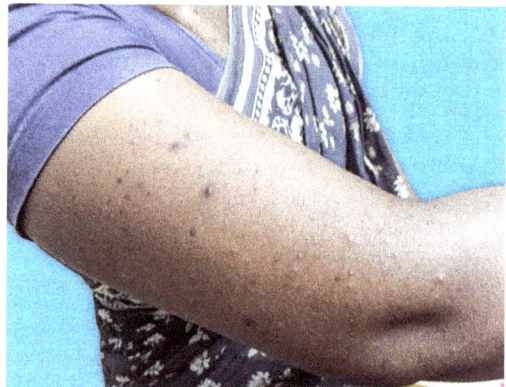

FIG. 24: Same patient as in Figure 23 showing lesions over the arm.

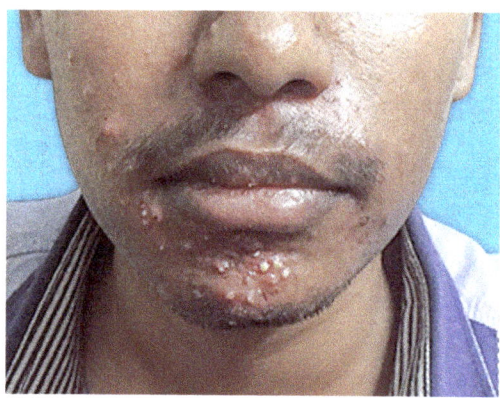

FIG. 25: Predominantly pustules; note the seborrhea.

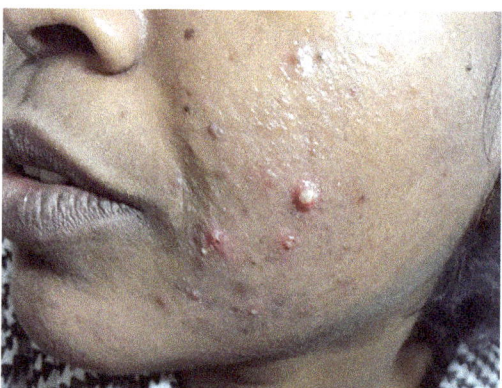

FIG. 26: V-zone acne with pustule.

CHAPTER 3: Clinical Features

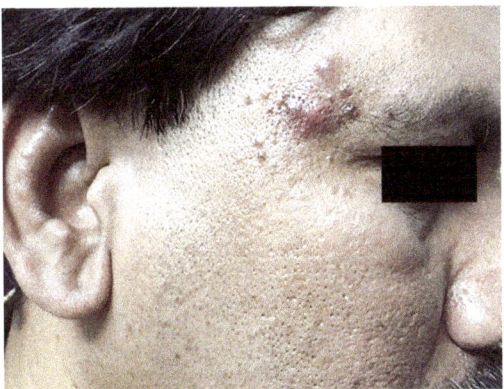

FIG. 27: Cystic lesion; temporal acne.

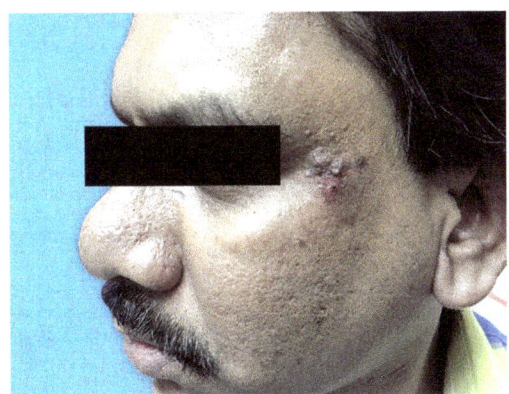

FIG. 28: Same patient as in Figure 27.

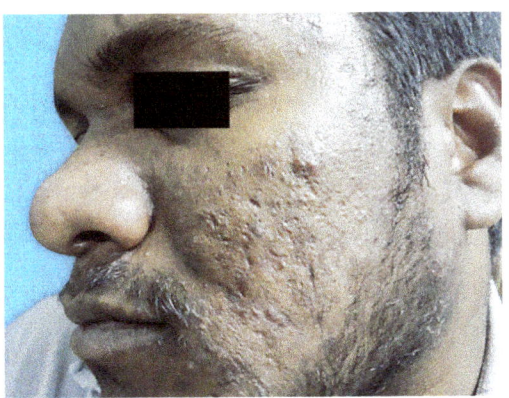

FIG. 29: Persistent nodular lesions of acne; note the resultant scars.

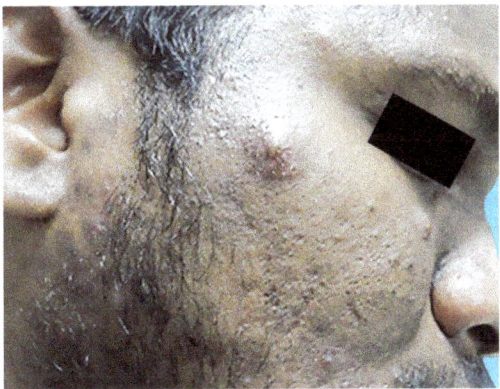

FIG. 30: Persistent nodular lesions of acne; same person as in Figure 29; note the resultant scars.

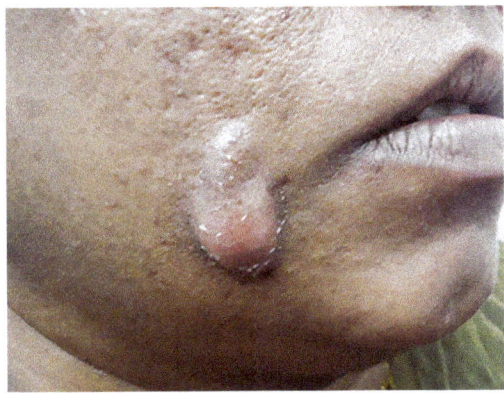

FIG. 31: Acne cysts are not true cysts as they are not lined by epithelium.

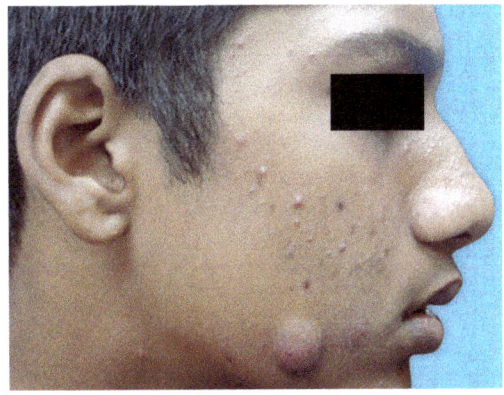

FIG. 32: Classical cystic lesion in a boy with acne.

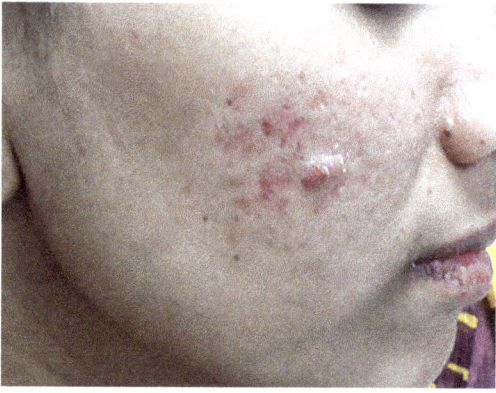

FIG. 33: Middle-aged woman with few nodulocystic lesions healing with scar.

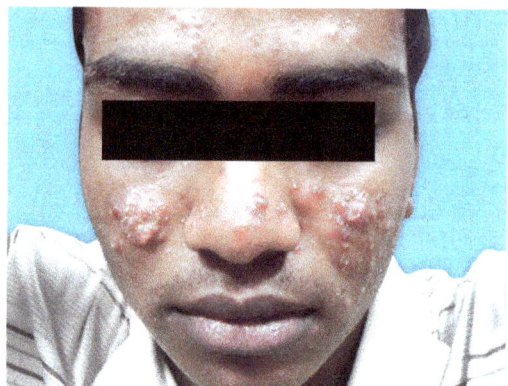

FIG. 34: Classical nodulocystic acne; note the androgenetic alopecia.

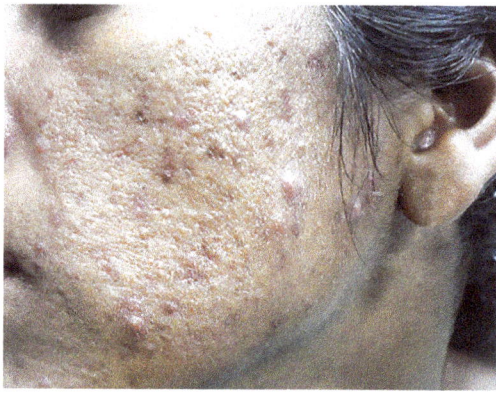

FIG. 35: Therapy-resistant acne with nodular lesions.

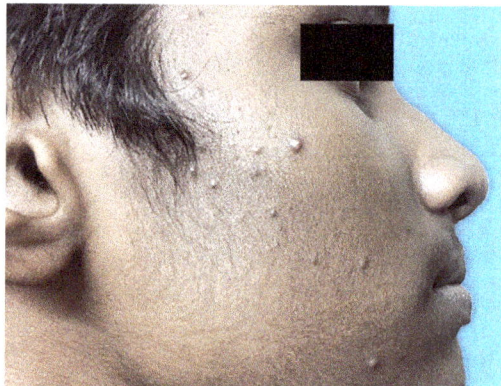

FIG. 36: Mild acne in a teenager.

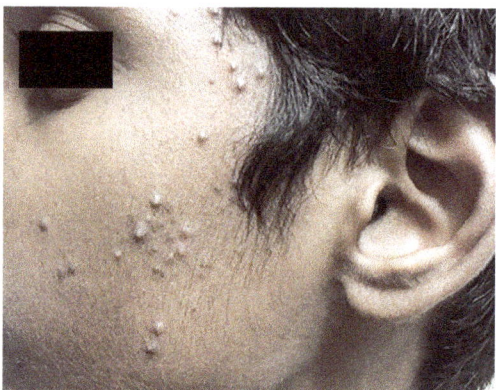

FIG. 37: Mild acne in a teenager; same patient as in Figure 36.

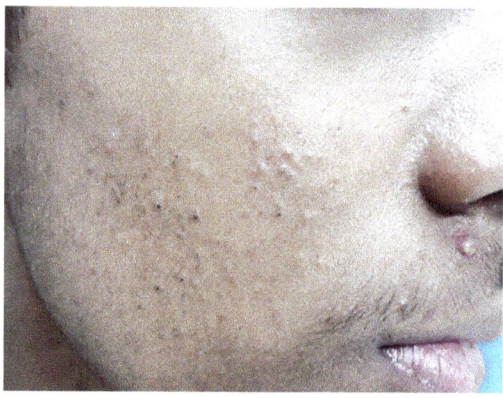

FIG. 38: Mild acne in a teenager; note that the open comedones are better seen than the closed ones.

CHAPTER 3: Clinical Features

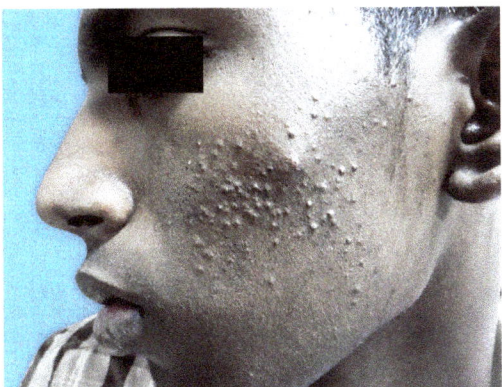

FIG. 39: Mild-to-moderate acne in a 15-year-old boy.

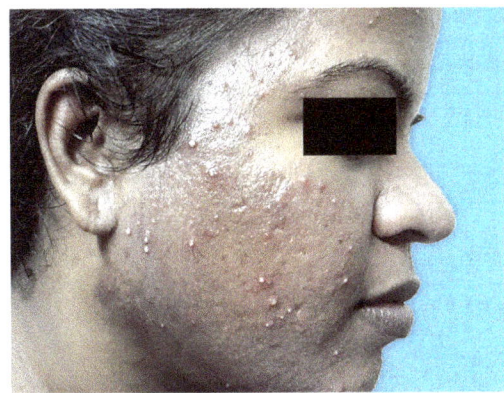

FIG. 40: Moderate acne showing predominantly pustules.

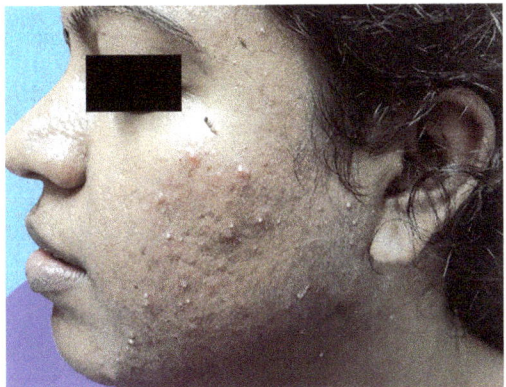

FIG. 41: Moderate acne showing predominantly pustules; same patient as in Figure 40.

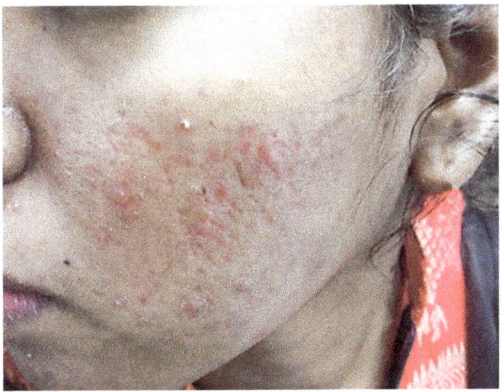

FIG. 42: Moderate acne with scar.

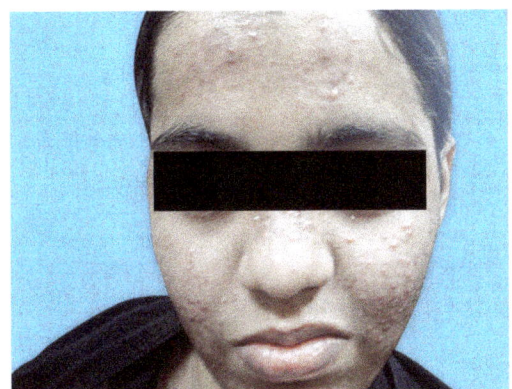

FIG. 43: Severe acne; it is not necessary to investigate unless there are other features of hyperandrogenism.

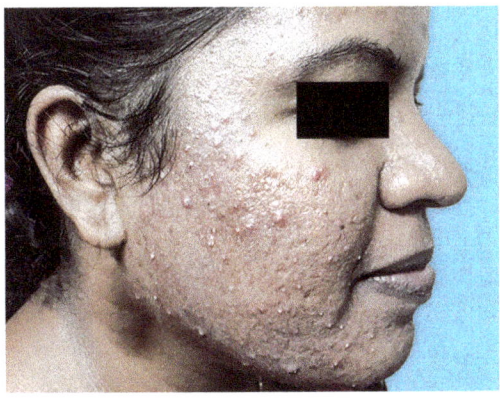

FIG. 44: Severe acne who also had polycystic ovary syndrome.

CHAPTER 3: Clinical Features

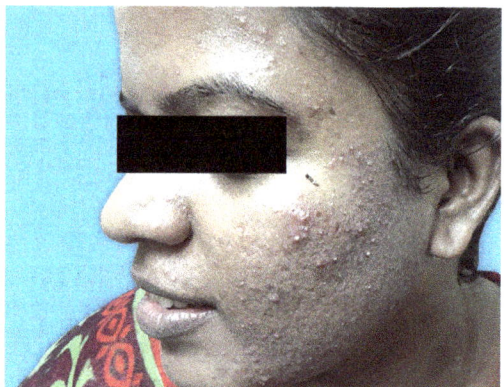

FIG. 45: Severe acne; same patient as in Figure 44.

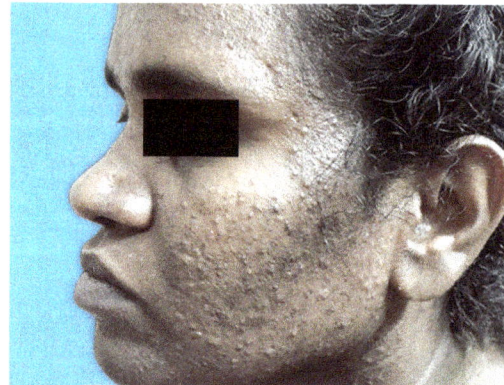

FIG. 46: Very severe acne, resistant to treatment will need hormone assessment.

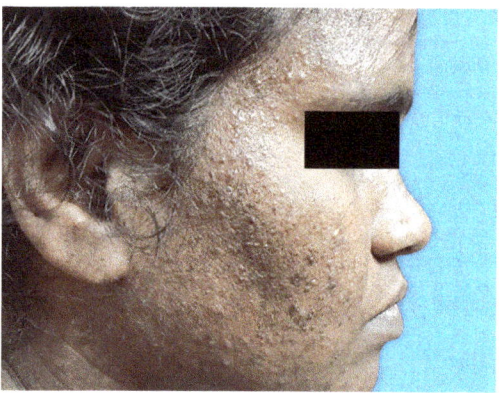

FIG. 47: Very severe acne, resistant to treatment; same patient as in Figure 46.

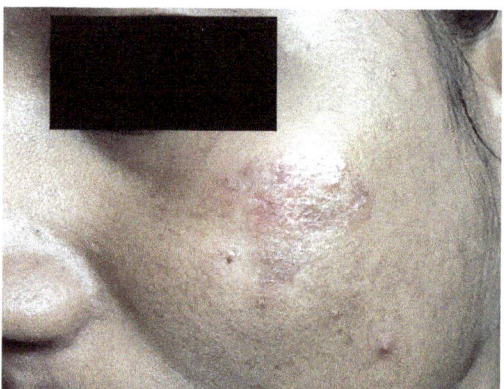

FIG. 48: Erythema is one of the major causes for concern in patients with acne.

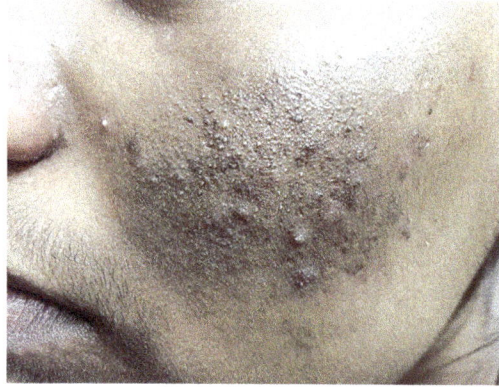

FIG. 49: Pigmentation is a common manifestation in acne.

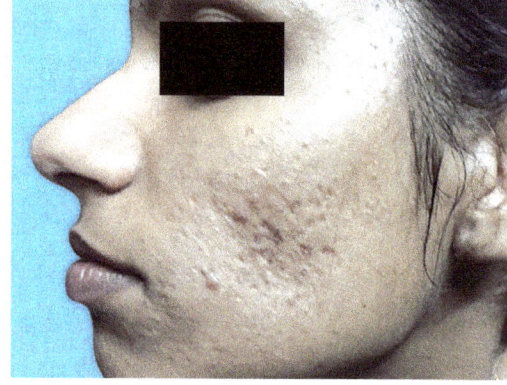

FIG. 50: Scarring and dilated pores are the telltale evidence of acne.

Symptoms

Acne vulgaris in majority of the patients is asymptomatic. However, increased sebum production which results in oily skin starts manifesting well before the clinical onset of acne. Thus, the first clinical presentation and complaint from the adolescents is that of an oily skin which is not uncommon in prepubertal children. Itching is not an uncommon symptom in patients with acne. According to some, the itching is possibly due to the release of histamine-like compound from *Cutibacterium acnes*. In some patients with itching, scratching and picking may lead to scarring if not attended appropriately. Thus, history of persistent scratching and picking should give a clue to elicit more details to rule out psychological stress in such persons. Repeated excoriation leading to itch–scratch cycle can only be detected and alleviated by proper history-taking. **Box 1** gives important points to include while eliciting history in acne patients and in those who are suspected to have drug-induced origin.

BOX 1 | **Points to be noted while eliciting history in drug-induced acne.**

- Occupation
- Dietary habits
- Duration of lesion
- Onset of drug intake in chronological order
- *Details of each drug*:
  ○ Dosage
  ○ Duration
- *Exacerbating factors*:
  ○ Hormonal therapy
  ○ Use of cosmetics (type, frequency, duration)
- Environmental factors
- *Relationship with the drug*:
  ○ Time interval between initiation of drug and onset of lesion
  ○ Time interval between improvement and withdrawal of drug

Signs

Even before development of acne lesions, many patients present with oily skin as a result of increased sebum production. Apart from seborrhea, the primary manifestations of acne include comedones, papules, pustules, cysts, and nodules. Secondary changes include erythema, scaling usually secondary-to-topical treatment, pigmentation, scarring, and keloid formation. Systemic association like fever is not uncommon in severe form of acne like acne fulminans.

Many clinical signs such as patterned hair loss, hirsutism, and acanthosis nigricans are seen in patients with endocrine acne.

Cutaneous Lesions

Face is the primary site of acne. Shoulders and front and back of chest are quite frequently involved in many patients. Men are more prone for involvement of the back. It is not surprising to see patients with severe involvement of trunk while face remains spared. Many lesions over the trunk tend to involve the interscapular region. The T- and V-zone distribution of facial acne is an important observation which may give a clue to the underlying endocrine abnormality. The T-zone of the face starts from the midpoint and sides of the forehead extending downward to include the nose and midportion of chin. This area is the most acne-prone zone of the face. The T-zone involvement or central face involvement is a common manifestation in acne vulgaris, while the V-zone involvement affecting the lower third of face involving the jaw line and chin is seen in adult-onset acne or acne associated with endocrine problems like polycystic ovarian syndrome (PCOS). Involvement of trunk is quite common in acne and severe inflammatory lesions with deep nodules over the trunk that are seen in acne fulminans and acne conglobata.

Acne is one disease where many types of skin lesions are seen in the same patient at a given point of time as it is characterized by several clinical lesions as mentioned earlier. Some patients may still have monomorphic lesions with few lesions of different morphology, particularly during the early stage of evolution of the disease. By and large, most patients present with polymorphic skin lesions.

The three important aspects to concentrate while inspecting an acne patient include:
1. Noninflammatory lesions
2. Inflammatory lesions
3. Signs of sequelae like pigmentation and scars

The skin type and presence of findings such as oily skin, excoriation marks, hirsutism, other features of hyperandrogenism, and insulin resistance have to be assessed before deciding on the treatment protocol.

Noninflammatory Lesions

Comedones are the noninflammatory lesions of acne and are pathognomonic of the disease. Comedones are of two types, namely the open and closed types. The open comedones are also referred to as the black comedones while the closed ones are called the white comedones. The dark appearance of the open comedone corresponds to the impacted keratin and/or lipid in the dilated follicular orifice which is seen at the summit of a slightly raised skin-colored papule. Because of this distinct brownish-black color, open comedones are easily visualized, whereas the closed comedones may not be easily visualized in the early stages. They are small skin-colored papules but do not have clinically visible follicular orifice. Stretching the skin will make the comedones slightly prominent and visible. Apart from the closed and open comedones, sandpaper comedones, macrocomedones, and submarine comedones are also described in acne patients. **Box 2** gives the list of various types of comedones seen in patients with acne.

BOX 2	Types of comedones in acne.
• Open comedones • Closed comedones • Sandpaper comedones • Macrocomedones • Submarine comedones	

Sandpaper comedones consist of multiple closed comedones predominantly distributed over the forehead. Macrocomedones are large, closed comedones seen over the forehead giving a rough, gritty feel. While submarine comedones are closed comedones of size greater than 0.5 cm in diameter and are placed deeply when compared to the other types of comedones. Presence of submarine comedones may indicate recurrence and evolution into a severe form of inflammatory nodular lesions.

Inflammatory Lesions

Inflammatory lesions of acne develop from the abovementioned comedones including the microcomedones. The inflammatory lesions of acne include small papules to large fluctuant nodules resembling abscesses. Papules, pustules, nodules, and abscess formation are seen in many patients during different stages of the diseases or all the lesions can be present in a patient at a particular time of examination. The term cyst should not be used to describe the large fluctuant nodules, as in acne, there is no true cyst formation. These are better referred to as nodular acne. Inflammatory lesions, if left untreated or inappropriately treated, may lead to disfiguring sequelae such as fistula, sinus tract formation, scars, and keloids.

Papules are usually skin-colored but may be erythematous. Sometimes, because of excoriation in psychologically disturbed patients, these papules may have central excoriation mark which can, sometimes bleed. In patients who are on topical treatment, especially keratolytic agents such as benzoyl peroxide and retinoic acid, and those using face wash containing peeling agents like salicylic acid may, in addition, show scaling. Location and extent of the inflammatory infiltrate in the dermis greatly determines the type of inflammatory lesion whether papule, pustule, nodule, or abscess.

Presence of grouped comedones and severe deep-seated inflammatory lesions should raise suspicion of acne conglobata.

Those with acne vulgaris are also more prone to develop chemical-induced acne. In some patients, in addition to the abovementioned lesions in the classical sites of T- or V-zone of the face, presence of comedones in the temporal region and retroauricular area, with a straw-colored cyst may indicate associated acne of chemical origin and will give a clue to the diagnosis of chloracne.

SEQUELAE

Pigmentary changes and scar formation are very common sequelae of acne often associated with excoriation in psychologically disturbed individuals to such an extent to lead on to development of prurigo nodularis. Patients may present at a given point of time with different stages of evolution of the disease and its complications.

Multiple excoriations, postinflammatory pigmentary changes, and scarring can be seen in a patient along with active lesions. The self-inflicted excoriations are mostly seen only over the accessible sights. Invariably the interscapular area will be spared as this anatomical region is unreachable by the patient. In some patients, excoriations can also be seen over not only acne lesions but also other lesions like that of folliculitis. It will be interesting to note that anxious patients with acne excoriee often spend many hours in a day in front of the mirror injuring the skin either by picking or traumatizing the lesions with instruments like tweezers in order to get temporary relief from their anxiety. In such anxious patients with acne, severely pruritic papulonodules of size up to 2 cm in diameter located preferentially on the extensor aspect of the extremities resembling prurigo nodularis are considered as an extreme variant of acne excoriee.

Scarring

Scarring is a frequent sequel of acne. Both inflammatory and noninflammatory acne can lead on to scar formation and is seen as a consequence of acne in majority of patients. It can present as atrophic scar resulting from loss of tissue or as hypertrophic scar or keloid due to excessive fibrous tissue laying.

Acne scars are broadly divided into four types namely ice pick scars, rolling scars, box scars, and hypertrophic scars.

Ice pick scars represent narrow, deep scars which are widest on the skin surface and taper as they go deeper into the dermis.

Rolling scars are shallow, wide scars that have an undulating appearance.

Box scars are wide, sharply demarcated scars. The width of box scar is same at the surface and at the base.

Hypertrophic scars are usually seen over the trunk and tend to be much elevated from the skin surface.

Keloids

These are not uncommon in patients with acne. Keloids are firm skin-colored papules or plaques seen over the healed acne lesions and extend beyond the original size of the lesion. They can be itchy and sometimes even painful.

GRADING OF ACNE

It is important to grade acne to plan appropriate therapy. Grading also helps in assessing treatment response, modification of therapy, and to convince the patient during follow-up. Severity of acne can be graded by different methods. Assessing the severity using standard assessment methods will help not only in the treatment and follow-up in individual cases but also in scientific studies and clinical trials.

Type, number of lesions, and distribution are taken into consideration for assessing the severity of acne. Most common grading system which is easily applicable in daily practice is grading acne as mild, moderate, and severe.

The evaluation of acne can be done by any of the following methods:
- Overall or global assessment
- Evaluation of individual lesions
- Evaluation according to the predominant lesion type

For academic purpose, Leeds photometric grading scale that uses a scale of 0–10 and includes face, chest, and back is the most commonly used method. However, severity of lesions is not taken into consideration in this method of grading.

Other methods adopted in the assessment of acne severity are listed below. Some of which also use the psychological effects and the QOL.
- The comprehensive acne severity system (CASS)
- Cardiff acne disability index (CADI)
- Assessment of the psychosocial effects of acne (APSEA)
- Acne quality of life scale (Acne-QOL)
- Acne quality of life four-item index (Acne-Q4)

The authors have personally experienced a better patient compliance by assessing the severity of acne and QOL. Therefore, they are of the opinion that every patient from prepubertal age onward should be assessed for both disease severity and QOL. **Table 1** gives the measures available to assess the QOL of acne patients.

A user-friendly grading system is given in **Box 3** for easy practical approach.

TABLE 1: Assessment of quality of life of acne patients.

Generic measures	• EuroQoL-5D • Short form 36 (SF-36)
General health questionnaire	• UK sickness impact profile • Preference-based measures of utility
Dermatology-specific measures	• Dermatology life quality index • Skindex • Dermatology quality of life scales • Dermatology-specific quality of life instrument • Children's dermatology life quality index
Acne-specific quality of life instruments	• Cardiff acne disability index • Acne-specific quality of life questionnaire • Acne quality of life scale • Acne quality of life index • Assessments of the psychological and social effects of acne

BOX 3 User-friendly grading system for acne.

- *Mild*: 0–5 lesions*
- *Moderate*: 6–20
- *Severe*: 21–50
- *Very severe*: >50

*Papules and pustules on one side of the face.

CHAPTER 4

Types and Variants of Acne

Acne vulgaris, as the name implies is the most common form of acne. *Acne* means prime of life and *vulgar* means common. Apart from acne vulgaris, a number of acne variants are recognized. In this section, features of the following will be discussed:
- Childhood acne
- Acne vulgaris
- Variants of acne
- Hormonal acne

CHILDHOOD ACNE (FIGS. 1 TO 30)

In children based on the age of onset, acne is classified as follows: onset at birth to 4–6 weeks; 6 weeks up to 1 year; 1–7 years; 7 years up to 12 years or menarche in girls; as neonatal, infantile, mid-childhood, and preadolescent or prepubertal acne, respectively.

Neonatal Acne

Neonatal acne is seen in the first 2 weeks of life in up to 20% of healthy newborns.

Nasal bridge and the cheeks are the most common sites involved. Other sites involved include scalp, eyelid, chin, neck, and rarely the trunk. The clinical lesions include erythematous papules and pustules. Comedones are conspicuously absent so are deep-seated nodules. The lesions resolve spontaneously within 1–3 months without any sequelae. Benign cephalic pustulosis is a hormonally mediated benign eruption now considered as variant of neonatal acne. These lesions develop within the first month of life and lack comedones papules and nodules. The eruption resolves spontaneously.

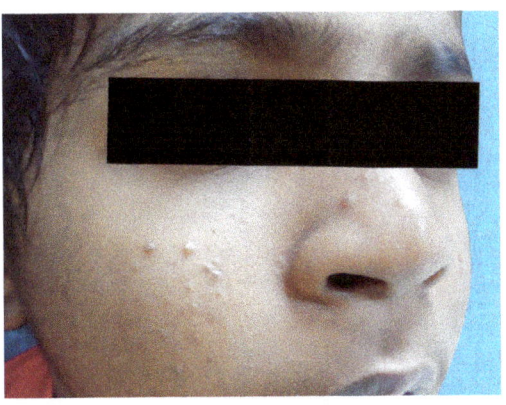

FIG. 1: Acne in a toddler; the production of proinflammatory cytokines by *Cutibacterium acnes* is not the primary pathogenic factor in acne.

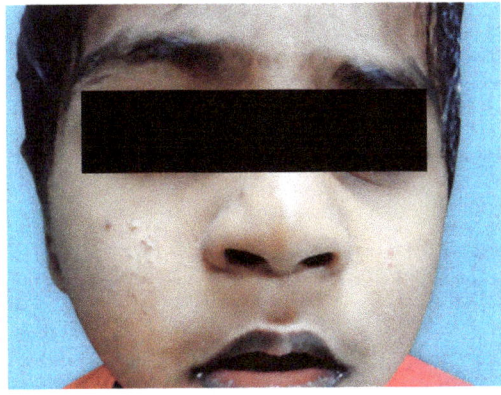

FIG. 2: Same patient as in Figure 1.

CHAPTER 4: Types and Variants of Acne

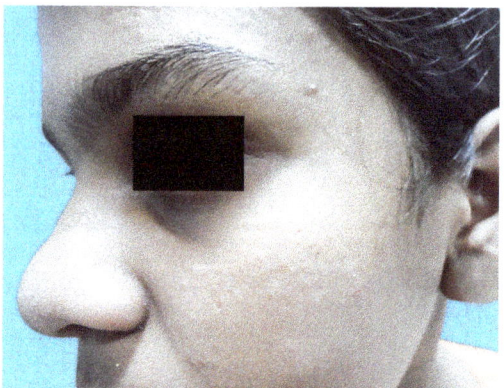

FIG. 3: Seborrhea—the initial manifestation in childhood acne.

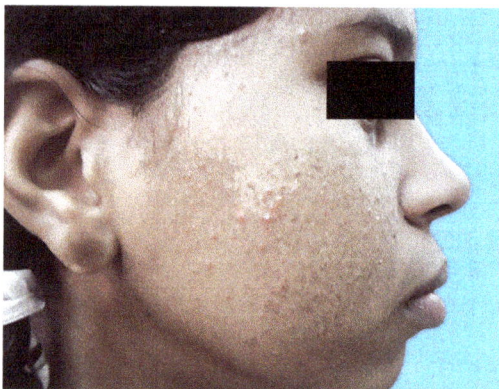

FIG. 4: Childhood acne with closed comedones in a prepubertal girl.

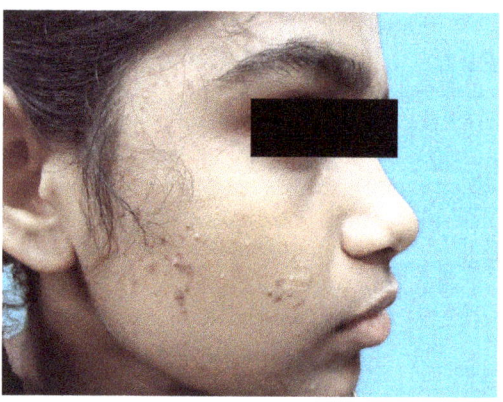

FIG. 5: Prepubertal acne with open and closed comedones.

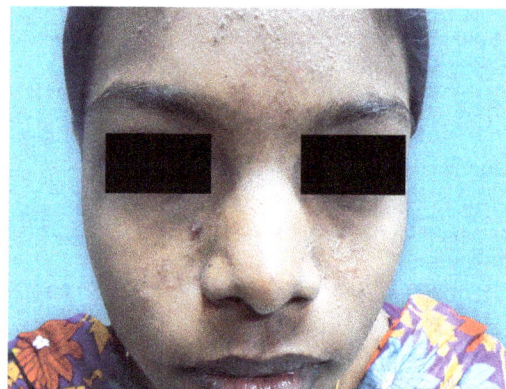

FIG. 6: Prepubertal acne involving T-zone.

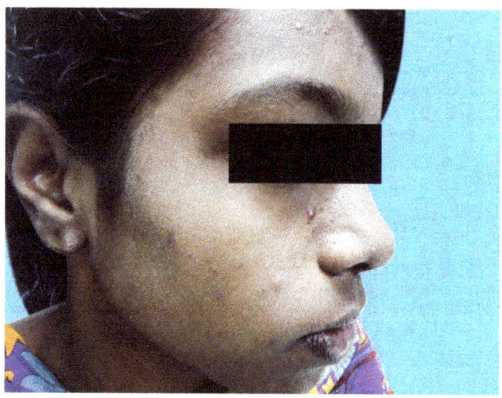

FIG. 7: Same patient as in Figure 6.

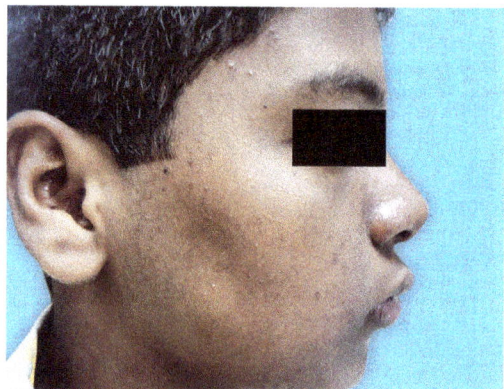

FIG. 8: A prepubertal boy with sandpaper comedones and few open comedones.

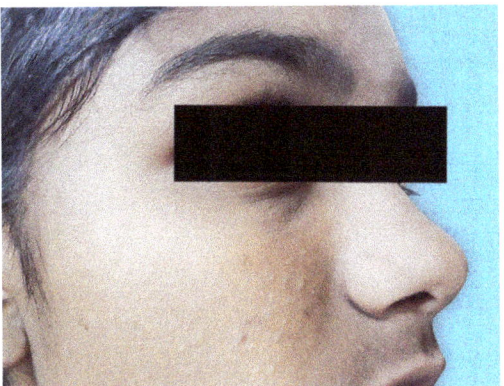

FIG. 9: Microcomedone in a 12-year-old girl.

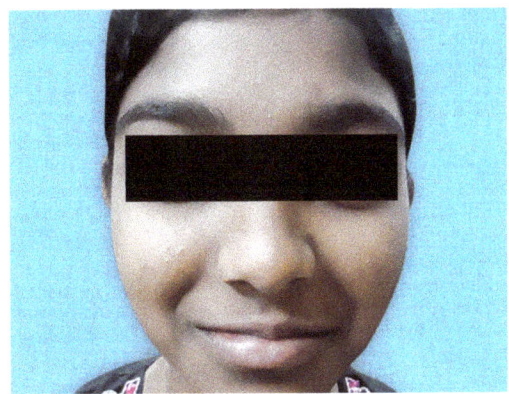

FIG. 10: Same patient as in Figure 9 with microcomedones.

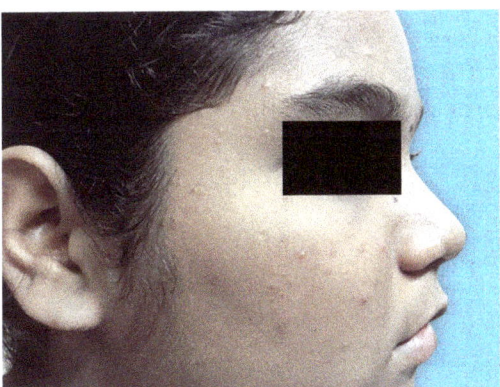

FIG. 11: Acne in a 7-year-old girl may indicate endocrine abnormality; note the mild hirsutism.

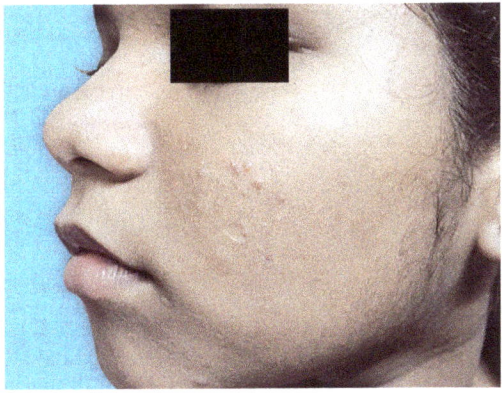

FIG. 12: Same patient as in Figure 11 with acne and hirsutism.

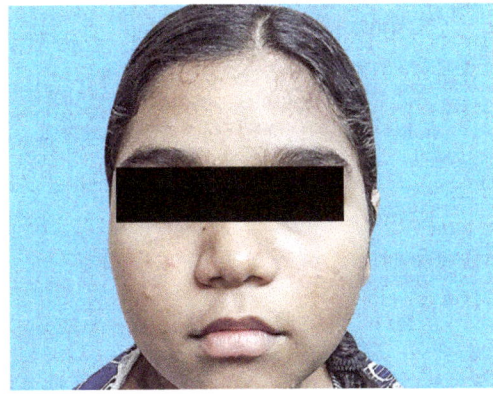

FIG. 13: Acne in an obese girl; same patient as in Figures 11 and 12.

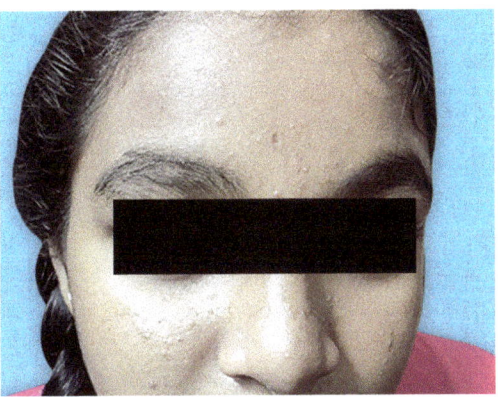

FIG. 14: Acne in a 13-year-old girl heralding the onset of puberty.

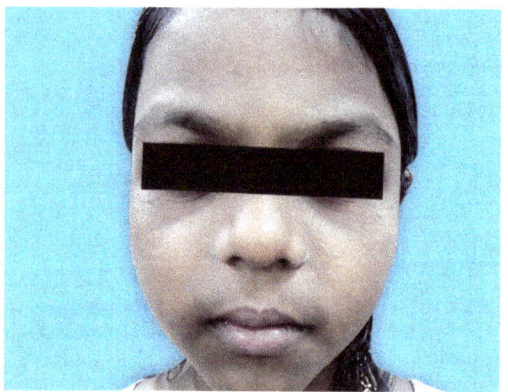

FIG. 15: Predominantly closed comedones in a prepubertal girl.

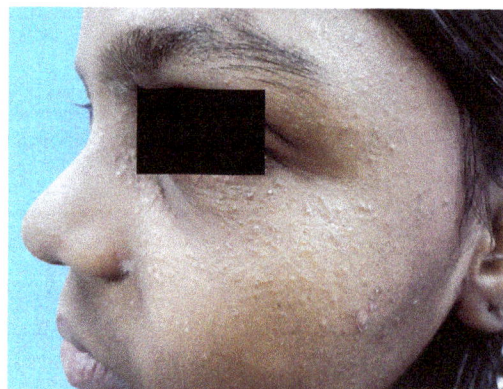

FIG. 16: Extensive lesions in prepubertal girl; better delineated by closer examination; same patient as in Figure 15.

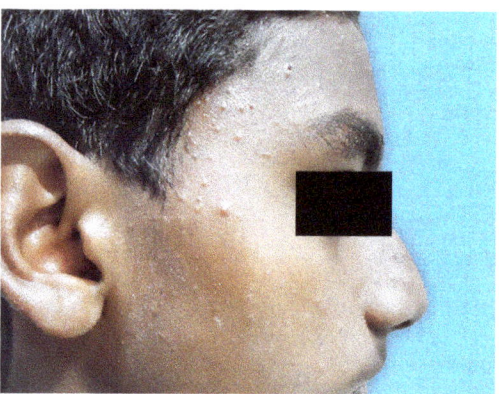

FIG. 17: Seborrhea and temporal acne in a preadolescent boy.

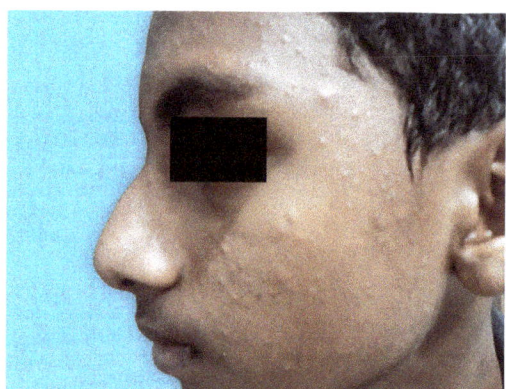

FIG. 18: Same boy as in Figure 17.

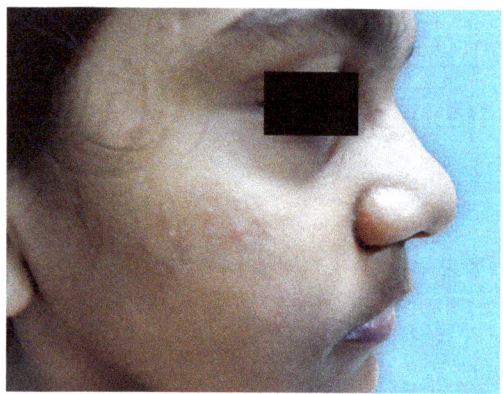

FIG. 19: Acne vulgaris in a preadolescent.

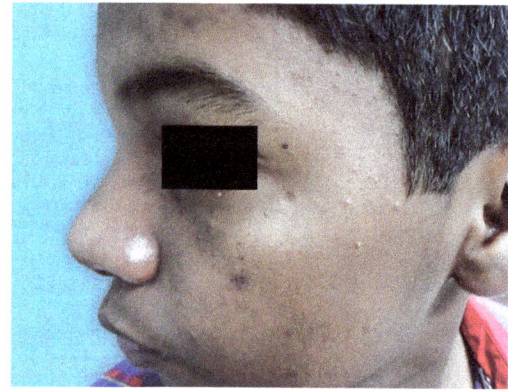

FIG. 20: Small open and closed comedones in a 10-year-old boy; note the milium near lower eyelid.

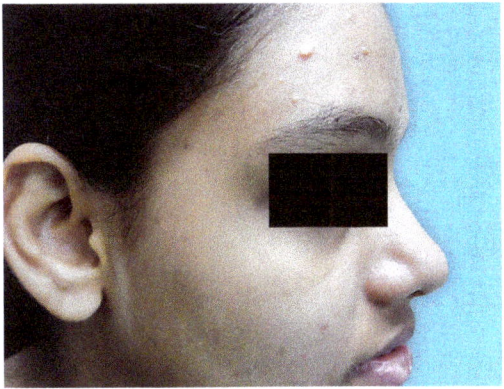

FIG. 21: Papules of acne marking the onset of puberty.

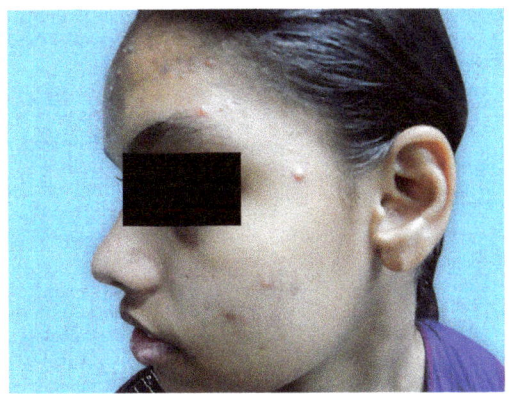

FIG. 22: Papules of acne in same girl as in Figure 12.

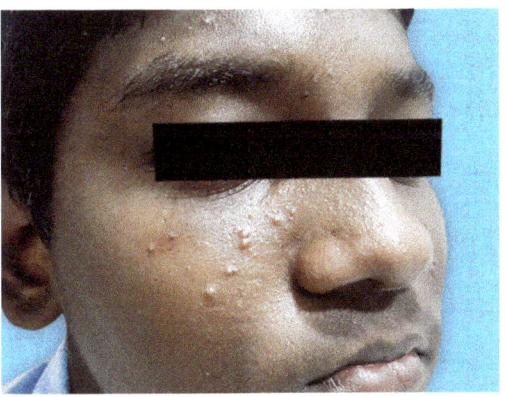

FIG. 23: Papules of acne in T-zone and oily skin in a 14-year-old boy.

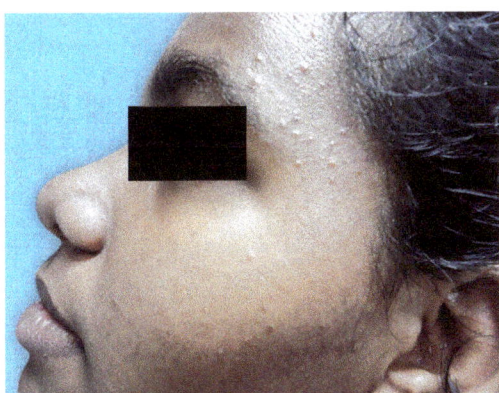

FIG. 24: Acne in a 7-year-old girl may either mark early menarche or an endocrine abnormality.

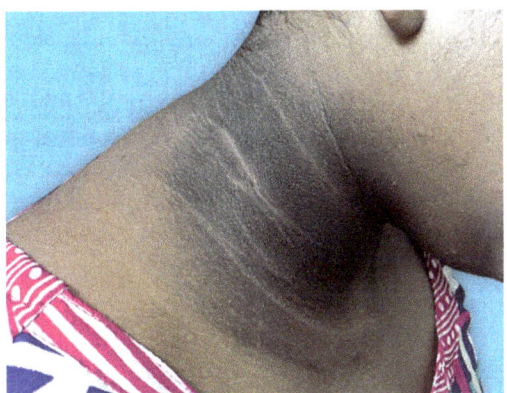

FIG. 25: Mid-childhood acne in an obese girl; note acanthosis nigricans; must evaluate for endocrine abnormality.

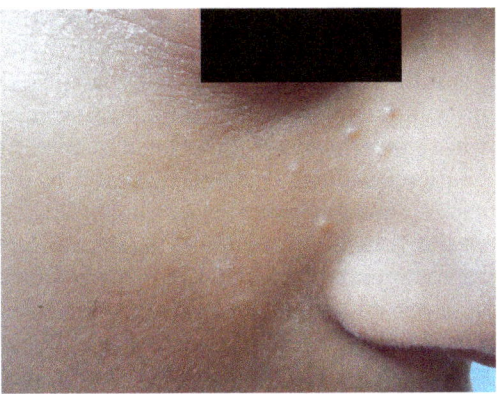

FIG. 26: Mild childhood acne may warrant endocrine evaluation, if child develops features of hyperandrogenism.

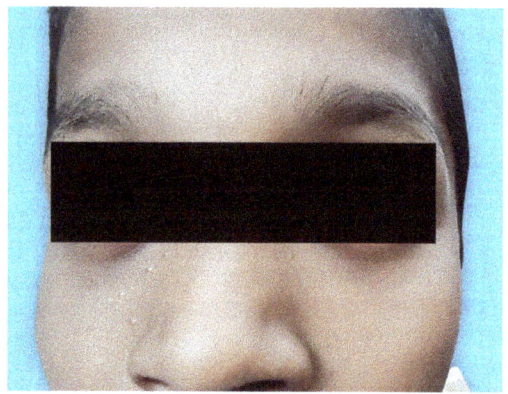

FIG. 27: Mild childhood acne; same patient as in Figure 26.

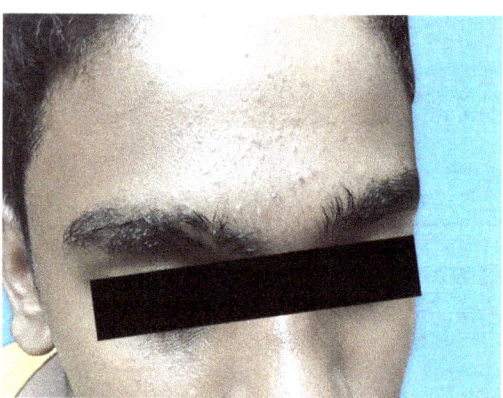

FIG. 28: Mild acne in a preadolescent.

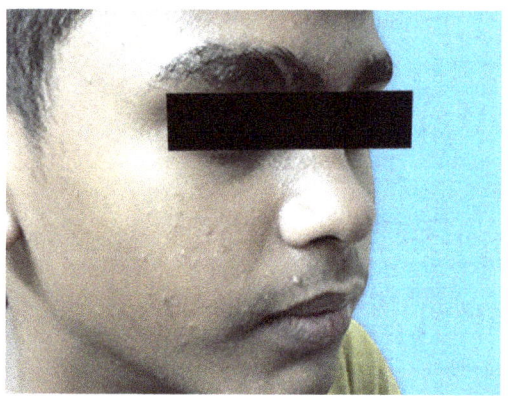

FIG. 29: Same preadolescent boy as in Figure 28 showing closed comedones.

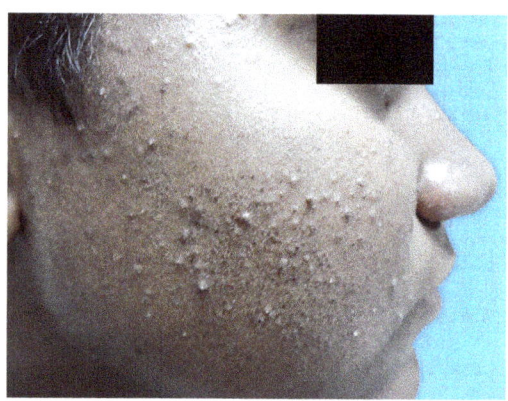

FIG. 30: Moderate acne in a 10-year-old boy; there is a correlation between the severity of acne and number and size of lesion.

Infantile Acne

Infantile acne is less frequently seen than neonatal acne and starts manifesting from 6 to 16 months of age. Boys seem to be more frequently affected when compared to girl babies. Unlike neonatal acne, in infantile acne, all classical lesions of acne vulgaris, namely comedones, both closed and open, papules, pustules, and nodules, can be demonstrated. The lesions resolve by 4-5 years of age with formation of scar in some children. If the lesions are very severe and persistent hyperandrogenemia should be thought of and evaluated for. In such infants, signs of precautious puberty, such as increased height, weight, and enlarged clitoris or penis should be looked for and if present, endocrine evaluation becomes mandatory. It should be remembered that children with infantile acne are prone to develop more severe acne during adolescence.

Mid-childhood Acne

Acne after infancy and before 8 years is extremely rare. Diagnosis of mid-childhood acne indicates hyperandrogenism. However, one has to remember that in the current days where the age of menarche has advanced, some children developing acne around 7 years may well be prepubertal acne which normally starts manifesting from 8 years of age. These children, especially born in acne-prone family, may develop such lesions which persist up to adolescence and adulthood indicating an early onset of acne vulgaris.

Mid-childhood acne is extremely rare, and a diagnosis warrants investigation to rule out hyperandrogenism.

> **BOX 1** **Evaluation in a child with acne suspected to have endocrinopathy.**
> - Family history of virilization
> - Age of menarche in girls
> - Tanner stage
> - Thelarche
> - Pubarche
> - Testicular enlargement
> - Clitoral enlargement
> - Growth chart
> - Height, weight, body mass index
> - Bone age by measurement

Prepubertal Acne

Acne developing in the age group 7-12 years is referred to as prepubertal acne. However, because of early puberty, acne occurring in this age group can well be adolescent acne in some children as 12 years of age is no longer the lower age limit for normal onset of adolescent acne. Therefore, earlier onset of acne should be considered as representation of first sign of onset of puberty in the above age group. Preadolescent acne clinically manifests as seborrhea and comedones.

Acne conglobata is a severe variant of acne and has been reported in infants presenting with severe inflammatory cystic lesion, sinus tracts, and scarring.

Grading of Acne

It is difficult to grade acne in children, as there are no validated systems available for grading childhood acne. However, conventionally acne can be graded as mild, moderate, or severe, and presence of scar be considered as poor prognostic sign. Associated endocrine abnormality should be viewed with diligence. Important findings to be noted in history and clinical examination in a child with acne suspected to have endocrinopathy are listed in **Box 1**.

The following clinical scenario may give a clue to suspect underlying problem in children with acne:
- *Up to 1 year*: Acne with accelerated growth and signs of virilization—adrenocortical tumor
- *1-7 years*: Acute onset, persistent severe acne with features of virilization—underlying endocrinopathy
- *7-12 years (boy)*: Recalcitrant severe acne—congenital adrenal hyperplasia
- *7-12 years and above (girl)*: Ovarian androgen excess is normally due to polycystic ovarian syndrome (PCOS), but may be from benign or malignant ovarian tumor.

However, studies indicate that in the absence of clinical symptoms and signs, the risk of true endocrinopathy in pediatric acne is relatively low, and hence, an elaborate investigation is seldom needed in these children. It will be generally acceptable that in quite a number of children, especially girls, after exclusion of underlying endocrine abnormality clinically, preteen acne nowadays can very well be considered as onset of menarche which will eventually continue as acne vulgaris.

ACNE VULGARIS (FIGS. 31 TO 60)

Acne vulgaris is a disorder of the adolescence. However, oily skin and microcomedones may herald the onset in the prepubertal stage starting from 8 years of age. In quite a few, it is mild and self-limiting. Nevertheless, acne lesions may persist beyond the teenage and may become severe in adulthood. Though acne is usually asymptomatic in some patients, itching, pain, tenderness, or redness may be the presenting symptom apart from seborrhea. Acne vulgaris *per se* does not present with systemic symptoms. Deep-seated lesions in severe acne present with pain and tenderness.

Site of Affection

In acne vulgaris, the lesions are invariably seen over the face in nearly 99% of patients. However, in many, the lesions extend to involve the neck, shoulders, chest, and back (60%). In those with severe disease, lesions are seen more extensively over the other body sites.

When the lesions start appearing, they are seen predominantly centering around the pilosebaceous units. This very well explains the sites of predilection over the face involving the T-zone which is rich in pilosebaceous units. It is worthy to note that not all patients have an oily skin involving the entire face. Rather the T-zone is oily while the rest of the face is dry in those individuals having a combination type of skin. At a given point of time, although one type of lesion predominates, detailed examination will reveal other types of lesions, both inflammatory and noninflammatory, in a patient based on which the treatment will vary.

The lesions are invariably polymorphous of variable extent and severity, except in the early stages. The superficial lesions include comedones, papules, and pustules. All types of comedones including open, closed, sandpaper, and macrocomedones can be seen at the same time. Early appearance of open comedones may indicate a poor prognosis. These frequently appear in the T-zone of the face. Since closed comedones are skin-colored and do not have visible follicular opening, they are likely to be missed unless the skin is stretched and examined under adequate lighting.

Papules and pustules are also classical inflammatory lesions of acne vulgaris and may develop *de novo* or from the preexisting comedones. Among the deeper lesions, submarine comedones are those of size greater than 0.5 cm in diameter and are placed deeply when compared to the other types of comedones. Presence of submarine comedones indicates possibility of recurrence and evolution into a severe form of inflammatory nodular lesions in future. Nodules and pseudocysts are deeper lesions of acne which invariably lead to disfiguring scars. It is not uncommon to see few excoriation marks, erythema over the treated or healed lesions, and pigmentary changes in patients with acne vulgaris. The erythema is more easily delineated in fair individuals. Those with darker skin color are prone to develop pigmentation following resolution of inflammatory lesions with or without treatment. Pigmentation is not uncommon after healing of noninflammatory lesions such as comedones.

Normal course of the disease in a self-limiting case takes 2 weeks to few months for comedones and papulopustules, respectively.

Grading in Acne Vulgaris

Acne vulgaris grading is important for both treatment point of view as well as for research purposes. Lesions of acne vulgaris can be graded as mild, if the number of comedones and inflammatory lesions is <20 and 15, respectively or <30 taking into consideration both the inflammatory and noninflammatory lesions put together.

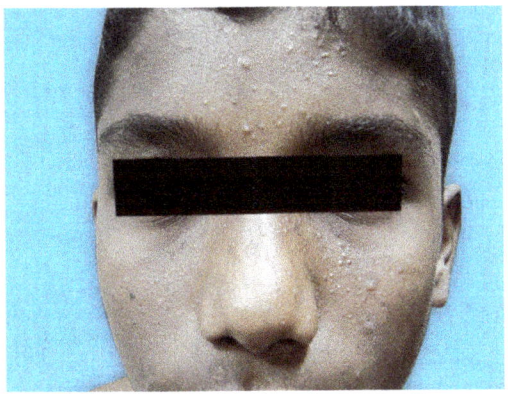

FIG. 31: Sudden onset of seborrhea and inflammatory lesions in an adolescent showing polymorphic lesions indicating poor prognosis.

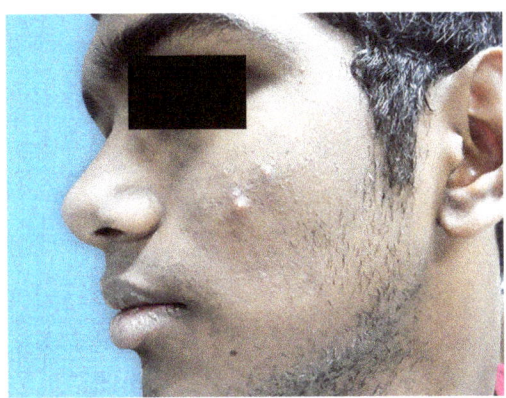

FIG. 32: Early pustular lesion of acne vulgaris.

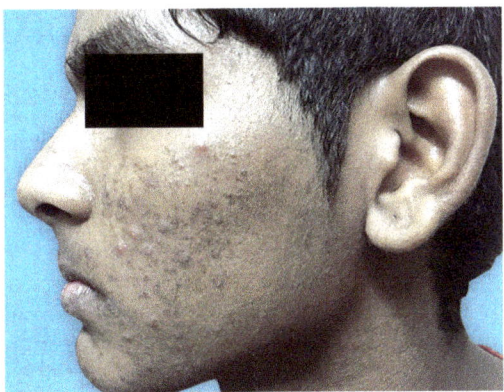

FIG. 33: Erythematous papules in an adolescent.

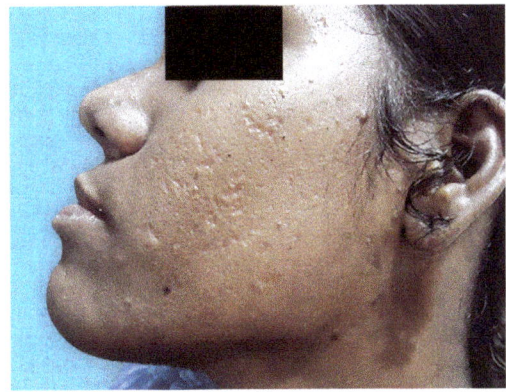

FIG. 34: Few papules and scars in an adolescent indicating genetic proneness for scaring.

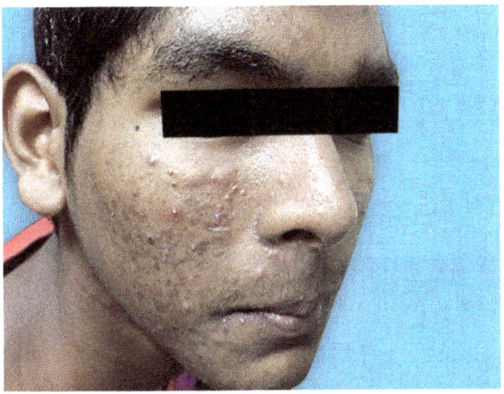

FIG. 35: Seborrhea, comedones, papules, pustules, and nodules in an adolescent.

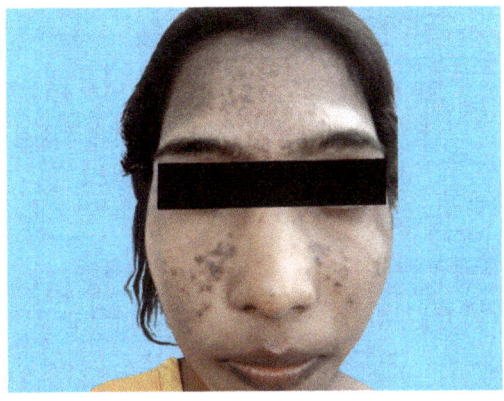

FIG. 36: T-zone involvement in an adolescent girl.

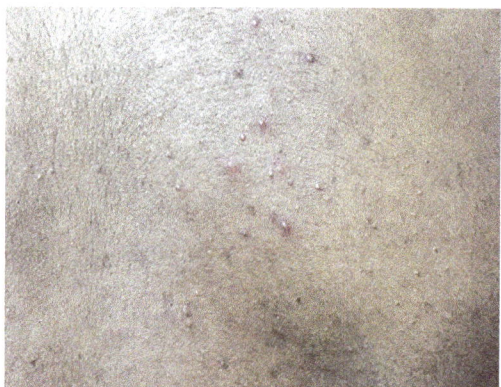

FIG. 37: Involvement of trunk an adolescent boy.

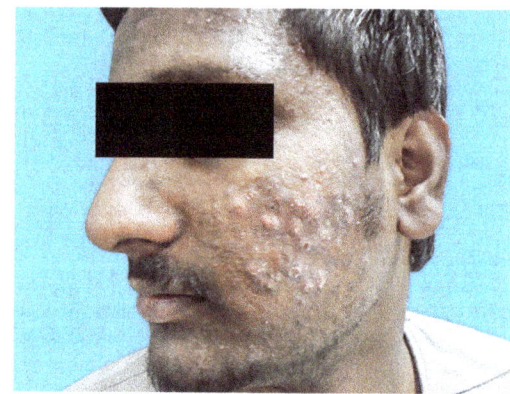

FIG. 38: Inflammatory lesions of acne.

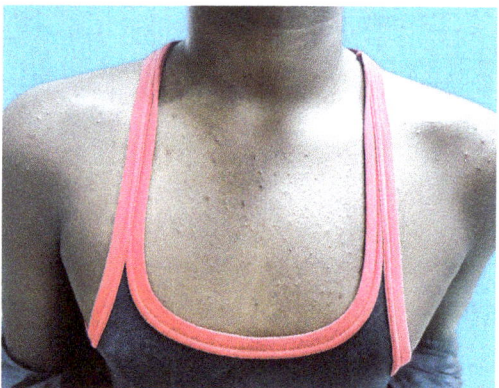

FIG. 39: Involvement of chest and shoulder in an adolescent boy.

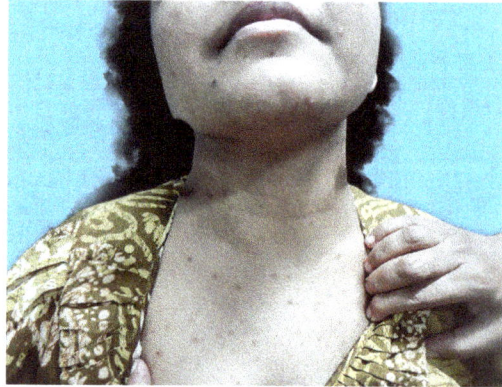

FIG. 40: Involvement of chest in an adolescent carries poor prognosis; note facial lesions as well.

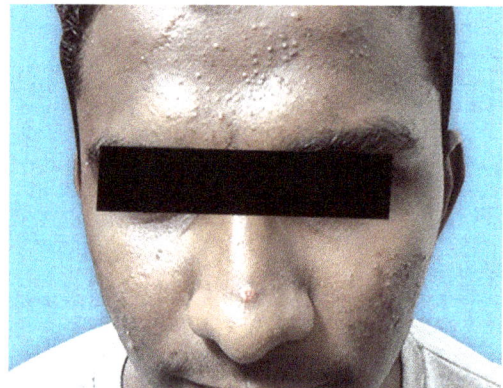

FIG. 41: Grade I acne vulgaris in an adolescent boy having T-zone distribution.

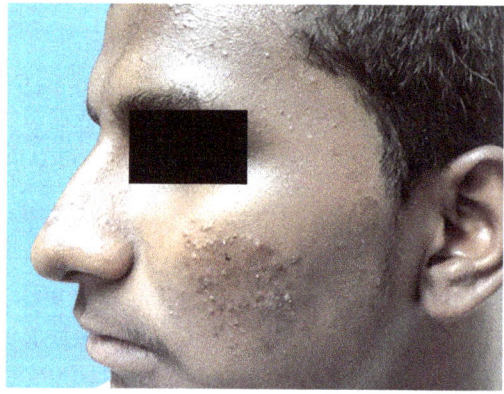

FIG. 42: Same boy as in Figure 41.

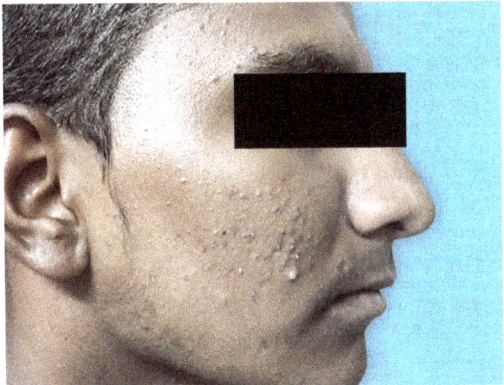

FIG. 43: Grade I acne vulgaris in an adolescent; same patient as in Figure 41; note the seborrhea and pustules.

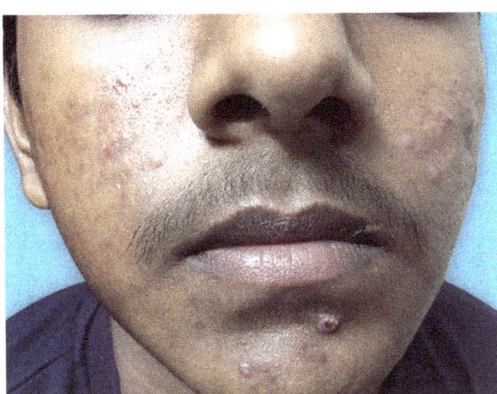

FIG. 44: Grade II acne vulgaris in an adolescent; note the scarring.

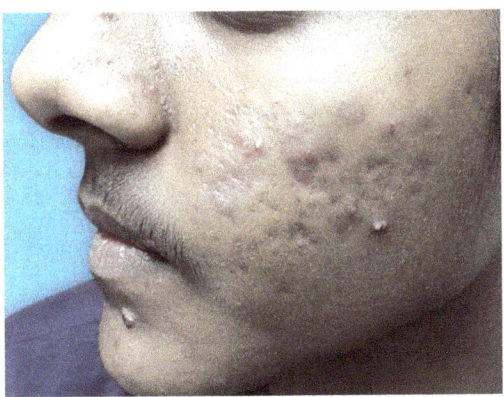

FIG. 45: Grade II acne vulgaris in an adolescent; same patient as in Figure 44.

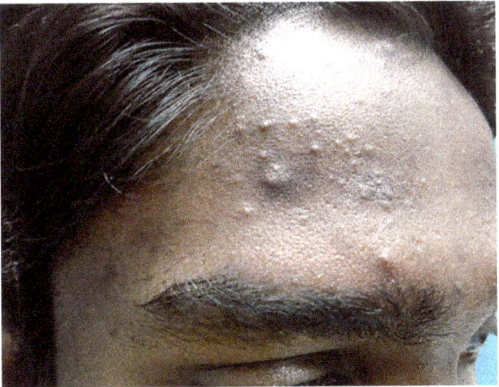

FIG. 46: Adolescent boy developing papular lesions over forehead.

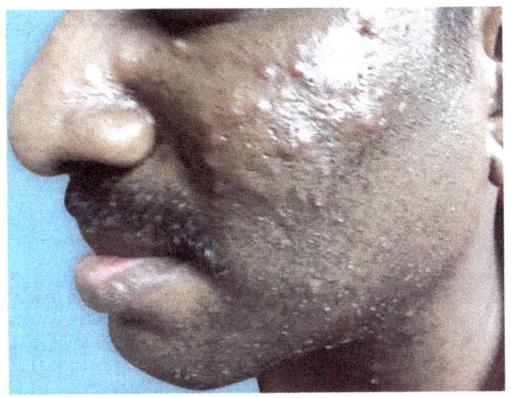

FIG. 47: Nodulocystic lesions in an adolescent male; note the seborrhea and scarring.

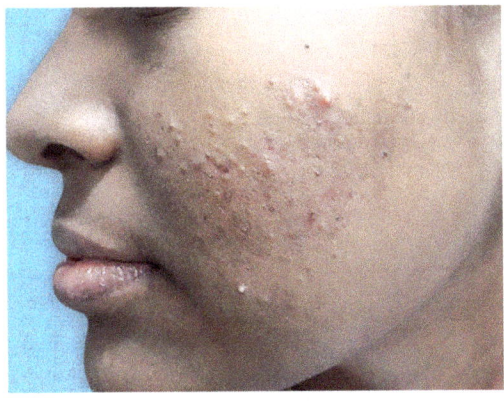

FIG. 48: Papulopustule of acne vulgaris in an adolescent.

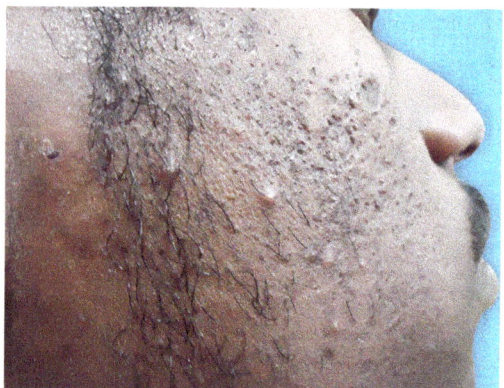

FIG. 49: Acne vulgaris with scarring.

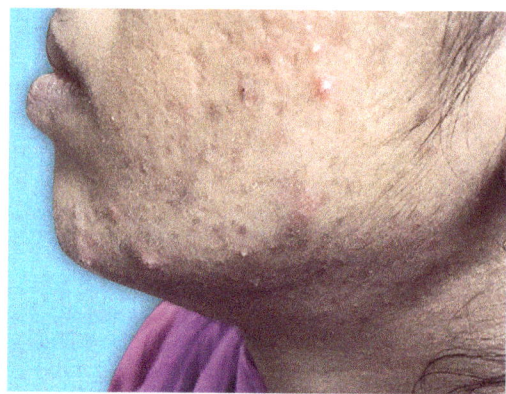

FIG. 50: Inflammatory lesions with features of hyperandrogenism in an adolescent girl.

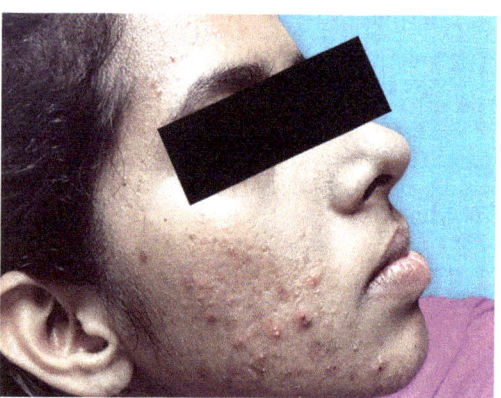

FIG. 51: Acne vulgaris with scars; same patient as in Figure 50.

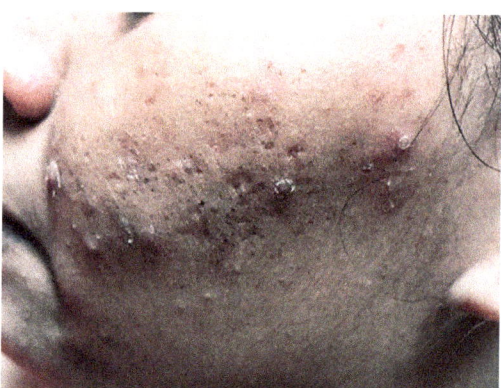

FIG. 52: Acne vulgaris with scaling following keratolytic application.

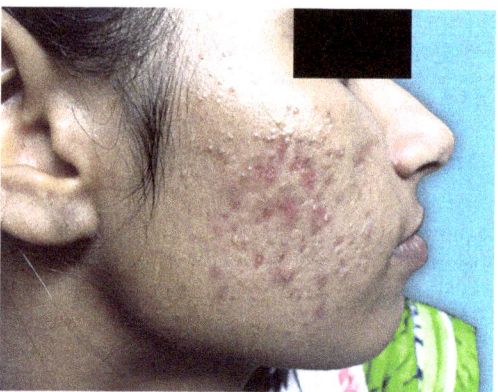

FIG. 53: Acne vulgaris with erythema and scarring.

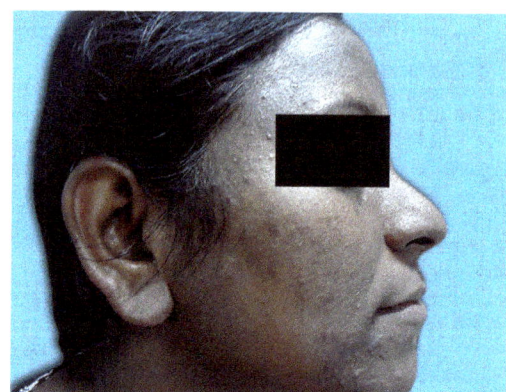

FIG. 54: Acne vulgaris with pigmentation.

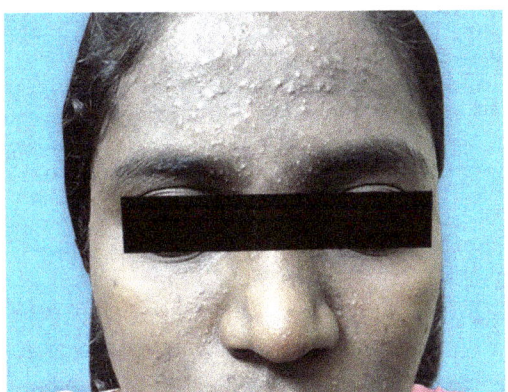

FIG. 55: Acne vulgaris with facial pigmentation in an adolescent.

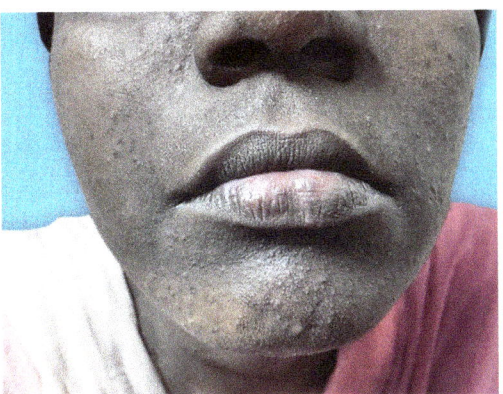

FIG. 56: Acne vulgaris with facial pigmentation in same patient as in Figure 55; note involvement of perioral area.

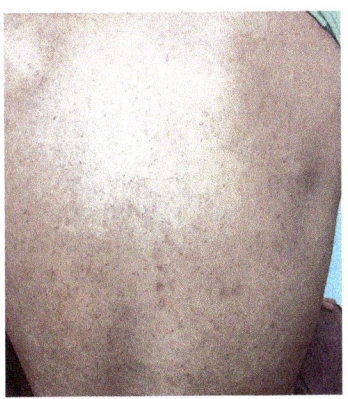

FIG. 57: Acne vulgaris with pigmentation over back.

FIG. 58: Acne vulgaris with multiple black and white comedones with pigmentation; same boy as in Figure 57.

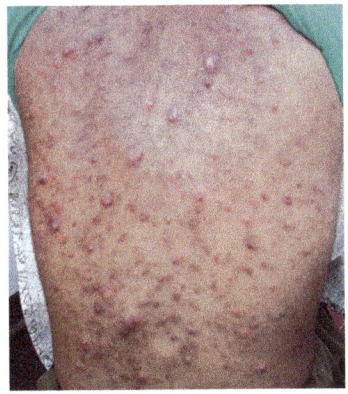

FIG. 59: Acne vulgaris with severe scarring in an adolescent; a few of them are keloidal.

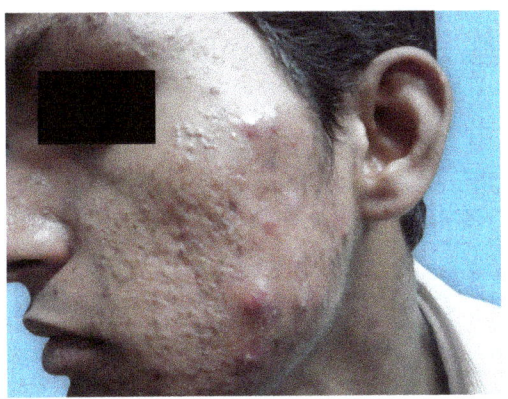

FIG. 60: Acne vulgaris nodulocystic lesions with disfiguring scar.

Whereas moderate acne is where the numbers of comedones and inflammatory lesions are 20–100 and 15–50, respectively, or 30–125 taking into consideration both the inflammatory and noninflammatory lesions put together. To label acne vulgaris severe, the patient must have a total lesion count >125 or 100 comedones and 50 papulopustules. He/she should have more than five deep-seated nodules or pseudocysts. Severe form of acne vulgaris is seen in patients with acne conglobata. Such patients also present with systemic symptoms like fever as in acne fulminans. Significant numbers of the patients with acne vulgaris have psychological impact regardless of the grade of disease. The affection is more with patients having facial acne than those with only truncal involvement. The impact further worsens with sequelae like pigmentation and scarring.

Sequelae

In majority of patients with inflammatory lesions, scars are evident in addition to the existing lesions and indicate sites of healed lesions. In severe forms of acne vulgaris, sinus tracts may develop between deep-seated pustules and nodules leading to highly disfiguring scars and even keloids in prone individuals.

ACNE VARIANTS (FIGS. 61 TO 110)

Clinical manifestation of acne is so variable due to various other associated factors. Many different types of acne and acne-related problems have been examined. The different forms of acne are listed in **Box 2**.

Adult-onset Acne (Acne Tarda)

Adult-onset acne, also known as late-onset acne, is defined as acne lesions that appear for the first time beyond the age of 25. It affects up to 15% of women and is rare in men. Drugs are known to induce acne in adulthood. The common drugs incriminated in the development of adult-onset acne are listed in **Box 3**.

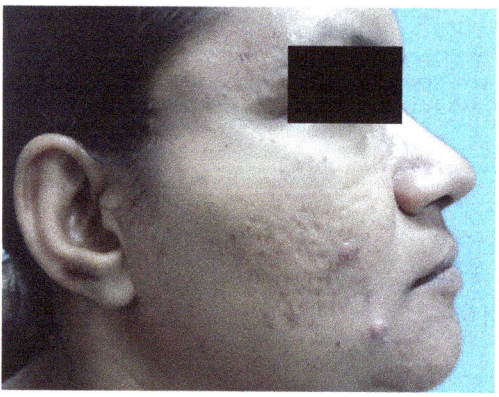

FIG. 61: Late-onset acne in a middle-aged woman.

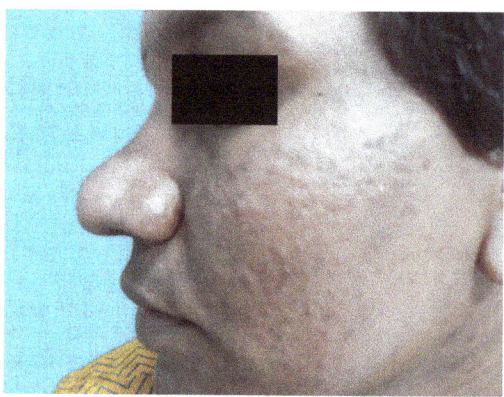

FIG. 62: Late-onset acne in a patient on replacement therapy.

CHAPTER 4: Types and Variants of Acne

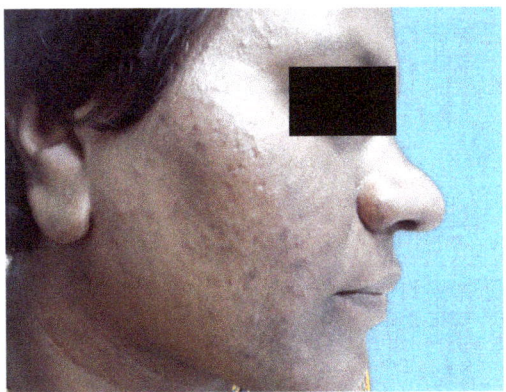

FIG. 63: Same lady as in Figure 62 on hormonal therapy.

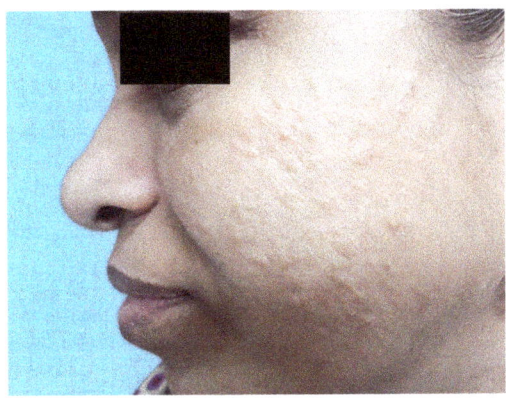

FIG. 64: Late-onset acne in a diabetic woman.

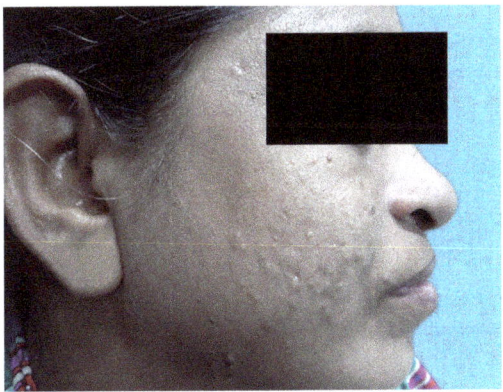

FIG. 65: Same woman as in Figure 64.

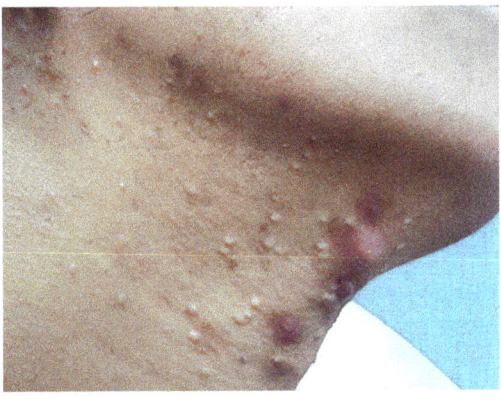

FIG. 66: Persistent acne in a woman; consider late-onset adrenal hyperplasia.

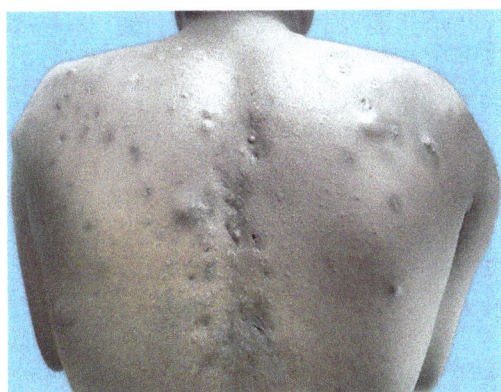

FIG. 67: Acne conglobata runs a chronic course and can last even up to the fifth decade.

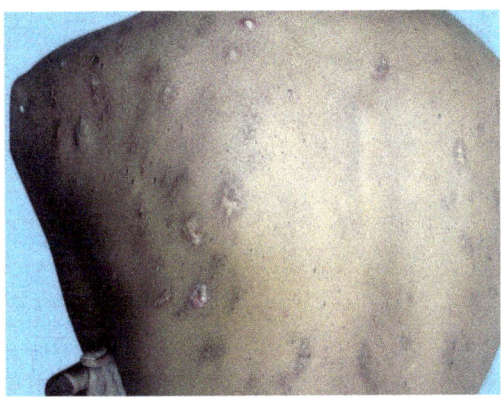

FIG. 68: Acne conglobata following treatment; note the deep irregular scars.

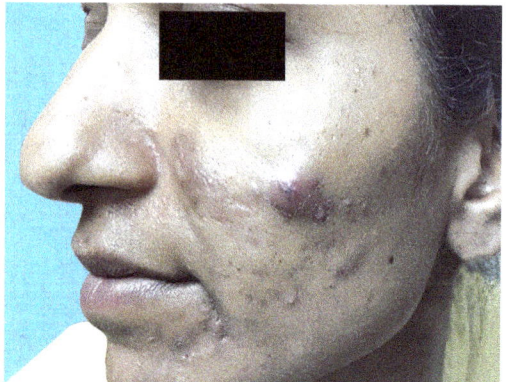

FIG. 69: Nodulocystic lesions in a woman with keloidal scar.

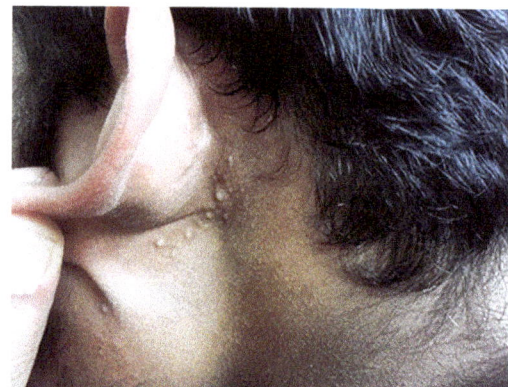

FIG. 70: Retroauricular yellowish papule is a marker of chloracne.

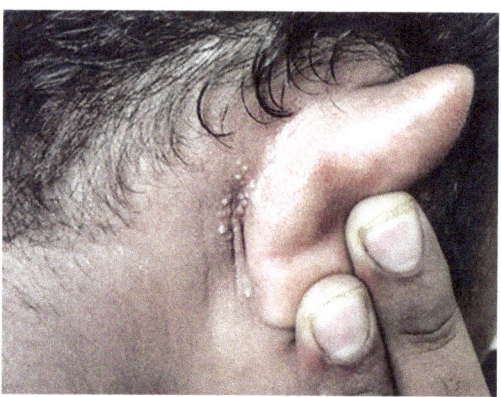

FIG. 71: Retroauricular papules; same patient as in Figure 70.

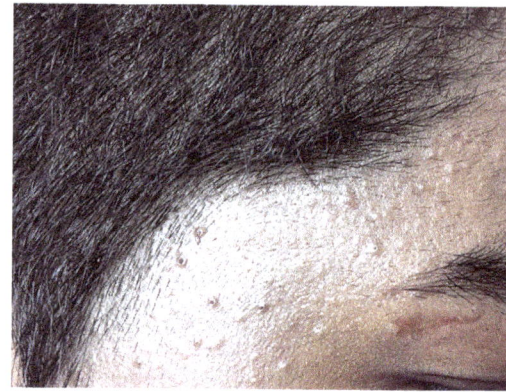

FIG. 72: Temporal lesions are seen in chloracne.

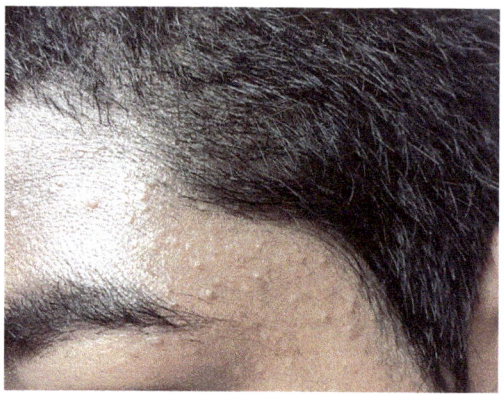

FIG. 73: Temporal lesions; same patient as in Figure 72.

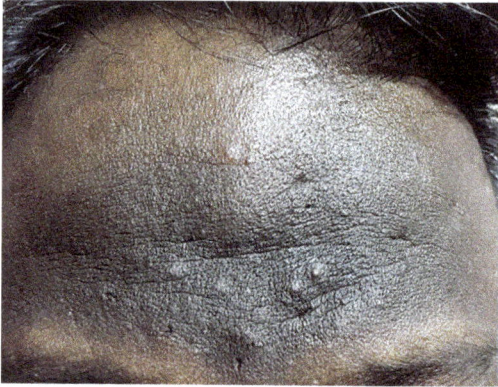

FIG. 74: Acne papules resulting from chronic friction; note lichenification.

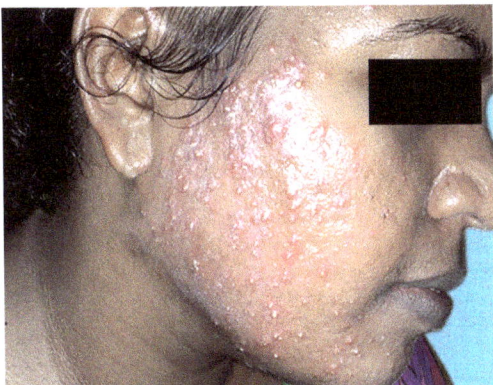

FIG. 75: Cosmetic acne.

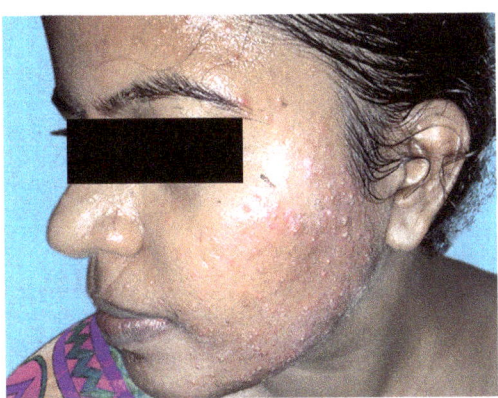

FIG. 76: Cosmetic acne; same patient as in Figure 75.

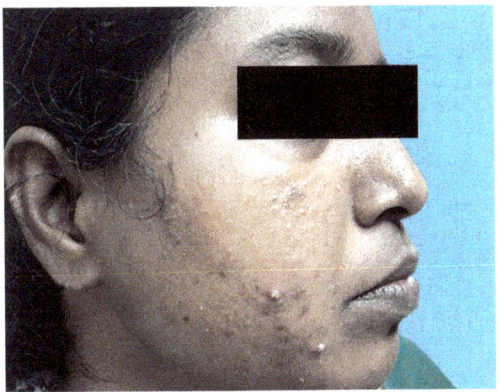

FIG. 77: Acne venenata; note the oily skin, closed comedones, and pustule.

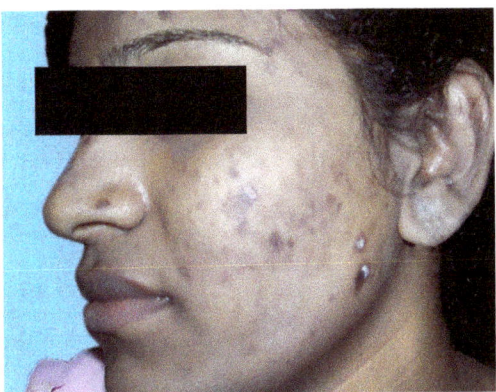

FIG. 78: Acne excoriée with pitted and pigmented scars.

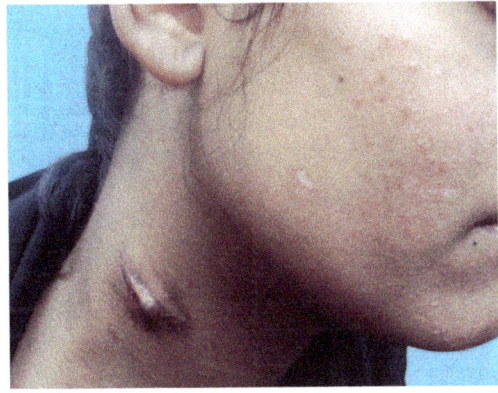

FIG. 79: Acneiform eruption in a patient on isoniazid (INH).

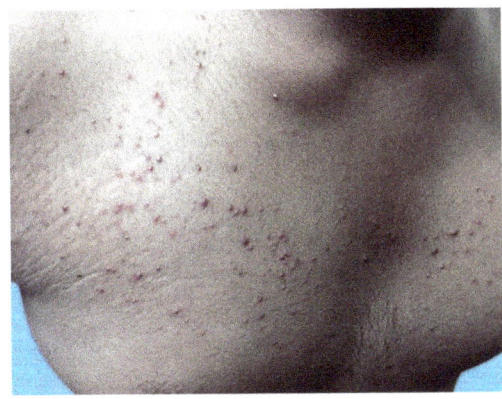

FIG. 80: Acneiform eruption; note absence of comedones and monomorphic papular eruption.

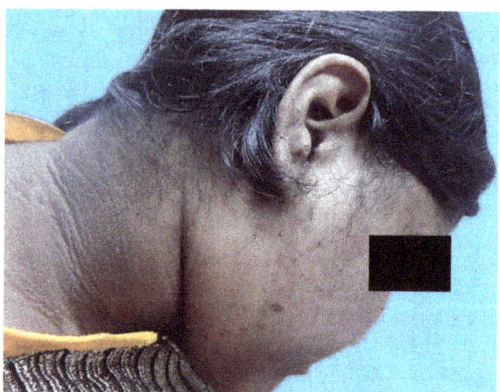

FIG. 81: Seborrhea, acne, hirsutism, and alopecia (SAHA) syndrome in an obese girl; note hirsutism.

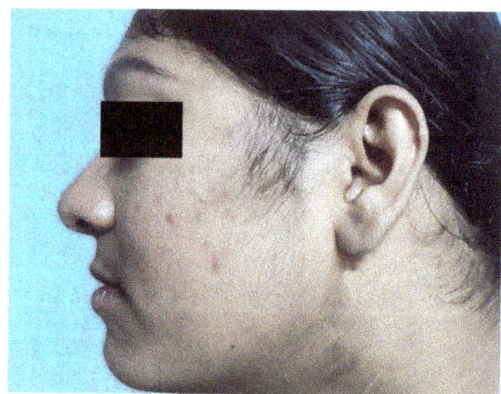

FIG. 82: Seborrhea, acne, hirsutism, and alopecia (SAHA) syndrome in a woman with polycystic ovarian syndrome.

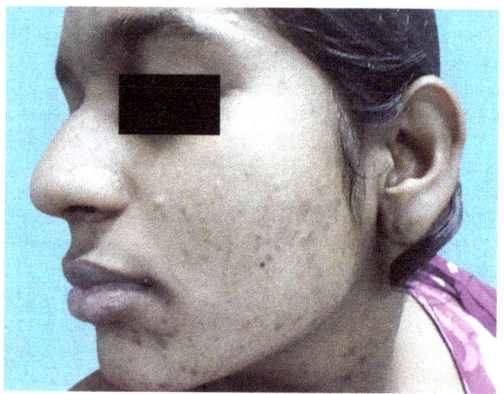

FIG. 83: Seborrhea, acne, hirsutism, and alopecia (SAHA) syndrome in a girl with acne and polycystic ovarian syndrome (PCOS).

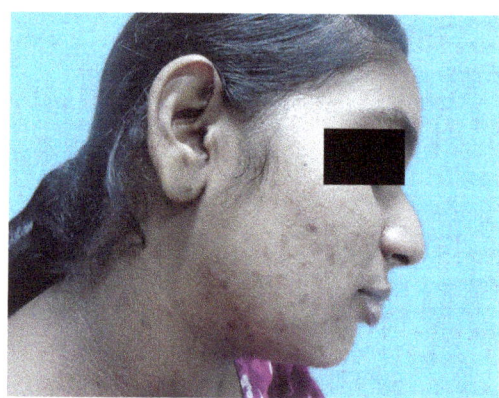

FIG. 84: Seborrhea, acne, hirsutism, and alopecia (SAHA) syndrome; same patient as in Figure 83.

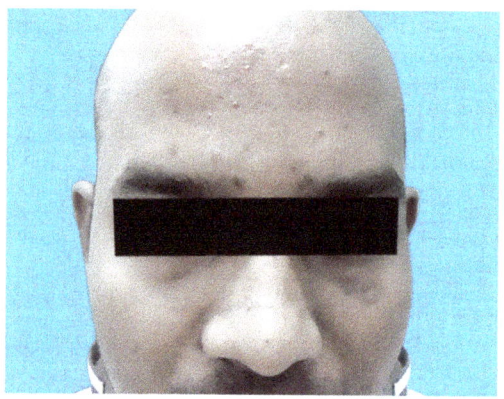

FIG. 85: Acne, patterned alopecia, acanthosis nigricans (APAAN) syndrome.

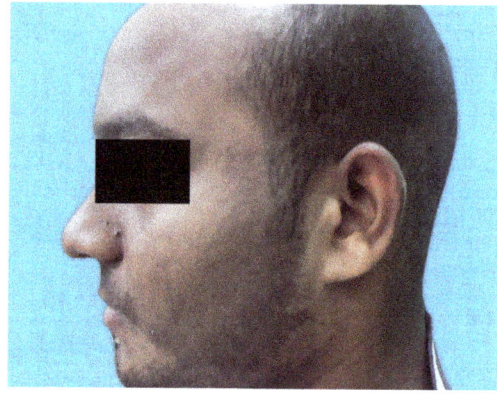

FIG. 86: Same man as in Figure 85.

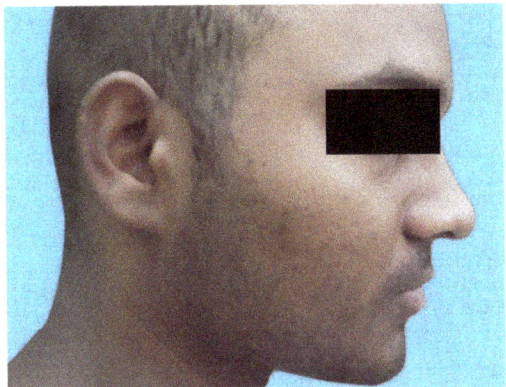

FIG. 87: Acne, patterned alopecia, acanthosis nigricans (APAAN) syndrome; same patient as in Figure 85.

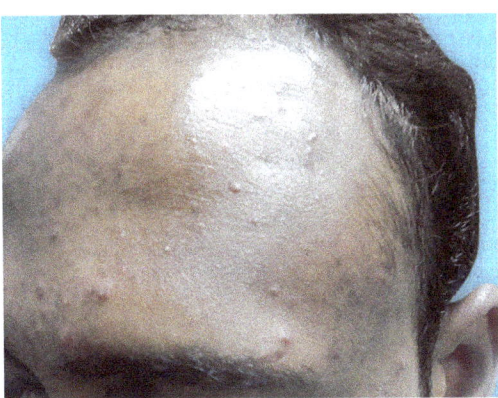

FIG. 88: Seborrhea, acne, and patterned hair loss in a man who also had acanthosis nigricans.

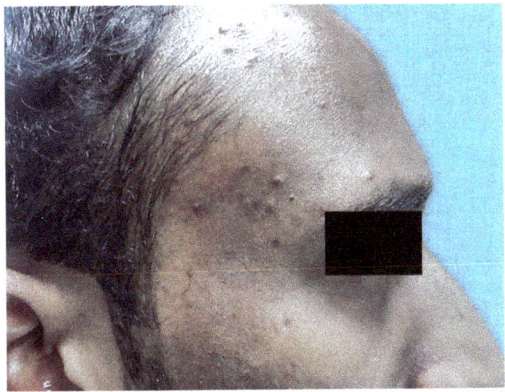

FIG. 89: Acne, patterned alopecia, acanthosis nigricans (APAAN) syndrome; same patient as in Figure 88.

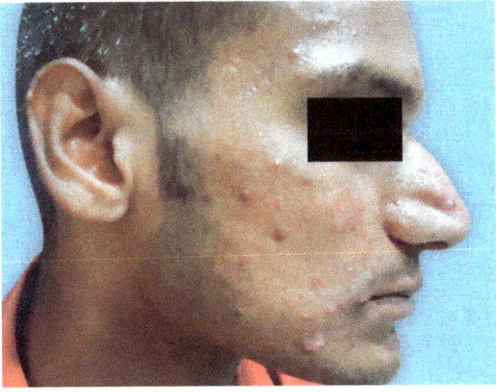

FIG. 90: Grade III acne in acne, patterned alopecia, acanthosis nigricans (APAAN) syndrome.

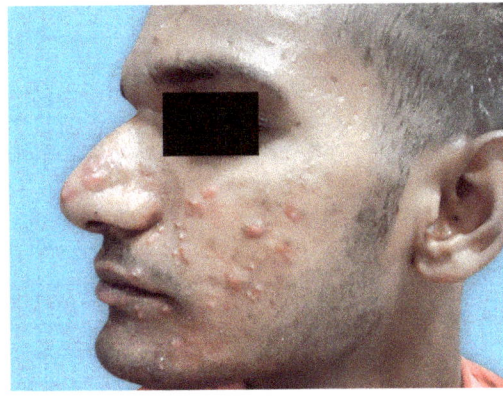

FIG. 91: Grade III acne in acne, patterned alopecia, acanthosis nigricans (APAAN) syndrome; same patient as in Figure 90.

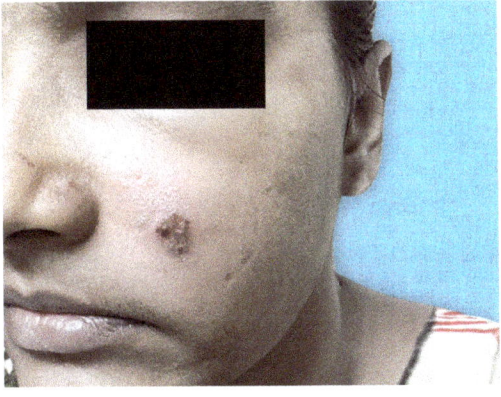

FIG. 92: Facial edema following self-inflicted trauma of an acne papule.

CHAPTER 4: Types and Variants of Acne

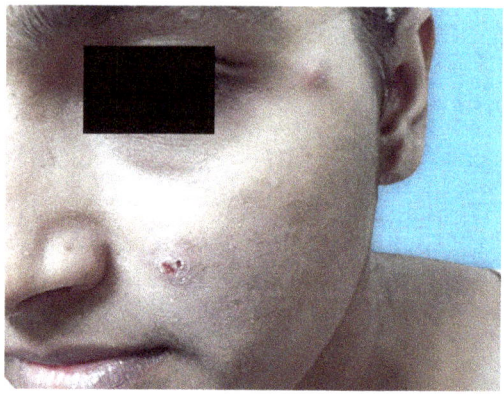

FIG. 93: Excoriation of acne papule leading to edema; same patient as in Figure 92.

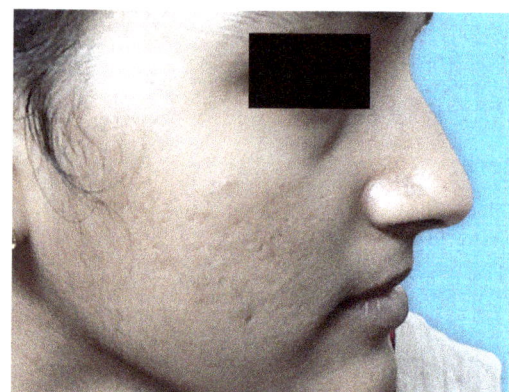

FIG. 94: Same patient with edema as in Figure 92.

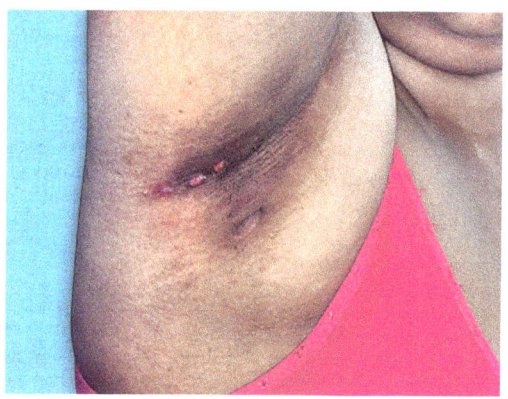

FIG. 95: Hidradenitis suppurativa in a woman with recurrent exacerbation.

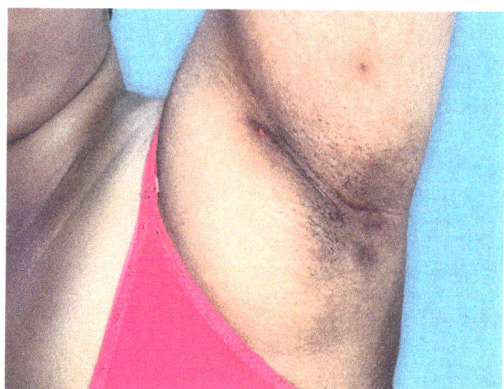

FIG. 96: Same patient as in Figure 95.

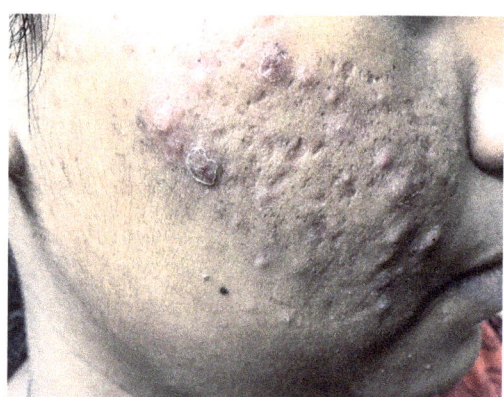

FIG. 97: Inflammatory acne of same patient as in Figure 96.

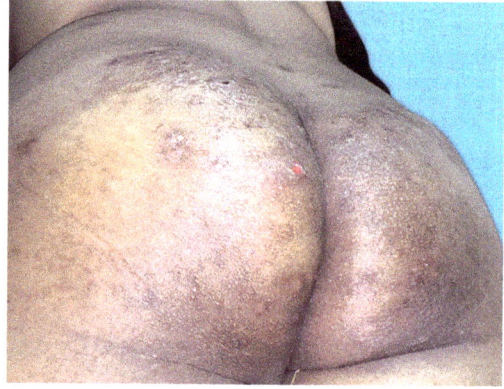

FIG. 98: Hidradenitis suppurativa affecting the gluteal region.

CHAPTER 4: Types and Variants of Acne

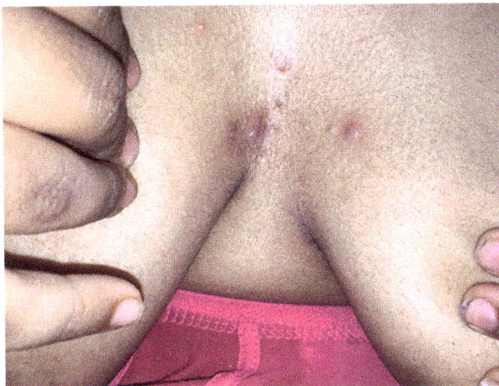

FIG. 99: Hidradenitis suppurativa involving anterior chest; same patient as in Figure 95.

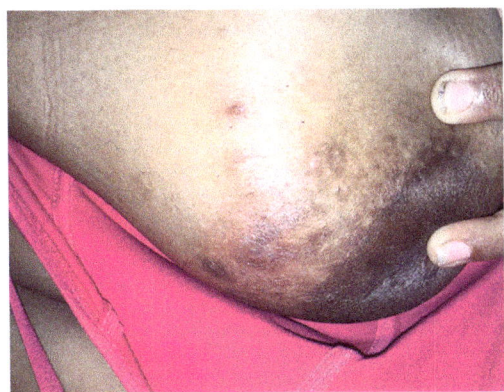

FIG. 100: Lesions over the breast tissue in same patient as in Figure 95.

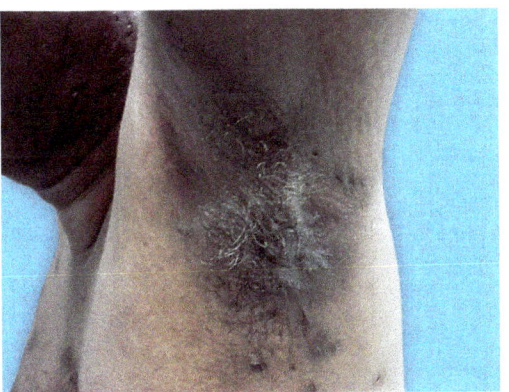

FIG. 101: Hidradenitis suppurativa.

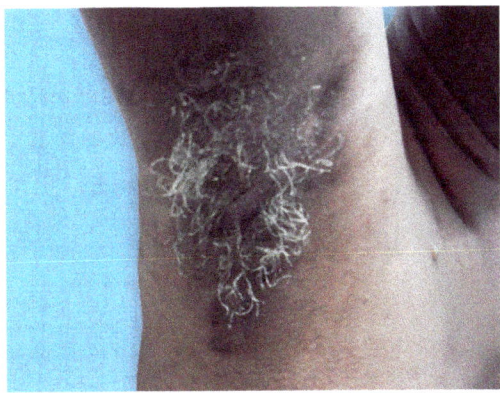

FIG. 102: Hidradenitis suppurativa; same patient as in Figure 101.

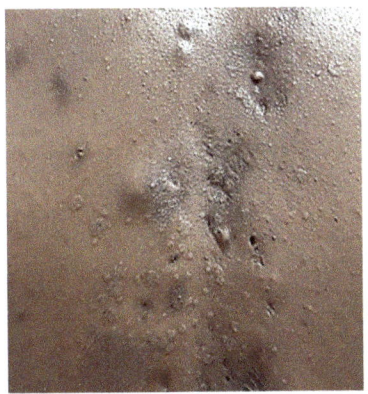

FIG. 103: Acne conglobata; close-up view of back; note the disfiguring scars.

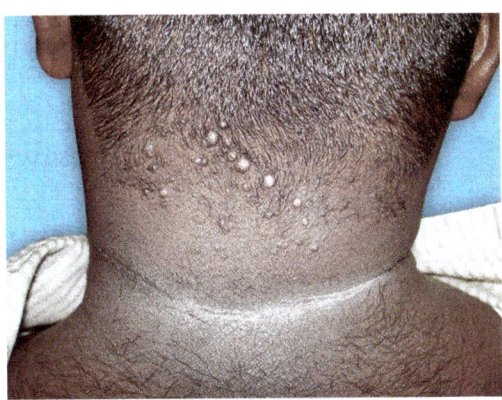

FIG. 104: Acne keloidalis nuchae.

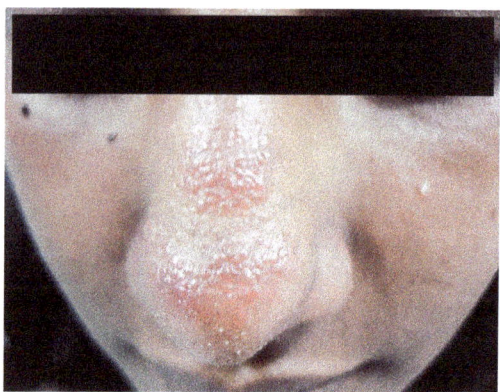

FIG. 105: Rosacea granulosa.

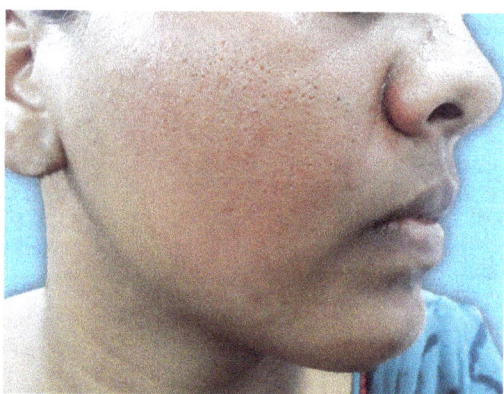

FIG. 106: Young lady developing solid facial edema progressing to rosacea.

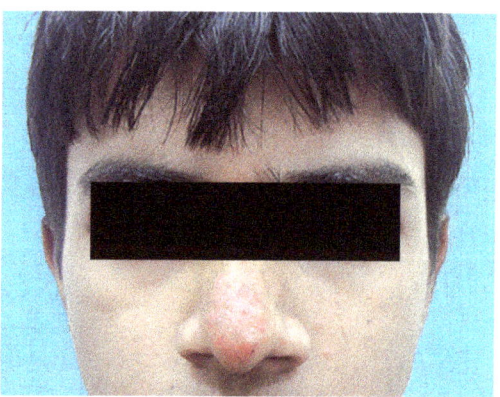

FIG. 107: Acne rosacea in a teenager.

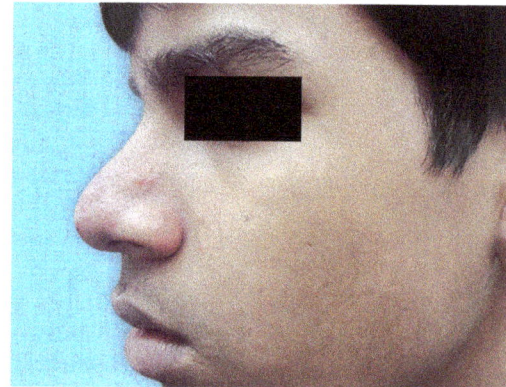

FIG. 108: Acne rosacea in a teenager; same patient as in Figure 107.

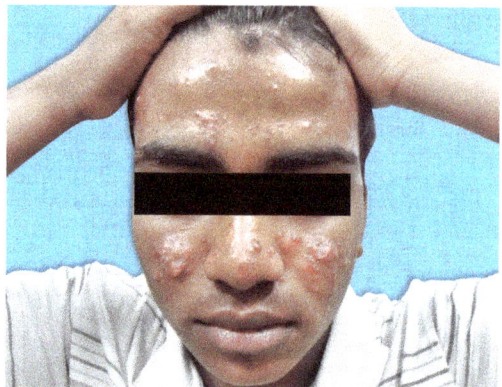

FIG. 109: Acne eruption; note the monomorphic lesions.

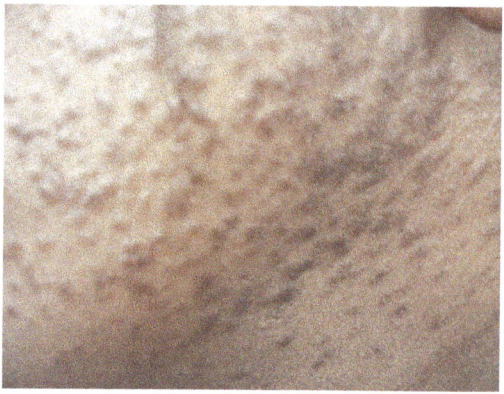

FIG. 110: Close-up view of patient as in Figure 109; note the monomorphic lesions.

> **BOX 2 Acne variants.**
> - Late/adult-onset acne
> - Acne conglobata
> - Acne fulminans
> - Occupational acne (chloracne, oil acne, coal tar, and pitch acne)
> - Acne mechanica
> - Gram-negative folliculitis
> - Radiation acne
> - Tropical acne
> - Acne aestivalis
> - Pseudoacne of the nasal crease
> - Acne cosmetica
> - Pomade acne
> - *Acne associated with psychological problems:*
>   - Acne excoriée
>   - Body dysmorphic disorder
>   - Eating orders
> - Granulomatous acne
> - Drug-induced acne
> - *Syndromes:*
>   - SAHA syndrome
>   - APAAN syndrome
>   - Apert's syndrome
>   - SAPHO syndrome
>   - PAPA syndrome
> - Acne with solid facial edema
> - Inverse acne and follicular occlusion triad/tetrad
> - Acne keloidalis nuchae and acne varioliformis
> - Acne rosacea
> - Penile acne
> - Acneiform eruptions
> - Acneiform nevi
> - Acne in pregnancy
> - Sensitive skin syndrome
>
> (APAAN: acne, patterned alopecia, acanthosis nigricans; PAPA: pyogenic arthritis, pyoderma gangrenosum, and acne; SAHA: seborrhea, acne, hirsutism, alopecia; SAPHO: synovitis, acne, pustulosis, hyperostosis, and osteitis)

> **BOX 3 Common drugs incriminated in the development of adult-onset acne.**
> - Corticosteroids
> - *Antiepileptics*: Phenytoin, carbamazepine
> - *Antidepressants*: Sertraline, lithium
> - *Antipsychotics*: Pimozide, risperidone
> - *Antitubercular*: Isoniazid, pyrazinamide
> - *Antiviral*: Ritonavir, ganciclovir
> - *Calcium channel blockers*: Nimodipine, nilvadipine
> - *Antineoplastic*: Dactinomycin
> - *Immunosuppressives*: Cyclosporine
> - *Vitamins*: Vitamin B12
> - *Miscellaneous*: Clofazimine

Face is the predominant site affected in women, and the role of cosmetics in the induction of clinical disease has been clearly excluded by studies. Lesions are predominantly seen in the V-zone of the face involving the jaw line and the neck but may be seen anywhere on face, chest or back. These women invariably complain of premenstrual flare of the lesions. Both inflammatory and noninflammatory lesions are seen and the comedones are predominantly that of closed type. Macrocomedones may evolve into inflammatory lesions including papules and pustules ultimately resulting in scar formation. The lesions tend to be persistent and are more prone for sequela like scarring. It is very important to realize that adult-onset acne has significant psychosocial implications when compared to acne vulgaris. Women are more significantly affected than men are, psychologically. Many adult women with acne who present with comedones are relatively older than their counterparts presenting with papulopustules. Those presenting with comedonal acne also have an increased incidence of smoking. There seems to be an increased prevalence of acne in patients with psychological disorders, such as anorexia and bulimia nervosa. The main differences between adolescent acne and adult-onset acne are given in **Table 1**.

Important findings in endocrine disorders associated with late-onset acne are given in **Table 2**.

TABLE 1: Differences between adolescent acne and adult-onset acne.

Features	Adolescent acne	Adult-onset acne
Family history	Very common	May be present
Premenstrual flare	May be present	Common
Age of onset (years)	12–18	>25
Gender	Male > female	Female > male
Sites involved	Face and trunk	Face; trunk involvement rare
Face	T-zone of face	V-zone of face
Types of lesion	Noninflammatory and inflammatory	Inflammatory lesions
Morphology: • Comedones • Papulopustule • Nodule	 • Common • Common • Sometimes seen	 • Rare • Characteristic • Frequently seen
Sequelae	Scarring depends on severity	Severe disfiguring scars
Response to treatment	Predictable and good	Unpredictable, resistant

TABLE 2: Important findings in endocrine disorders associated with late-onset acne.

Findings	PCOS	CAH	NCAH	CS	AST
History	Dysmenorrhea; decreased fertility	Early onset of acne; infertility; accelerated growth	Decreased fertility; dysmenorrhea	Menstrual abnormality (oligomenorrhea)	Fever; weight loss; abdominal pain; oligomenorrhea/amenorrhea
General examination	Insulin resistance	Ambiguous genitalia; hypertension	Ambiguous genitalia; hypertension	Central obesity; insulin resistance	Features of Cushing's syndrome; signs of virilization (deepening of voice, reduced muscle mass, decreased breast mass, clitoromegaly)
Dermatological examination	Hirsutism; alopecia; acne	Hirsutism; acne	Hirsutism; alopecia; acne	Hirsutism; acanthosis nigricans; striae acne	Hirsutism; acne

(AST: androgen secreting tumor; CAH: congenital adrenal hyperplasia; CS: cesarean section; NACH: nonclassic congenital hyperplasia; PCOS: polycystic ovarian syndrome)

Acne Conglobata

Acne conglobata is a relatively rare but not uncommon type of severe acne. The word "conglobate" refers to rounded mass. Boys are more commonly affected than girls. The onset of acne conglobata is during the teens but the lesions tend to continue and extend into adulthood. The disease involves face, neck, and trunk, and in severe cases may extend to the thighs and arms. Patients present with painful deep-seated nodules which are tender to touch. The nodules are large, tender, and dusky in color unlike the nodules of acne vulgaris which are skin-colored. Other acne lesions, such as comedones, papules, and pustules, can be seen in the same patient. The comedones are open comedones with multiple pores.

Some patients give a history of mucoid/serous/purulent discharge from the nodules. Multiple sinus tracts are almost hallmark of this disease which are the result of subcutaneous dissection of inflammatory nodules. These lead to irregular and disfiguring scars requiring surgical management. However, there will be no systemic symptoms, such as fever as seen in acne fulminans.

Acne Fulminans

Acne fulminans is also called as acne maligna. This is the most severe form of acne with systemic symptoms mostly seen in males. Unlike other forms of acne, here trunk is more severely affected than face. It was Plewig and Kligman, who emphasized that sudden onset, severe lesions, and systemic upset are characteristic features of acne fulminans. In some patients, the distinctive systemic symptom like fever may be absent. These cases are described as sine fulminans.

Acne fulminans has been found to be associated diseases, such as ulcerative colitis and Crohn's disease and syndromes, such as synovitis, acne, pustulosis, hyperostosis, and osteitis (SAPHO) and pyogenic arthritis, pyoderma gangrenosum, and acne (PAPA) syndromes.

In many patients, the disease starts as acne vulgaris during adolescence and runs a course of mild-to-moderate acne for about 2 years (ranges from 6 months to 5 years). There will be a sudden onset of fever, arthralgia, and severe painful necrotic and ulcerative nodules. In addition to the fever and arthralgia, patients may also present with other inflammatory signs and symptoms, such as erythema nodosum and bone pain.

Skin lesions include papule, pustules, and nodules. The characteristic lesions are inflammatory, painful, and tender ulcerative friable plaques and nodules with hemorrhagic crusts predominantly distributed over the shoulders, upper chest, and back. Some lesions may resemble pyogenic granuloma. Comedones are usually inconspicuous. Majority of patients present with fever, malaise, myalgia, arthralgia, and swelling of the joints. Some may even have anorexia and lose weight. Clinically, there may be pallor and in such patients, and anemia and leukemoid reaction should be suspected. Painful hepatosplenomegaly should be looked for in such individuals. Bone pain especially over the anterior chest, clavicle, and sternum may indicate focal osteolysis and there have been reports of aseptic osteolysis in acne fulminans.

Ankles, hips, and sacroiliac joints are other sites of osteolytic lesions. Thus, it is extremely important to examine every patient with sudden onset of painful nodules with a tendency to ulcerate thoroughly with special attention paid to the bones and joints. In all cases with a diagnosis of acne fulminans associated with syndromes such as SAPHO and PAPA should be ruled out. Acne conglobata which also presents with tender nodules can be easily differentiated from acne fulminans by the presence of comedones and absence of systemic symptoms in the former. Failure to respond to antibiotic therapy is a feature of acne fulminans.

Occupational Acne

Occupational acne is defined as development of acne-like lesions after exposure to occupational agents in persons not prone to develop acne and who have not had acne before engaging in the said occupation. Acne venenata is the term used by some authors to denote acne and acneiform lesions induced by external contact with chemicals. Hence, it is also referred to as contact acne. These may include halogenated organic compounds, insoluble cutting oil, detergents, and coal tar derivatives. Occupational acne results not only from direct occupational exposure but also nonoccupational exposure to the industrial wastes and consumption of contaminated food products. Accidental exposure to dioxin was identified as one of the most important causes in the development of acne-like lesions. Occupational acne is also referred to as chemical acne and chloracne. The following variants are included under occupational acne:

- Chloracne
- Pomade/oil acne
- Coal/pitch acne

Chloracne

Chloracne was first described by von Bettman and named by Herxheimer as early as 1899. It was identified to be caused by chlorine present in the environmental pollution. The common chemicals causing chloracne include chloronaphthalene, chlorobiphenyls, and chlorodiphenyl oxide. Exposure to halogenated organic compounds can also lead to clinical disease. This is commonly from exposure to fungicides, insecticides, and wood preservatives containing chlorinated hydrocarbons.

Contact to these chemicals not only causes acne-like lesions but also leads to affection of ophthalmic, nervous, and hepatic systems. Hence, these patients should be diagnosed early and treated appropriately.

The classical distribution of lesions is over the malar prominence and mandibular line. Involvement of retroauricular area is pathognomonic of chloracne. Retroauricular involvement is not seen in acne vulgaris. Another significant finding is the sparing of nose even in patients with facial involvement. In extensive cases, comedones are seen also over neck, trunk, extremities, and genitals in men. Some patients also demonstrate mucocutaneous and nail pigmentation. Differentiating features between chloracne and acne vulgaris are enlisted in **Table 3**.

TABLE 3: Differentiating features between chloracne and acne vulgaris.

Features	Chloracne	Acne vulgaris
History	Exposure to chloracne genes	Family history of acne
Age of onset	Any age depending on exposure	Adolescent
Seborrhea	Uncommon	Usual
Xerosis	Common	Not a feature
Comedones	Predominant	Present
Site	Malar, mandibular–temporal, and retroauricular	Midfacial (T-zone)
Nose involvement	Spared	Common
Other sites	Axillae, scrotum, penis	Chest, back
Papules pustules	Uncommon	Common
Cyst-like lesions	Common, straw-colored	Rare, skin-colored
Other findings	• Palmoplantar hyperhidrosis • Mucosal/nail pigmentation	• Features of insulin • Resistance
Systemic findings	Ophthalmic, nervous, hepatic	Rare

Oil Acne

Oil acne is also referred to as pomade acne. The lesions are essentially folliculitis developing after prolonged contact with oil. Those working in the industries and workshops dealing with heavy industrial oils are more prone to develop oil acne. The sites involved are those areas covered by oil-soaked clothing which include arms and thighs, and to some extent, the trunk. However, exposure to airborne oil mist can also induce oil acne which can manifest on exposed sites. With improvement in the working atmosphere and better education, the incidence of oil acne has significantly come down in the recent years.

Coal Acne

Coal acne is seen in persons engaged in road maintenance, tar plant, and construction. Coal tar oils and pitch produce acne-like lesions predominantly involving the exposed areas. Comedones are predominantly seen over the face. Coal tar melanosis, a phototoxic reaction, is a common finding observed in these patients due to the photosensitizing property of the tar.

In addition to the pigmentary changes and comedones, tar papilloma keratosis, and acanthoma should also be looked for in these patients. One must also keep in mind that very prolonged exposure is hazardous to health because of the carcinogenic potential of coal tar.

Exclusive involvement of face is invariably a feature of acne venenata and coal acne. Involvement of buttocks is seen in tropical acne and pomade acne. Involvement of hands in addition to the face is seen in detergent acne while retroauricular involvement is pathognomonic of chloracne.

Regarding the clinical lesions, comedones are present only in chloracne and acne venenata and are absent in tropical acne, detergent acne, and pomade acne. Salient features of different types of occupational acne are summarized in **Table 4**.

Acne Mechanica

As the name implies, these are lesions that result from prolonged mechanical trauma to the skin. Occlusion, pressure, and friction are common physical insults resulting in acne mechanica. In certain occupations, where facemasks and other occlusive clothing, including straps and belts are used, acne mechanica is a common

TABLE 4: Salient features of occupational acne.

Type	Causative agent	Site		Lesions			
		Face	Others	Comedone	Papule and pustule	Nodules	Pseudo cysts
Chloracne	Halogenated organic compounds	✓	Retroauricular	Closed	✗	✗	✓
Acne venenata/cosmetica	Cosmetics	✓	✗	Closed	✗	✗	✗
Tropical acne	Heat and humidity	✗	Neck, back, extremities, buttocks	✗	✗	✓	✓
Pomade acne	Oil	✗	Arm, thigh, buttocks	✗	✓	✗	✗
Detergent acne	Detergents	✓	Hands	✗	✓	✗	✗
Coal acne	Tar	✓	✗	Open	✗	✗	✗

problem. The eruptions are inflammatory papules and pustules and occasionally deep-seated nodules appearing in crops. Sometimes, in a person already having acne lesions such as microcomedones, heat, or pressure may lead to its rupture causing an inflammatory lesion. A meticulous examination will reveal a pigmented, lichenified plaque interspersed with comedones. Fiddler's/violinist's neck is a clinical variant of acne mechanica. According to some authors, acne mechanica is a complication due to external physical force which exacerbates the underlying pathology.

Gram-negative Folliculitis

Treatment of acne with continuous long-term administration of oral antibiotics may lead a condition called gram-negative folliculitis. The commonly reported antibiotic causing gram-negative folliculitis is oral tetracycline. Patients using antibiotic initially show improvement of acne lesion which is transient only to be followed by worsening of the disease. The occurrence of gram-negative folliculitis is to be suspected, whenever there is worsening of acne lesions following prolonged antibiotic therapy where the new lesions appear more over the nose and presence of deep-seated nodules along with papulopustules. The diagnosis can be proved by doing a culture.

Radiation Acne

Both ultraviolet (UV) radiation and ionizing radiation can induce acneiform eruptions. Following acute face radiation, dermatitis, comedo-like papules develop over the sites of external beam radiation therapy. Favre–Racouchot syndrome is seen in old people who have had excessive exposure to sunlight. These are called solar or senile comedones and nodular elastoidosis. Solar comedones are observed in persons above the age of 50 years. Clinically, the lesions manifest as yellow plaque studded with large open comedones, the common site affected being temporal and periorbital area. Symmetry is a striking feature in this disease though few may manifest with asymmetric lesions depending on the UV exposure. Some individuals present with giant comedones and cysts.

Tropical Acne

Persons working in extreme heat and those working in the tropical climates develop follicular lesions which may really be disabling. Tropical acne is common in those working in the furnace where they have to work in scorching heat or those who work in tropical zones with thick clothing. Follicular inflammatory lesions develop which can easily become infected with coagulase-positive staphylococci. Painful large deep-seated nodules develop mainly over the trunk and buttock. In some persons, the inflammation may be so severe to result in big swelling with multiple discharging sinuses. This may closely mimic acne conglobata. However, absence of previous history of acne during teenage and lack of facial involvement may give a clue toward diagnosis of tropical acne in a person coming from tropical country or working in hot environment.

Acne Aestivalis

Acne aestivalis is also known as Mallorca acne as it was reported from Mallorca in Europe. The lesions start as monomorphous eruption consisting of erythematous papules of uniform size occurring soon after exposure to sun. Comedones are not seen in acne aestivalis. This condition has a female predilection and is seen commonly in the age group 20–30 years. The sites affected include arms, neck, and chest. There will be remission following months of protection from UV light. However, the lesions promptly recur on re-exposure.

Pseudoacne of the Nasal Crease

Development of acneiform papules over the transverse nasal crease is common in the preadolescent children. These are not due to dilated pilosebaceous orifices filled with keratin plug. However, instead they represent ruptured milium with a microscopically demonstrable granulomatous reaction to keratin plug. These lesions are often confused with prepubertal acne which they actually are not.

Acne Cosmetica

Acne cosmetica is a general term that refers to any acneiform eruption caused by the use of cosmetics. This will include products that are both comedogenic and acneigenic. Comedogenic products are those that can induce only follicular keratinous impaction leading to comedones, whereas acneigenic products can induce both papule and pustule formation. Products, such as isopropyl myristate in petrolatum even in low concentrations are comedogenic. Whether a product is purely comedogenic or acneigenic is difficult to determine as the response observed in animal experiment is quite variable from that of the human response. Similarly, the concentration at which the comedogenicity or acnegenicity is demonstrable also varies. For example, sodium lauryl sulfate, a common emulsifier, is acneigenic and produces papulopustules in a dose-related manner. Most of such cosmetics can produce lesion under occlusion much earlier and at lower concentrations. These lesions are histologically demonstrated to have microcomedones.

Acne Associated with Psychological Problems

One of the most frequent psychocutaneous disorders is acne. Although acne vulgaris affects up to 85% of teenagers, not all of them have a psychological condition. Acne excoriée is a classic case of acne linked to a psychological issue.

Acne is one of the common psychocutaneous disorders. Though acne vulgaris is seen in as high as 85% of teens, not all have psychological problem. Nevertheless, associated reduction in quality of life is observed in most of them. Acne excoriée is a classic example of acne associated with psychological problem. Body dysmorphic disorder (BDD) and eating disorders are two common psychological disorders that are closely associated with acne. Acne was found to be the presenting feature in a small percentage of people with BDD. Anorexia nervosa may develop in acne patients having psychological problem.

Acne Excoriée

Acne excoriée is seen predominantly in adolescent girls. However, adolescent boys and mature women are also reported to suffer from this common disorder. Acne excoriée is frequently associated with stress and considered as a self-inflicted condition. The affected individual is said to be compulsively picking acne lesions. The common site affected is the face. The disease may represent a personality problem, obsessive–compulsive disorder, and/or bodily focused anxiety. The lesions present in many stages of evolution of the disease, including papulopustules, excoriation, crusts, and pigmentation. These patients develop and frequent scarring. A meticulous history may reveal that these teenagers (even the matured women) spend long hours in front of the mirror injuring their acne lesions and even normal appearing skin, with locally available instruments, such as forceps or tweezers. It is said that such self-inflicted trauma temporarily relieves anxiety. Some patients even in the absence of a lesion, the patients tend to pick the skin overlying imaginary acne lesions. The clinical lesions are of two types, namely the round irregular small but deep excoriation marks over the acne lesions and linear erosions or vibeces. These findings clearly indicate self-mutilation and give a clue to the underlying psychiatric problem. Distinctly these findings are seen on the face and accessible sites. If lesions are present over the interscapular area, they are usually unaffected by external trauma. Persistent mutilation may result in unacceptable scarring. Contact dermatitis should be excluded in all cases before contemplating on acne excoriée and labeling of a psychological problem. In such patients, an underlying BDD should also be suspected. Atopic background has been documented in some patients with acne excoriée.

Body Dysmorphic Disorder

In patients with BDD, the acne perceived and projected by the patient is out of proportion to the physical signs observed by the physician. These patients may show signs of depression or anxiety. Some may even have obsessive–compulsive behavior. This is one of the dermatological conditions with a significant risk of suicidal tendency. It should be understood by the treating dermatologists that these patients may have a global mental disorder and require psychiatric management as well.

Eating Disorder

It has been reported that acne and anorexia nervosa are associated. These two conditions can complement each other adversely. In teenage children, acne itself can act as a predisposing factor for anorexia in vulnerable group of adolescents. Some adolescents with acne in the process of controlling diet in an attempt to reduce calories end up with anorexia nervosa. Real disorder can be confirmed with investigations, such as serum growth hormone and insulin-like growth factor-1.

Granulomatous Acne

Granulomatous acne also referred to as acne agminata is commonly seen in young adults though any age can be affected. Clinically, acne agminata is characterized by the presence of deep-seated nodules commonly involving the cheeks. The other sites affected include forehead, eyelids, and chin. The absence of comedones and involvement of eyelid will differentiate acne agminata from acne vulgaris. Many terminologies were used to describe this condition. Some of them include lupus miliaris disseminatus faciei, tuberculoderma of the face, acne telangiectodes of Kaposi, and facial idiopathic granuloma with regressive evolution. However, there is no clear-cut evidence for its association with tuberculosis despite the microscopic presence of epithelioid granuloma and caseation. If left untreated, these lesions may resolve after 2–3 years with ugly scars. In every resistant deep-seated acne without comedones involving the eyelids, acne agminata should be considered as a possibility.

Drug-induced Acne

The most common of all drug-induced acne, "steroid acne" tops the list. The other drugs causing acneiform eruptions are given in **Box 4**.

Steroid Acne

Prolonged treatment with corticosteroid both topically applied and systemically taken including oral, nasal, and parenteral routes of administration ends up in acneiform eruption. Steroid acne is much more common with usage of potent topical steroids used with occlusion. Steroid acne is not seen in all patients treated with corticosteroids. It is said to occur in those having high level of circulating corticosteroids.

According to some authors, steroid acne and pityrosporum folliculitis are one and the same. However, pityrosporum folliculitis which manifests as itchy superficial follicular papulopustules, whereas steroid acne is invariably asymptomatic. The occurrence of pityrosporum folliculitis in individuals not on corticosteroid therapy is an indicator that both steroid acne and pityrosporum folliculitis are different entities. The duration between starting on treatment and occurrence of lesions are variable. In some individual, acneiform lesions develop much earlier than others who

> **BOX 4** **Drugs-inducing acneiform eruptions.**
>
> - *Hormones:*
>   - Corticosteroid in all forms, such as oral, parenteral, topical and inhaled
>   - ACTH/synthetic ACTH
>   - Anabolic steroid/synthetic androgen:
>   - Danazol
>   - Nandrolone
>   - Stanozolol
>   - Medroxyprogesterone
> - *Anticonvulsants:*
>   - Carbamazepine
>   - Phenytoin
>   - Phenobarbitone
>   - Troxidone
>   - Gabapentin
>   - Topiramate
> - *Antidepressants:*
>   - Lithium
>   - Sertraline
> - *Neuroleptics/antipsychotics:*
>   - Pimozide
>   - Risperidone
> - *Antitubercular:*
>   - Isoniazid
>   - Pyrazinamide
> - *Antineoplastics/EGFR antagonists:*
>   - Dactinomycin
>   - Pentostatin
>   - Cetuximab
> - *Antiviral:*
>   - Ritonavir
>   - Ganciclovir
> - *Calcium antagonists:*
>   - Nilvadipine
>   - Nimodipine
> - *Halogen:*
>   - Sodium fluoride
>   - Potassium iodine
> - *Antimalarial:*
>   - Quinine
> - *Immunosuppressives:*
>   - Cyclosporine
>   - Sirolimus
>   - Tacrolimus
> - Genetically engineered human growth hormone
> - Vitamin B12
> - *Miscellaneous:*
>   - Buserelin
>   - Cabergoline
>   - Clofazimine
>   - Dantrolene
>   - Disulfiram
>   - Famotidine
>   - Follitropin alfa
>   - Isosorbide mononitrate
>   - Mesalazine
>   - Ramipril
>   - Sulfur
>   - Thiouracil
>   - Thiourea
>
> (ACTH: adrenocorticotropic hormone; EGFR: epidermal growth factor receptor)

take a longer time to clinically manifest with acne-like lesions.

Steroid acne is characterized by eruption in crops of dense inflammatory lesions predominantly papulopustules. The sites affected include face, chest, and back. Apart from presenting as steroid acne, these lesions can be seen as steroid rosacea and perioral dermatitis in addition to the preexisting skin condition. Steroid acne is characterized by development of crops of dense-inflamed papulopustules. The main difference in the clinical presentation is the absence of comedones. Monomorphous appearance of lesions as against polymorphous lesions seen in various stages of evolution in acne vulgaris and the sites of distribution not limiting to the seborrheic areas are other clues to the diagnosis of steroid acne. Steroids can worsen preexisting acne or induce new lesions of acne

TABLE 5: Differences between acne vulgaris and steroid acne.

Features	Acne vulgaris	Drug-induced acne
Family history	Very common	Uncommon
Premenstrual flare	May be present	Not seen
History of drug intake	Very rare	Always present
Age of onset	12–18 years	Any age
Gender	Male > female	Any gender
Sites involved	Face and trunk	Trunk more common
Face	T-zone of face	No zone preference
Types of lesion	Noninflammatory and inflammatory	Inflammatory
Morphology: • Comedones • Papulopustule • Nodule	 • Common • Common • Sometimes seen	 • Never seen • Monomorphous • Never seen
Other findings	Syndrome association, if any	Disease for being treated
Sequelae	Scarring depends on severity	Resolves without scarring
Response to treatment	Predictable and good	Disappears on withdrawal of offender

in a person prone to develop acne. Though steroid acne is a separate entity which has to be differentiated from acne vulgaris in many patients both can coexist. Unless the steroids are withdrawn, any amount of anti-acne treatment will not give complete clearance of lesions. The major differences between acne vulgaris and steroid acne are given in **Table 5**.

Syndromes Associated with Acne

Acne can occur in some individuals with endocrine abnormality and certain other disorders presenting as definite syndromes. Many such syndromes where acne is a component have been documented. The list of syndromes associated with acne is provided herein:
- SAHA (seborrhea, acne, hirsutism, alopecia) syndrome
- APAAN (acne, patterned alopecia, acanthosis nigricans) syndrome
- Apert's syndrome
- SAPHO syndrome
- PAPA syndrome
  - PASH (pyoderma gangrenosum, acne, and hidradenitis suppurativa) syndrome
  - PAPASH (pyogenic arthritis, pyoderma gangrenosum, acne, and hidradenitis suppurativa) syndrome
  - PAC (pyoderma gangrenosum, acne, and ulcerative colitis) syndrome
  - HAIR-AN (hyperandrogenism, insulin resistance, and acanthosis nigricans) syndrome

The features of each syndrome are listed below:
- *SAHA syndrome (dermatological androgenization syndrome)*:
  - Seborrhea
  - Acne
  - Hirsutism
  - Alopecia
- *APAAN syndrome*:
  - Acne
  - Patterned alopecia
  - Acanthosis nigricans

- *Apert's syndrome*:
  - Acne
  - Synostosis of the cranium vertebral bodies hands and feet
  - Cleft palate
  - Bifid uvula
- *SAPHO syndrome*:
  - Synovitis
  - Acne
  - Pustulosis palmoplantaris
  - Hyperostosis
  - Osteitis
- *PAPA syndrome*:
  - Pyogenic arthritis
  - Pyoderma gangrenosum
  - Acne
- *PASH syndrome:*
  - Pyogenic arthritis
  - Acne
  - Suppurative hidradenitis
- *PAPASH syndrome:*
  - Pyogenic arthritis
  - Pyoderma gangrenosum
  - Acne
  - Suppurative hidradenitis
- *PAC:*
  - Pyoderma gangrenosum
  - Acne
  - Ulcerative colitis
- *HAIR-AN syndrome:*
  - Hyperandrogenism
    - Hirsutism
    - Patterned hair loss (vertex/crown area)
    - Masculinity
    - Clitoromegaly
    - Menstrual irregularity
  - Acne
  - Insulin resistance
  - Acanthosis nigricans

Polycystic ovarian syndrome and Cushing's syndrome are common disorders in which acne can be the presenting symptom. Many patients with PCOS and Cushing's syndrome are clinically diagnosed first by the dermatologists. This further asserts the need to be aware of endocrine acne and its features.

SAHA Syndrome

The SAHA syndrome also known as dermatological androgenization syndrome was first described in the year 1982. It is characterized by acne and features of androgenism. The clinical components include seborrhea, acne, hirsutism, and alopecia. This condition is most frequently associated with PCOS, cystic mastitis, obesity, and infertility.

APAAN Syndrome

The APAAN syndrome is a counterpart of SAHA syndrome observed in men. It is characterized by acne, patterned alopecia, and acanthosis nigricans.

Apert's Syndrome

The Apert's syndrome is also known as acrocephalosyndactyly. It is a genetic disorder with autosomal dominant inheritance. It is caused by mutation in the gene encoding fibroblast growth factor receptor 2 (*FGFR-2*) and amino acid substitution of exon 7 of chromosome 10. The skin lesions are due to increased androgen receptor sensitivity than an increase in the circulating androgen levels.

The clinical features are distinctive and include synostosis of the cranium, vertebral bodies, hands, and feet. Cleft palate and bifid uvula are other findings observed and reported in these patients. The skin lesions manifest as diffuse acneiform eruptions of papulopustules involving arms, buttock, and thighs. Lesions tend to be inflammatory with severe presentation at times. Seborrhea, nail dystrophy, and oculocutaneous hypopigmentation are other cutaneous findings reported.

SAPHO Syndrome

It was Chamot, a rheumatologist, who first introduced SAPHO syndrome in 1987. The exact etiology of SAPHO syndrome is not known. It has been postulated that the clinical presentation could be due to an autoimmune response to unknown antigen probably of bacterial origin. The acne component is different from that of acne vulgaris in having a sudden onset in addition to the presence of hemorrhagic lesions. The other findings of SAPHO syndrome are synovitis, pustulosis palmoplantaris, hyperostosis, and osteitis. As per the European Rare Disease Database, the clinical manifestations are categorized as very frequent, frequent, and occasional findings. **Table 6** gives the frequency of clinical findings in SAPHO syndrome.

Sternoclavicular and sternocostal joints are the most commonly involved joints in SAPHO syndrome. Swelling over these joints can be easily made out and gives a clue to the diagnosis. Sacroiliac, hip, knee, and ankle joints are also affected in patients with SAPHO syndrome.

Pain over the chest wall is another finding observed by some investigators, which is caused by hyperostosis of the anterior chest wall. The lesions do not easily respond to conventional acne treatment. Treatment of bone pain and disease will require special drugs.

Typical skin lesions seen in SAPHO syndrome include palmoplantar pustulosis (PPP) and acne. PPP is seen more commonly in women and whereas men present with acne more frequently than women. Acne of SAPHO syndrome takes a severe form manifesting as acne conglobata, acne fulminans, or inverse acne (hidradenitis suppurativa). Skin lesions vary in severity and may either precede, coexist, or follow arthritis. In nearly half the patients, skin lesions tend to precede arthritis. Sweet syndrome and Sneddon–Wilkinson disease have been reported in patients with SAPHO syndrome. Diagnosis of SAPHO syndrome is not difficult in the presence of all the components of the acronym. However, not all cases present with classic features of the syndrome. There are many diagnostic criteria published for SAPHO syndrome, the most precise and user-friendly criteria being the modified Kahn criteria. However, according to these criteria, presence of one inclusion criterion is sufficient for diagnosing SAPHO syndrome, which may lead to over diagnosis of the condition as there is no gold standard test to confirm the finding. The diagnostic criteria of SAPHO syndrome are given in **Box 5**.

Nevertheless, the diagnosis of SAPHO syndrome is an exclusion diagnosis and presence of skin manifestations especially acne makes the diagnosis much easier. The disease resolves spontaneously in only a minority of patients. In majority of them, the disease either runs a prolonged course with remissions and exacerbations or takes a chronic indolent course with involvement of new sites.

TABLE 6: Findings in SAPHO (synovitis, acne, pustulosis, hyperostosis, and osteitis) syndrome and their frequency.

Very frequent	Frequent	Occasional
• Arthralgia	• Acne	• Chronic diarrhea
• Bone pain	• Arthritis	• Cranial nerve paralysis
• Chest pain	• Edema	• Large intestine inflammation
• Craniofacial osteosclerosis	• Osteomyelitis	• Recurrent fracture
• Enthesitis	• Palmoplantar pustulosis	• Recurrent skin infections
• Hyperostosis	• Psoriasis	
• Neoplasm of the skeletal systems	• Sacroiliac joint abnormality	
• Osteolysis		
• Synovitis		

> **BOX 5** — Modified Kahn's criteria for the diagnosis of SAPHO (synovitis, acne, pustulosis, hyperostosis, and osteitis) syndrome.
>
> - *Inclusion criteria*:
>   - Bone and joint involvement associated with severe acne
>   - Bone and joint involvement associated with PPP and psoriasis vulgaris
>   - Bone and joint involvement associated with chronic bowel disease
>   - Isolated sterile hyperostosis/osteitis in adults
>   - Chronic recurrent multifocal osteomyelitis in children
> - *Exclusion criteria*:
>   - Infectious osteitis
>   - Tumoral conditions of the bone
>   - Noninflammatory condensing lesions of the bone
>
> (PPP: palmoplantar pustulosis)

Female gender, first episode involvement of anterior chest wall in addition to peripheral arthritis and skin lesions along with greatly elevated levels of inflammatory parameters are indicators of chronicity and poor prognosis.

PAPA Syndrome

The PAPA syndrome is a rare syndrome with autosomal dominant inheritance. Other than acne, components of PAPA syndrome include pyogenic arthritis and pyoderma gangrenosum, and hence, also referred to as PAPGA syndrome.

The genetic origin of PAPA syndrome is recently documented to be mutation related to chromosome 15.

Arthritis is the first component to manifest very early in life and then followed by acne at around puberty. The juvenile arthritis is often precipitated by trauma and with repeated episodes, the disease results in a mutilating joint.

In PAPA syndrome, acne is seen in most individuals but the presentation and degree of severity is variable. In many of them, it takes a severe form and course. The lesions begin just before or during adolescence and persist into adulthood. The lesions are inflammatory papulopustules and cystic nodules when severe, manifest as acne conglobata. They are resistant to treatment and eventually result in cosmetically unacceptable scarring.

Mayer-Rokitansky-Küster-Hauser syndrome is a Müllerian duct anomaly characterized by congenital absence of uterus and upper vagina with normal ovaries and fallopian tubes. Acne and PCOS are less frequent in women with Mayer-Rokitansky-Küster-Hauser syndrome despite a high rate of hyperandrogenemia.

Acne with Facial Edema

Acne with facial edema is also referred to as Morbihan's disease, a rare variant of acne, which is one definite indication for systemic corticosteroids. This is a disfiguring condition, clinically manifests with a woody edema of the mid-third of the face. There is always an accompanying erythema and acne, thus closely mimicking rosacea or Melkersson-Rosenthal syndrome. Though the intensity of edema fluctuates, spontaneous remission has never been reported.

Hidradenitis Suppurativa

Hidradenitis suppurativa is primarily a poral occlusion disorder. It is a chronic, debilitating recurrent inflammatory disorder of the apocrine glands. The disease starts during adolescence and presents as a symptomatic disease only after puberty. Prepubertal onset indicates premature adrenarche. Females are two and a half times more frequently affected than males. The common sites affected are the apocrine gland bearing location of the body, namely the axillae, groin, and the anogenital area. The most common sites of affection include genitofemoral and submammary areas in females while it is perianal and gluteal regions in males. Axillary involvement

TABLE 7: Clinical features of different stages of hidradenitis suppurativa.

Stage	Abscess	Sinus	Scar
1	Recurrent, individual	Nil	Nil
2	Recurrent, individual	+; widely separated	+; widely separated
3	Recurrent, multiple, interconnected	+; multiple, interconnected	Diffuse, involving the entire region

is the most common site of affection in both genders. Less commonly involved sites include retroauricular, preauricular, and occipital areas. Rarely, truncal lesions have also been reported.

The symptomatic lesions are always inflammatory papulopustules, which ultimately evolve into deep seated painful nodules. In many patients, there is a seropurulent discharge from these nodules. Sinus tracts are usual sequelae in spite of treatment in some. The resulting scar is invariably irregular and few patients may even develop keloid over these sites. Other lesions seen in hidradenitis suppurativa include follicular papules, pustules, pyogenic granuloma at the opening of sinus tracts, indurated plaques over the above-mentioned apocrine areas. Some patients may present with epidermoid cysts over the face, thorax, and external genitalia.

Diagnosis can be easily missed during early stages as folliculitis and rarely mistaken for scrofuloderma. The diagnostic criteria based on the San Francisco modification of the Dessau criteria include following:
- Typical lesions (painful deep-seated blind boils to start with, evolving to abscesses, draining sinuses, bridged scars, multiheaded open pseudocomedones)
- Typical sites (axillae, groin, perineal and perianal region, buttocks, infra- and intermammary folds)
- Recurrence and chronicity

All the three criteria should be fulfilled for the diagnosis of hidradenitis suppurativa. The three clinical stages of hidradenitis suppurativa based on severity of disease include stages 1, 2, and 3. The features of different stages of hidradenitis suppurativa are given in **Table 7**.

There are two variants of hidradenitis suppurativa apart from the classical presentation. In the variant that is part of follicular occlusion triad, patients give a family history of hidradenitis suppurativa, and is characterized by additional involvement of ears, chest, back, legs, and comedones with multiple openings. The variant where predominant gluteal involvement is seen is common in men. This clinical variant of hidradenitis suppurativa shows papules and folliculitis in addition to comedones.

Follicular Occlusion Tetrad

This is conglomeration of clinical findings seen in patients with acne conglobata. The components include acne conglobata, hidradenitis suppurativa, dissecting cellulitis of scalp, and pilonidal sinus. Earlier the first three components were described as follicular occlusion triad to which in the year 1975, pilonidal sinus was added and named as follicular occlusion tetrad. The condition may affect any age group without gender or racial predilection. However, it is more commonly seen in older adults. Positive family history, smoking obesity, and a carbohydrate rich diet seem to favor the disease, and so is living in humid conditions. For each of the components of this entity certain specific predisposing factors have been documented. The predisposing factors for each of the components are given in **Table 8**.

Not all patients present with all the four components of follicular occlusion tetrad at

TABLE 8: Predisposing factors for follicular occlusion tetrad.

Condition	Predisposing factors
Acne conglobata	• A dysfunctional immune system • Poor hygiene • Hormonal influence
Hidradenitis suppurativa	• Anabolic steroid • Testosterone-producing tumors
Dissecting cellulitis of scalp	Associated spondyloarthropathy
Pilonidal sinus	Excessive coarse body hair

a given point of time. For details about acne conglobata and hidradenitis suppurativa, readers may please refer to the earlier portion of this chapter. Dissecting cellulitis of the scalp like acne conglobata presents with deep-seated nodules and cysts with interconnecting sinuses. This is followed by secondary bacterial infection. The disease runs a chronic course resulting in irregular scarring and permanent alopecia.

Pilonidal sinus presents as erythematous painful nodule with a sinus tract. Recurrent infection of the sinus may result in cyst formation. In a long-standing case, the patient develops pain while sitting and even seropurulent discharge in some of them.

Acne Keloidalis Nuchae and Acne Varioliformis

Acne keloidalis nuchae and acne varioliformis are misnomers and are not related to acne vulgaris. Acne keloidalis nuchae presents as skin-colored papules, pustules, and keloid scar in the occipital area and is a cause for cicatricial alopecia.

Acne varioliformis or acne necrotica is a very are condition seen in adults. Clinically, presenting with pruritic painful papules over the frontoparietal area of the scalp and seborrheic area of the face, and hence resembling acne. Papules show central umbilication and eventually undergo central necrosis leaving behind varioliform scar.

Acne Rosacea

Acne rosacea is a common inflammatory disorder presenting in the early stages with simple flushing to be followed by a wide variety of other manifestations.

Clinical Features

The clinical manifestations of rosacea are variable and evolve slowly.

Based on the evolution of lesions, this can be observed as four phases, namely:
1. Prerosacea
2. Vascular rosacea
3. Inflammatory rosacea
4. Phymatous rosacea

Prerosacea: Rosacea may begin as a simple tendency to flush or blush easily, and then progress to a persistent redness in the central portion of face, particularly nose.

Vascular rosacea: As signs and symptoms worsen, vascular rosacea may develop, showing telangiectasia (dilatation of the end vessels).

Inflammatory rosacea: Small, red papules and pustules may appear and persist, spreading over the nose, cheeks, forehead, and chin.

Symptoms vary from stage to stage and patient to patient. One or more of the following symptoms should arouse suspicion of rosacea
- Redness of the face
- Blushing or flushing easily
- Burning or stinging feeling in the face
- Watering and irritation of the eyes
- Telangiectasia (dilated end vessels) over the face
- Red nose (bulbous nose)
- Acne-like papulopustules that may ooze or crust

> **BOX 6** | **Subtypes of rosacea.**
> - Erythematotelangiectatic rosacea
> - Papulopustular rosacea
> - Phymatous rosacea
> - Ocular rosacea
> - Granulomatous variant
> - Rosacea fulminans

Phymatous rosacea: This form of the disease, where there is hypertrophy of the soft tissue, commonly involves the nose (rhinophyma). Changes can also affect the chin (gnathophyma), ears (otophyma), forehead (metophyma), and eyelids (blepharophyma).

Based on the clinical finding, rosacea is further classified, which also helps in deciding on the treatment. Different subtypes of rosacea are listed in **Box 6**.

Erythematotelangiectatic Type

Central facial flushing, often accompanied by burning or stinging, is the predominant sign in erythematotelangiectatic rosacea (ETR). The redness usually spares the periocular skin. These patients typically have skin with a fine texture that lacks a sebaceous quality characteristic of other subtypes. The erythematous areas of the face at times appear rough and scaly due to chronic, low-grade dermatitis. Frequent triggers to flushing include acutely felt emotional stress, hot drinks, alcohol, spicy foods, exercise, cold or hot weather, and hot baths and showers. These patients also report that the burning or stinging is exacerbated when topical agents are applied. In all suspected cases of acne rosacea, following signs and symptoms help in the diagnosis:
- Facial redness, flushing, visible blood vessels
- Flushing and redness in the center of the face
- Visible broken blood vessels (spider veins)
- Dry, rough, scaling edematous skin
- Skin may be very sensitive, sting and burn
- Tendency to flush or blush more easily than other people

Papulopustular Rosacea

Papulopustular rosacea (PPR) is the classic presentation of rosacea. It is seen in middle-aged women who invariably give history of flushing. They present with erythematous papules surmounted by pinpoint pustules over the center of the face. Telangiectasias are likely to be present. They should be looked for carefully in the presence of erythema. The small telangiectatic vessels may not be clearly visible and may be difficult to distinguish from the erythematous background. The clinical findings include:
- Erythema and telangiectasia, punctuated by papules and pustules
- Oily skin with acne-like breakouts, having remissions and exacerbations
- Skin may be very sensitive, sting, and burn

Phymatous Rosacea

Phymatous rosacea is defined as marked skin thickenings and irregular surface nodularities of the nose, chin, forehead, one or both ears, and/or the eyelids. With increasing awareness and improving therapeutic facilities, this subtype is now becoming rare.

Phymatous rosacea is characterized by:
- Bumpy texture to the skin
- Skin feels oilier and skin pores look wide and large.
- There is gradual thickening of skin, especially over the nose. Skin may thicken on the chin, forehead, cheeks, and ears.
- Presence of telangiectasia

Ocular Rosacea

Ocular manifestations may precede the cutaneous signs by years and the patient can present with both for the first time.

The ocular manifestations include eye stinging or burning, dryness, irritation with light, or foreign body sensation, blepharitis, conjunctivitis, inflammation of the lids and Meibomian glands, interpalpebral conjunctival hyperemia, and conjunctival telangiectasias. Every patient with rosacea should be carefully examined for ocular involvement.

Signs and symptoms: Patients with ocular rosacea may have one or more of the following:
- Watery or bloodshot appearance
- Feel dry, gritty, often feels like sand in the eyes
- Eyes itch, burn, or sting, and sensitive to light
- Blurry vision
- Visible broken blood vessels and cysts on eyelid

Granulomatous Rosacea

This variant is characterized by monomorphic firm, yellow, brownish or reddish, papules or nodules on relatively normal-appearing skin affecting the cheeks and the periorificial areas. Diascopy reveals the lupoid character of the infiltrations. Acne agminata, otherwise known as lupus miliaris disseminatus faciei, is a rare caseating granulomatous variant of rosacea with discrete inflammatory erythematous papules involving the upper part of the face. Granulomatous rosacea is sometimes associated with scarring and may be resistant to conventional treatment.

Rosacea Fulminans

In rosacea fulminans, there is sudden onset of coalescent papules, pustules, and nodules and may occur with pregnancy, thyroid diseases, rheumatoid arthritis, depression, emotional stress. It has been reported to occur following high dose vitamin B6 and B12. Oral contraceptive pills, interferon alfa-2b, and ribavirin are other drugs that can precipitate rosacea fulminans.

Rosacea is associated with significant effect on the psychological well-being of the patient. Psychological effects of rosacea may manifest as one or more of the following:
- Feelings of frustration and embarrassment
- Worry
- Low self-esteem
- Work-related problems
- Anxiety and depression

Penile Acne

Penile acne is a poorly documented entity, seen in young men who present with comedones, papules, pustules, and inflammatory nodules involving the proximal penile shaft. Normally, follicular lesions develop along the pubic hairline. In some men, these lesions may involve the proximal portion of the shaft as well. Secondary infection and inflammation may give rise to pain and difficulty during sexual activities.

Acneiform Eruptions

Acneiform eruptions are dermatoses that resemble acne vulgaris. Lesions may be papulopustular, nodular, or cystic. While acne vulgaris typically consists of comedones, acneiform eruptions (such as acneiform drug eruptions) usually lack comedones clinically. Acne-like eruptions develop as a result of infections, hormonal, or metabolic abnormalities, genetic disorders, and as a manifestation of drug reactions.

The list of conditions giving rise to acneiform eruption is given in **Box 7**.

Occurrence of acneiform lesions has no age, gender, and racial predilection. It can present from as young as newborn to as old as over 80 years of age. Acne-like lesions constituting papules, pustules, and nodules are seen in these patients while comedones are conspicuously absent. Trunk is the most common site involved. On rare occasions, face may be involved in addition or rarely as the only site of involvement. Even if the face is involved, there is no preference for the

> **BOX 7** **Conditions giving rise to acneiform eruption.**
>
> - *Chemicals*:
>   - Cosmetics
>   - Chloracne C
>   - Other halogens
> - *Drug-induced*:
>   - Steroids
>   - Other drugs (see Box 7 in Chapter 2)
> - *Inflammation*:
>   - Eosinophilic pustular folliculitis
>   - Eruptive hair cyst
>   - Perioral dermatitis
> - *Genetic and congenital causes*:
>   - Nevus comedonicus
>   - Tuberous sclerosis complex
> - *Infections*:
>   - Bacterial: Gram-negative folliculitis
>   - Fungal: Pityrosporum folliculitis, coccidioidomycosis, sporotrichosis
>   - Treponemal: Secondary syphilis
> - *Neoplastic condition*:
>   - Lymphoma

seborrheic areas, T- or V-zones of the face. The physical location may be seen outside the area in which acne vulgaris commonly occurs.

Acneiform eruptions can be distinguished from acne vulgaris by a history of sudden onset, monotonous lesion morphology, and development of the eruption at an age outside the range typical of acne vulgaris. In the case of drug-induced acneiform eruptions, the eruption resolves with discontinuation of the medication.

Another classical finding is the monomorphic appearance of lesion that is seen in patients with acneiform eruption. In most of the patients, the cause of the condition can be identified. Removal of the cause wherever possible is the simple best successful method of treatment. The process can however be hastened with topical medications.

Acneiform lesions have been reported with cytotoxic drugs, such as methotrexate, cyclophosphamide, actinomycin D, and cisplatin. Cytotoxin-induced eruptions present as folliculitis over the face and trunk and mimic acne. The lesions begin as erythematous macules, followed by papulopustules. The entire episode resolves in 2 weeks of time. However, comedones may rarely present and persist for a longer period and resolve with pigmentation.

Papulopustular eruptions induced by newer targeted agents: Recently with the advent of antimitotic drugs, and their increasing usage, more and more incidences of papulopustular eruptions due to these targeted agents have been reported. As with any drug, the severity of cutaneous reactions varies. The monoclonal antibodies produce more severe reactions compared to epidermal growth factor receptor-tyrosine kinase (EGFR-TK) inhibitors. The papulopustular eruptions following EGFR inhibitors tend to wax and wane and resolves within 2 weeks followed by pigmentation. It has been observed that severity of the skin eruption may correlate with improved tumor response. According to the grading scale proposed by National Cancer Institute Common Terminology Criteria for Adverse events (CTCAE), the severity has been classified into four grades, the clinical features of which is given in **Table 9**.

It is important to be aware of the grading pattern of these cutaneous manifestations as studies have shown that the skin eruption is the best surrogate marker for clinical response to EGFR inhibitors. The papulopustular eruptions related to EGFR inhibitors, tyrosine kinase inhibitors, and protein kinase inhibitors typically start within the first 2 weeks of initiation of therapy. Patients with skin types I and II are more prone to develop reactions to EGFR inhibitors. Some patients complain of preceding pruritus and burning sensation before the commencement of follicular papulopustules over the seborrheic areas mainly the scalp, face, chest, and back. There

TABLE 9: The common terminology criteria for adverse events: grading of severity of papulopustular eruptions induced by newer targeted agents.

Grade	Body surface (area % involved)	Pruritus	Tenderness	Psycho-logical	Infection	Daily activity	Life-threatening
1	10	±	±	Nil	Nil	Unaffected	No
2	10–30	±	±	+	Nil	Affected	No
3	>30%	±	±	+	Local	Affected	No
4	Any %	±	±	+	Extensive	Affected	Yes

TABLE 10: Grading of papulopustular eruption to epidermal growth factor receptor inhibitors.

Grade	Number of papule/pustules	Areas of edema/erythema <1 cm	Pruritus/Pain	Daily work	Emotional disturbance
1A	<5	1	–	Unaffected	Nil
1B	<5	1	+	Unaffected	+
2A	6–20	2–5	–	Unaffected	Nil
2B	6–20	2–5	+	Affected	+
3A	>20	>5	–	Unaffected	Nil
3B	>20	>5	+	Affected	+

is also involvement of extremities, abdomen, and buttocks. Comedones are distinctly absent and the pustules are sterile. However, there can be secondary bacterial infection which can be localized to begin with that may soon become extensive. The entire course of event passes through four phases in succession. To begin with in phase I, there is sensory disturbance, erythema, and edema of upper trunk followed by papulopustular eruption in phase II. Crusting ensues in phase III followed by persistent xerosis, erythema, and telangiectasia in the last phase. According to the Multinational Association of Supportive Care in Cancer, the papulopustular eruption to EGFR inhibitors has been given a separate grading score **(Table 10)**.

Acneiform Nevi

Acneiform nevi is a condition where there is nevoid area of normal skin with acne lesions within the nevoid zone. This condition is usually seen over the back in persons with severe acne. The normal appearing skin can be bilateral or be localized to one side of the back. Reduced sebum excretion and bacterial load has been documented over the normal appearing nevoid skin. The real pathogenesis is not delineated.

Acne in Pregnancy

It has been observed that acne improves during first trimester and worsens during last trimester of pregnancy. The lesions tend to be more inflammatory. Noninflammatory lesions are relatively few in number. There is invariable truncal involvement in pregnant women. It has also been observed that patients who had acne during adolescence tend to have more severe acne during pregnancy those who have not.

Skin Sensitivity and Cosmetic Intolerance Syndrome

It is a common complaint from patients with acne that they have a "sensitive skin". It is of relevance to know about sensitive skin syndrome in connection to acne and its management. In a study of patients attending a dermatologist, it was observed that nearly 40% reported of having sensitive skin. The sensitive skin may be the skin of face, body, or genital skin. Facial skin was found to be the most commonly affected site. Females are far more affected than men. Among females, healthy women of childbearing age comprise the majority complaining of skin sensitivity. The incidence falls as the age advances. Cosmetic intolerance syndrome is just a continuum of sensitive skin syndrome and is more severe than sensitive skin. Variants of sensitive skin include acne type, rosacea type, stinging type, and allergic type.

- *Acne type*: These individuals are prone to develop acne and present with lesions that are predominantly comedones, both black and the white comedones.
- *Rosacea type:* Persons with rosacea type of sensitive skin have a tendency toward recurrent flushing and facial erythema.
- *Stinging type:* These persons have a predilection for developing stinging or burning sensation.
- *Allergic type:* Those with allergic types of sensitive skin exhibit itching, erythema, and scaling.

Some individuals may manifest with more than one type of sensitive skin.

Inflammation being the common underlying pathogenic process in sensitive skin, it is important to identify these individuals and treat them appropriately.

HORMONAL ACNE

It is important to understand hormonal acne has led to a paradigm shift in the management of acne at large. Hormonal acne refers to conditions where, during periods of hormonal excess or imbalances, acne flares up due to the combined effects of excess sebum or oil secretion and higher androgen levels in the body. Endocrine, paracrine, juxtacrine, autocrine, and intracrine pathways are ways by which hormones can exert their actions. On account of its capacity to synthesize miscellaneous hormones and express diverse hormone receptors, the pilosebaceous unit can be considered an endocrine organ in the skin. Among these hormones, androgen is clinically significant. The cutaneous features of hyperandrogenism are due to overexpression of androgenic enzymes or hyperresponsiveness of receptors. Exacerbation with relation to menstrual cycle, features of hyperandrogenism, and late onset are some of the important features to hormonal acne.

DIFFERENTIAL DIAGNOSIS OF ACNE (FIGS. 111 TO 140)

A number of conditions may be considered in the differential diagnosis of acne vulgaris.

The most important features differentiating acne vulgaris from all other types include:
- *Age of onset:* Adolescent age group
- *Site of affection:* Seborrheic sites of face and trunk
- Sparing of periorbital and preauricular sites gives a clue in many cases
- *Clinical lesion:* Comedones—pathognomonic of acne

The following are some of the diseases mimicking acne at various stages. This list does not include the conditions discussed under acne variants.
- *Comedones*:
  - *Closed comedones*:
    - Milia
  - *Open comedones*:
    - Dilated pore of Winer
    - Favre-Racouchot syndrome
    - Trichostasis spinulosa
    - Seborrheic keratosis

CHAPTER 4: Types and Variants of Acne

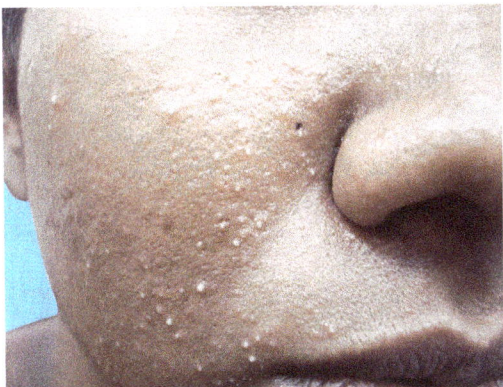

FIG. 111: Bacterial pustular eruption mimicking acne.

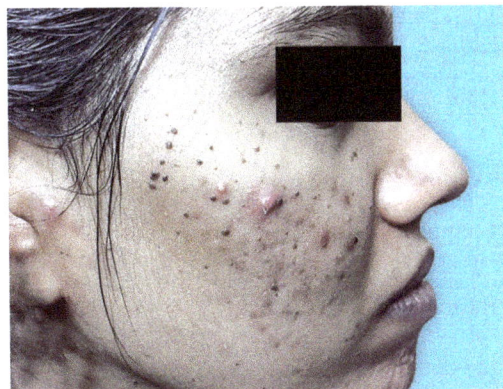

FIG. 112: Dermatosis papulosa nigra with acne; note the inflammatory papules of acne.

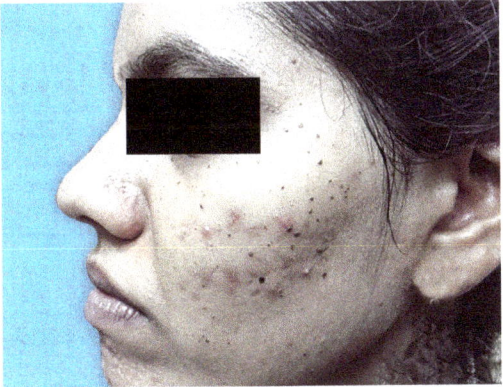

FIG. 113: Acne with dermatosis papulosa nigra; same patient as in Figure 112.

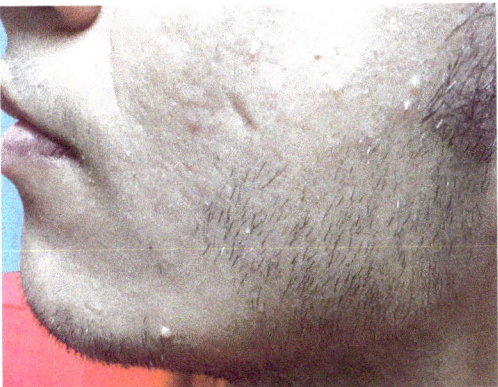

FIG. 114: Pearly papules of molluscum contagiosum mimicking papules of acne.

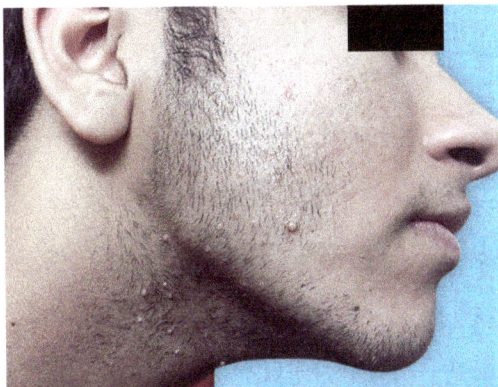

FIG. 115: Same man with acne as in Figure 114.

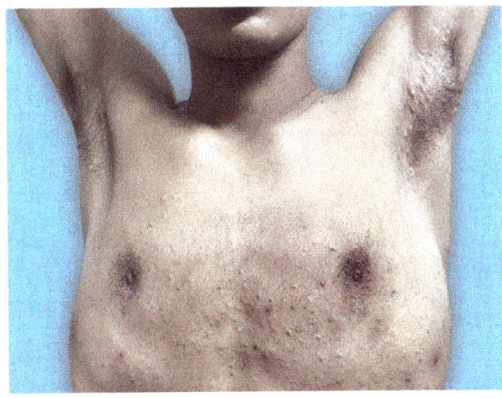

FIG. 116: Steatocystoma with acne; note the axillary involvement.

CHAPTER 4: Types and Variants of Acne

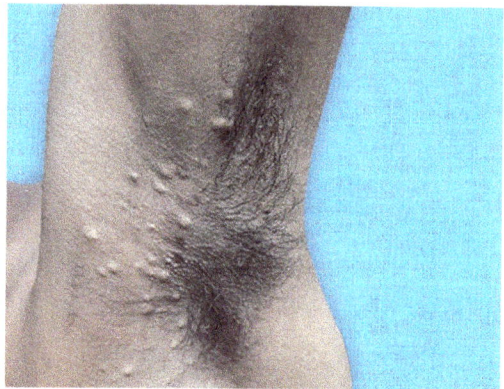

FIG. 117: Steatocystoma with acne; same patient as in Figure 116.

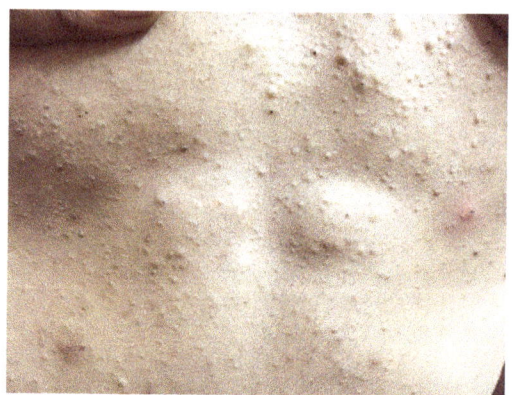

FIG. 118: Steatocystoma with acne; note the skin colored papules of steatocytoma.

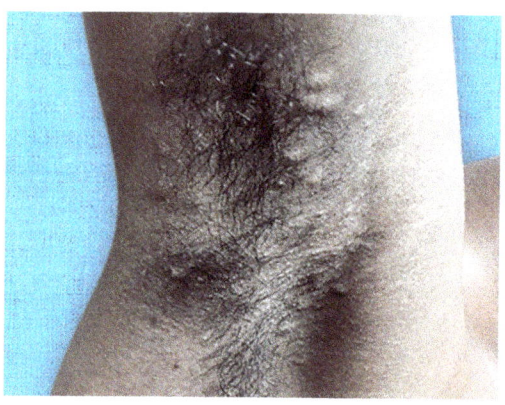

FIG. 119: Cystic lesions in the axilla mimicking hidradenitis suppurativa; same patient as in Figure 116.

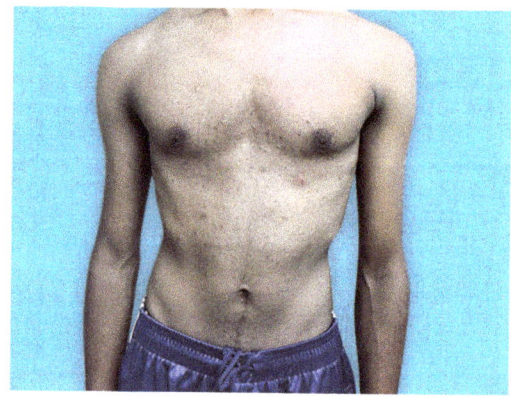

FIG. 120: Adolescent with acne lesions and cystic lesions of steatocystoma.

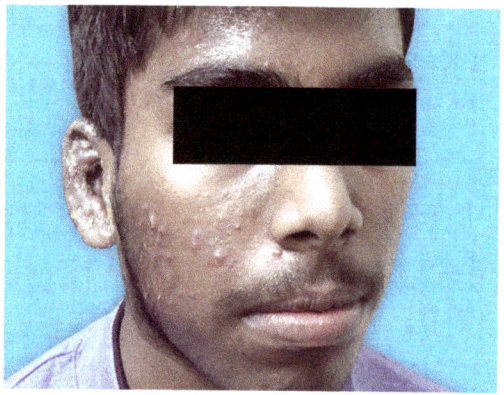

FIG. 121: Bacterial pustules can often be mistaken for acne pustules. Acne lesions are follicular and do not involve the pinna.

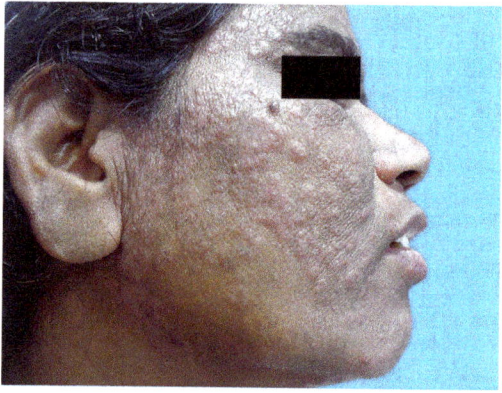

FIG. 122: Tinea faciei in a diabetic mimicking acne.

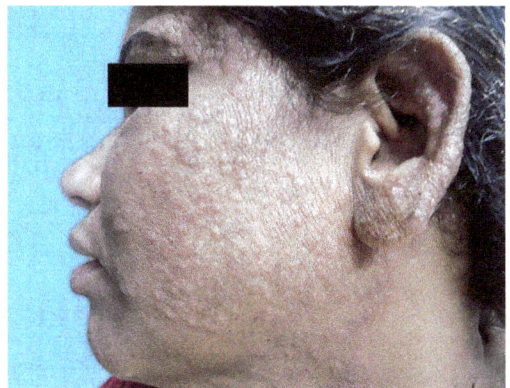

FIG. 123: Same as in Figure 122.

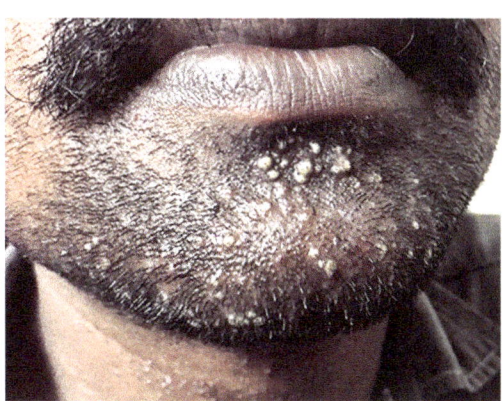

FIG. 124: Folliculitis mimicking pustular acne.

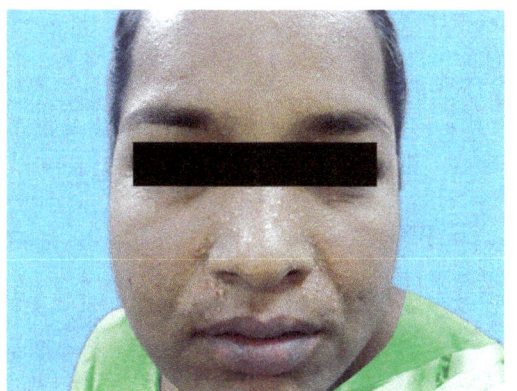

FIG. 125: Milia mimicking acne papules.

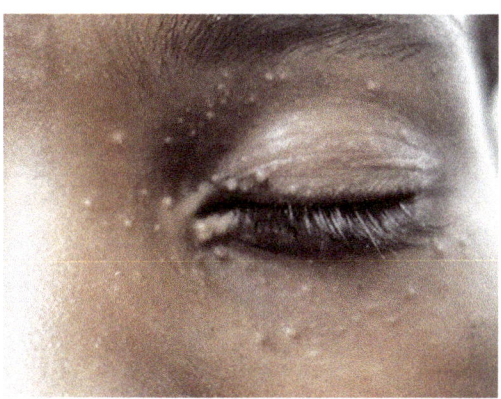

FIG. 126: Skin-colored papules of milia and syringoma; can be mistaken for early acne lesions.

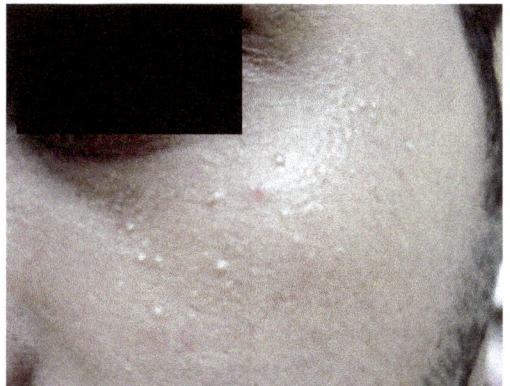

FIG. 127: Milia resembling closed comedones but are more prominent.

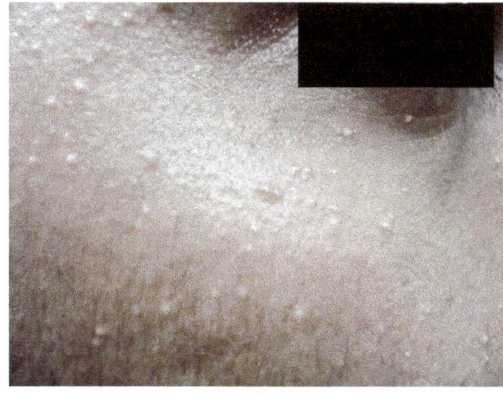

FIG. 128: Close-up view of milia closely mimicking acne.

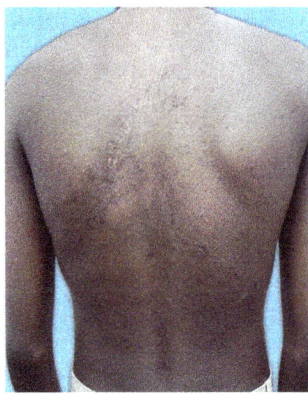

FIG. 129: Papules of Darier's disease; it may masquerade as acne.

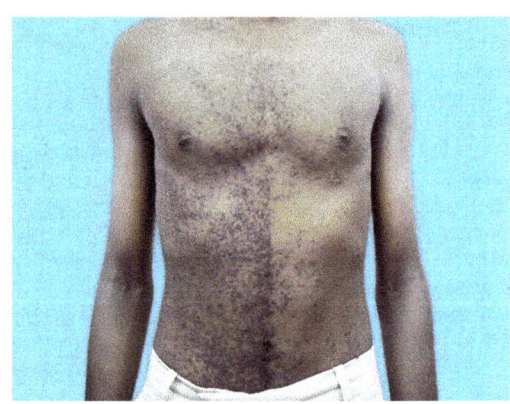

FIG. 130: Unilateral Darier's who also has acne; same patient as in Figure 129.

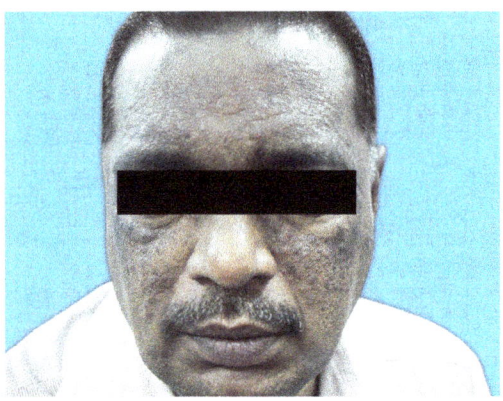

FIG. 131: Involvement of forehead in a man with Darier's disease mimicking comedones and papules of acne.

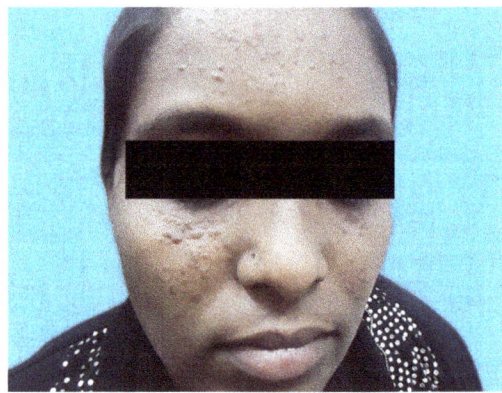

FIG. 132: Syringoma can mimic or coexist with acne.

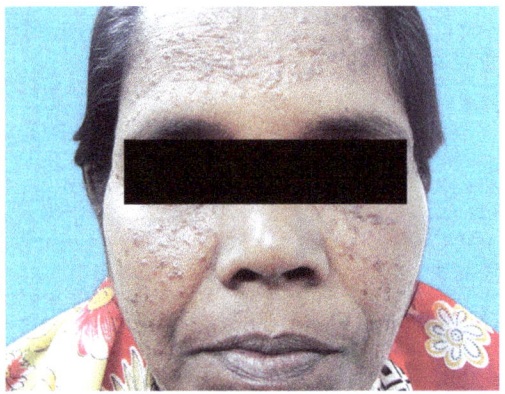

FIG. 133: Elderly lady with syringoma.

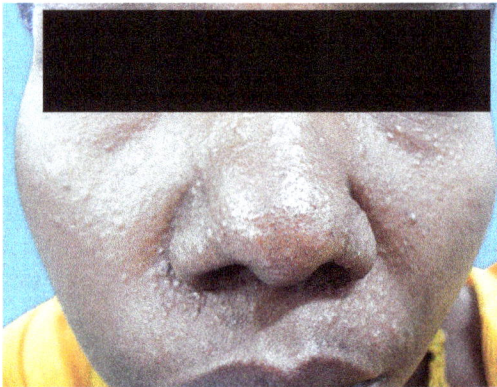

FIG. 134: Trichostasis spinulosa.

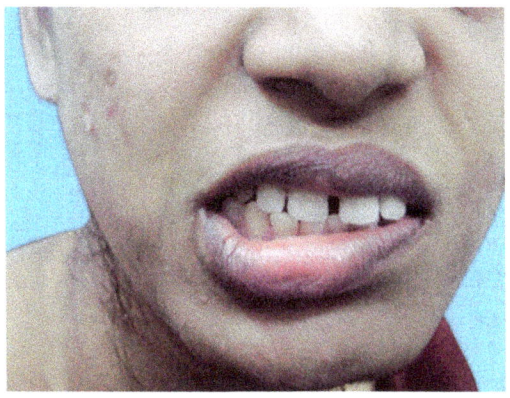

FIG. 135: Unilateral acne in patient with facial palsy I.

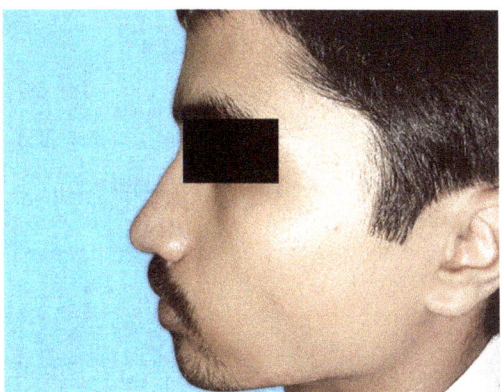

FIG. 136: Unilateral acne in patient with facial palsy II.

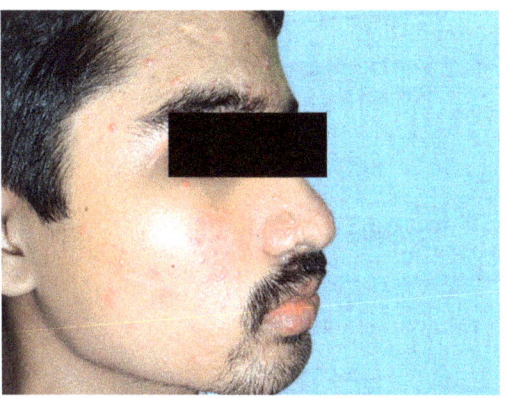

FIG. 137: Unilateral acne in patient with facial palsy; same patient as in Figure 136.

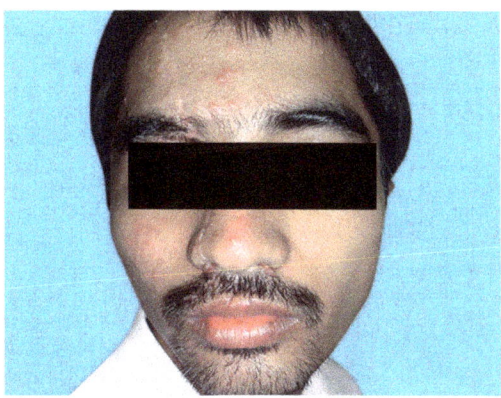

FIG. 138: Unilateral acne in patient with facial palsy; same patient as in Figure 136.

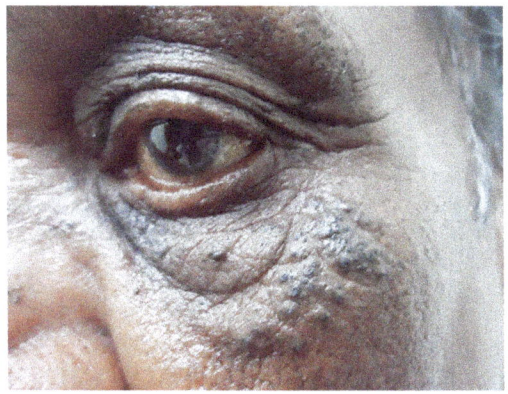

FIG. 139: Senile comedones I.

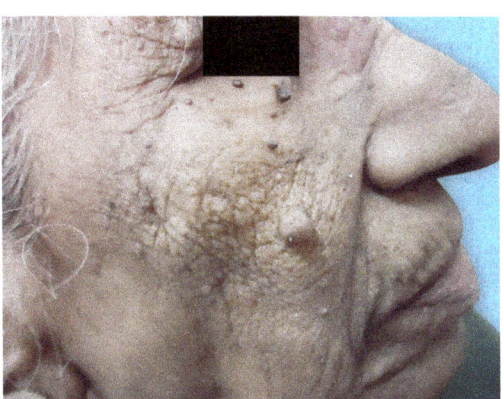

FIG. 140: Senile comedones II.

- *Papules*:
  - Pityrosporum folliculitis
  - Plane warts
  - Colloid milia
  - Keratosis pilaris
  - Darier's disease
  - Miliaria rubra
  - Pseudofolliculitis barbae
  - Candidiasis
- *Pustules*:
  - Bacterial folliculitis
  - Eosinophilic pustular folliculitis of Ofuji
  - Candidiasis
  - Periporitis
- *Nodules and cysts*:
  - Furuncle
  - Carbuncle
  - Multiple epidermoid cysts
  - Scrofulodermas (mimicking hidradenitis)
- *Scars*:
  - Chickenpox
  - Deep folliculitis
  - Scrofuloderma (mimicking hidradenitis)
- *Neoplastic conditions mimicking acne*:
  - Angiofibroma of tuberous sclerosis complex
  - Comedo nevus
  - Eruptive vellus hair cysts
  - Fibrofolliculoma
  - Steatocystoma multiplex
  - Syringoma
  - Trichodiscoma
  - Trichoepithelioma

The following conditions are to be thought of as differentials while seeing a patient with subtypes of rosacea:

- *Erythematotelangiectatic type*:
  - Seborrheic dermatitis
  - Contact dermatitis
  - Chronic photodamage
  - Lupus erythematosus
- *Papulopustular type*:
  - Acne vulgaris
  - Perioral dermatitis
  - Dermatophytosis
  - Demodicosis
  - Jessner's lymphocytic infiltrate
  - Lymphocytoma cutis
- *Phymatous type*:
  - Solid facial lymphedema
  - Lupus pernio
  - Cutaneous tuberculosis

CHAPTER 5

Course and Complications

DISEASE COURSE AND PROGNOSIS (FIGS. 1 TO 20)

As the name implies, acne vulgaris is a common disorder of the teens, the prime of life (acne meaning prime of life and vulgaris meaning common). In a significant portion of the adolescents, the disease is self-limited and fades as they overgrow the adolescent period. Though acne is considered as a "rite of passage" at this period of life, there is yet another significant number of adolescents in whom the disease takes a more severe and chronic course, leading to unwanted sequelae, both organic and psychosocial. In general, the course of acne is one of several years' duration followed by spontaneous remission in majority of patients by the end of teens or early 20s. However, in some individuals, the disease shows spontaneous fluctuations in the severity and extends well beyond the third decade.

Similarly, acne in children also takes its own course and has prognostic variations. In this chapter, the course and prognosis of childhood acne and acne vulgaris will be briefly discussed.

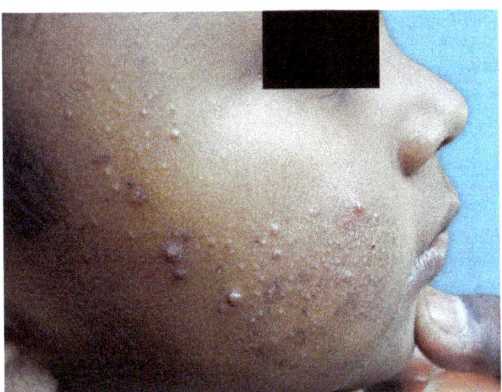

FIG. 1: Childhood acne in an infant. This child may develop acne vulgaris, which may run a difficult course.

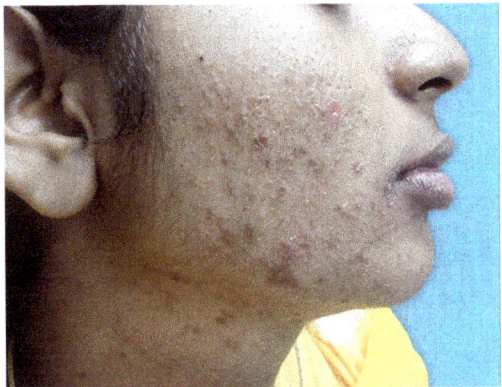

FIG. 2: A girl having acne with history of acne in sister and mother carries poor prognosis. Note the involvement of neck.

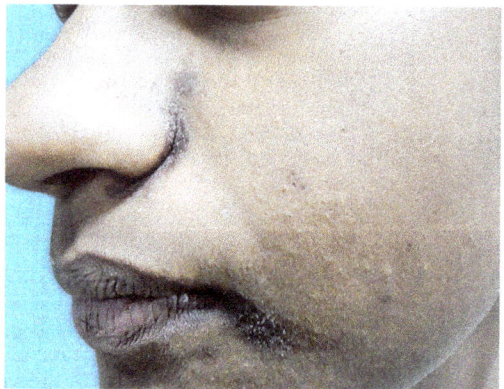

FIG. 3: Early-onset acne is a poor prognostic sign.

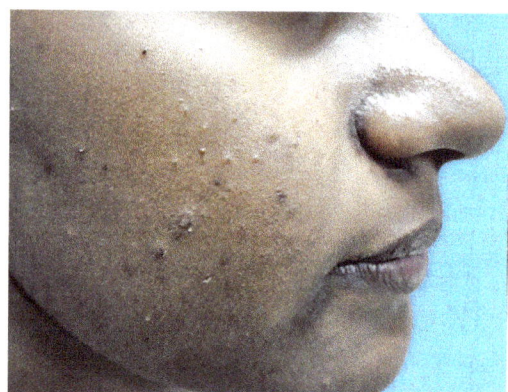

FIG. 4: Early-onset acne is a poor prognostic sign. Same patient as in Figure 3.

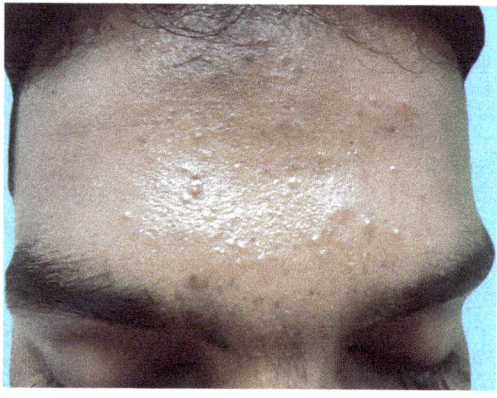

FIG. 5: Seborrhea is a poor prognostic factor. Note the oiliness of the skin.

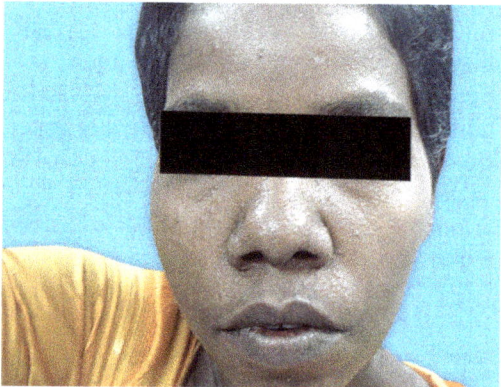

FIG. 6: Seborrhea, acne with polycystic ovary syndrome carries poor prognosis.

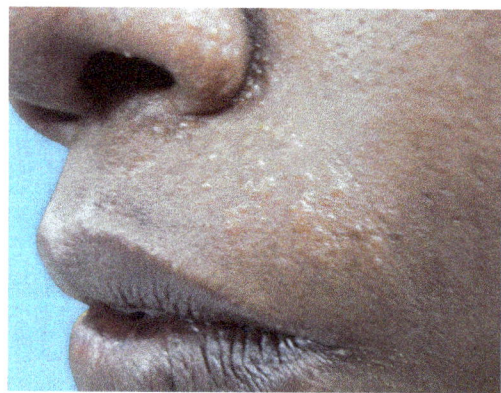

FIG. 7: Seborrhea, acne with polycystic ovary syndrome (PCOS) carries poor prognosis. Same patient as in Figure 6.

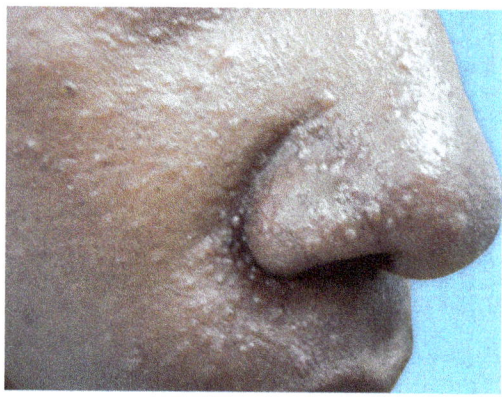

FIG. 8: Seborrhea, acne with polycystic ovary syndrome (PCOS) carries poor prognosis. Same patient as in Figure 6.

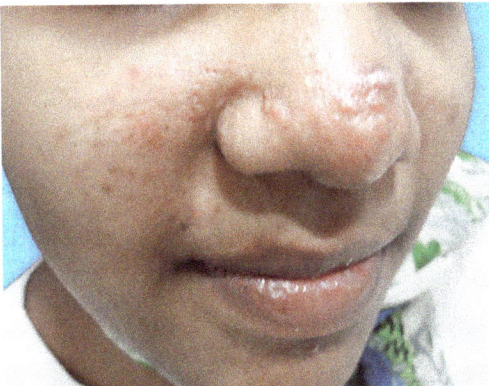

FIG. 9: Early onset with positive family history, both indicate poor prognosis.

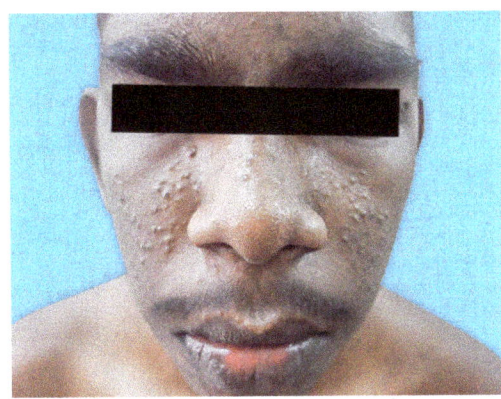

FIG. 10: A young boy with midfacial comedones, who carries relatively poor prognosis early in the course of the disease.

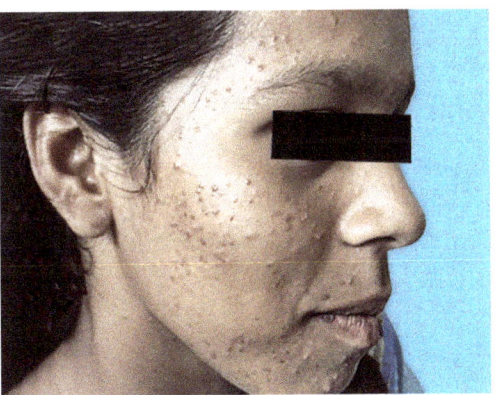

FIG. 11: Sudden onset of more number of lesions in a 13-year-old girl carries poor prognosis.

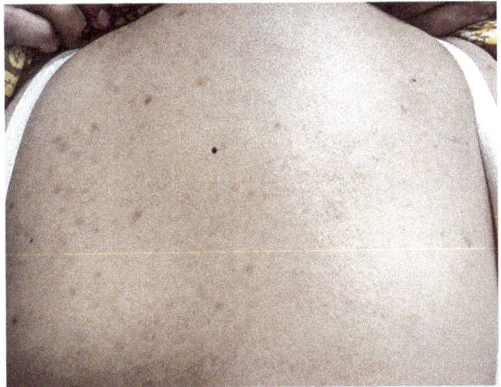

FIG. 12: Involvement of trunk in females carries poor prognosis.

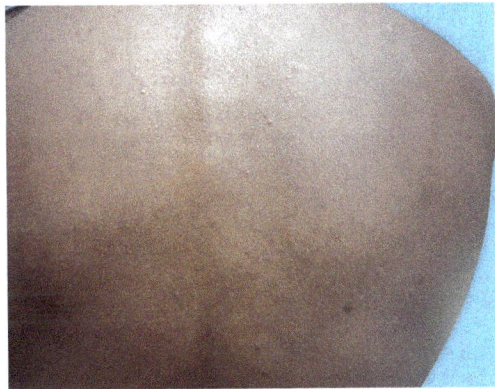

FIG. 13: Involvement of the back in a 12-year-old boy—a poor prognostic finding.

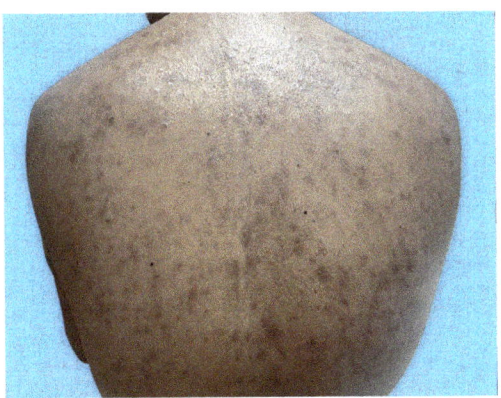

FIG. 14: Truncal acne carries poor prognosis.

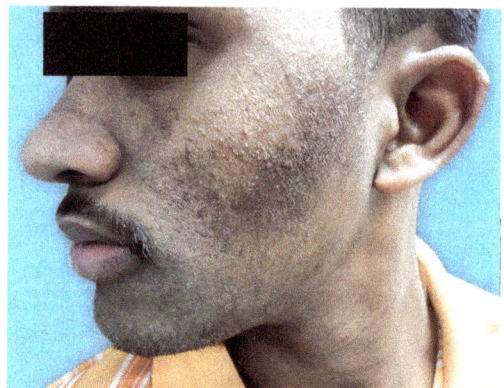

FIG. 15: This patient had frequent exacerbations of the disease, indicating poor prognosis.

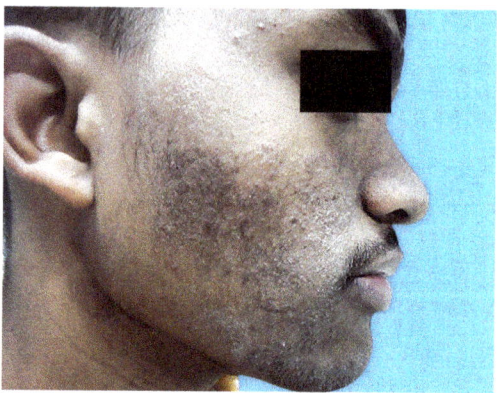

FIG. 16: This patient had frequent exacerbations of the disease, indicating poor prognosis. Same patient in Figure 15.

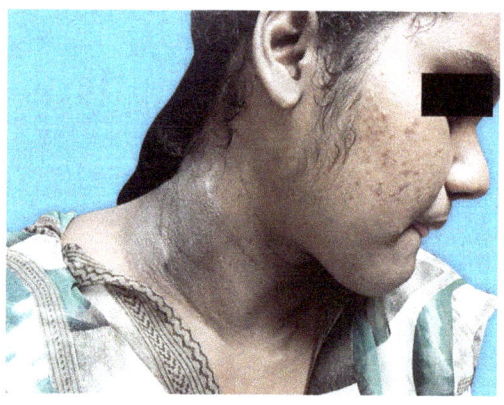

FIG. 17: Acne in a teenager with insulin resistance carries poor prognosis.

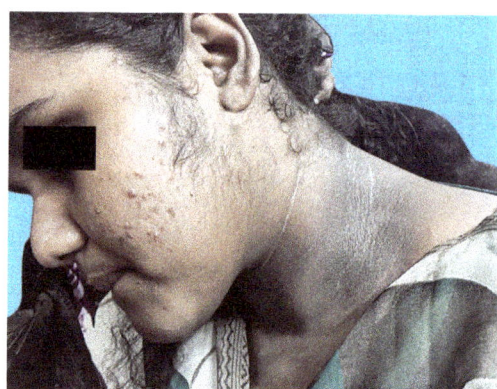

FIG. 18: Same patient as in Figure 17.

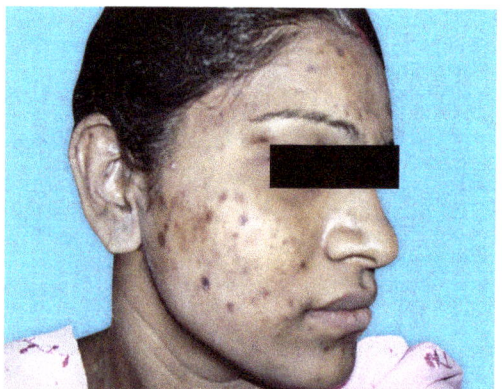

FIG. 19: Acne excoriée; psychological impact also plays a major role in the treatment outcome and prognosis.

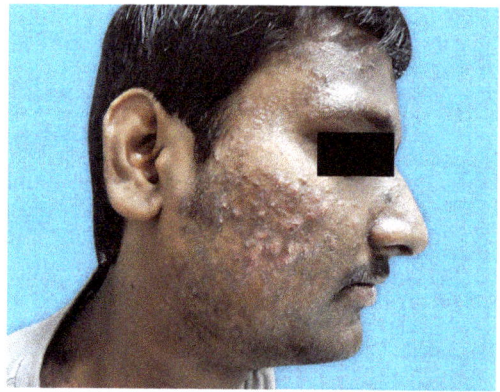

FIG. 20: Acne with insulin resistance tends to run a prolonged course.

Childhood Acne

Neonatal acne in most newborns settles without any sequelae and has a good prognosis.

Infantile acne: This acne is less common than neonatal acne. Nevertheless, unlike neonatal acne, infantile acne has a more persistent and variable course. Majority resolves by 5 years of age and in few infants and children, it persists until puberty. Since deep-seated lesions are not common, scarring is also not common in this age group.

Mid-childhood acne: Acne is very rare between 7 and 12 years of age (considering the age of menarche as after 12). Manifestation of acne in this age group indicates prolonged course and poor prognosis.

It is important to remember that the children who develop acne after 1 year of age may develop the disease during puberty as well. Certain poor prognostic signs include midfacial distribution of comedones in high numbers, increased levels of dehydroepiandrosterone sulfate (DHEAS) and total testosterone, and earlier menarche in females.

Acne Vulgaris

The course and prognosis vary from individual to individual. **Box 1** gives the list of poor prognostic signs in acne vulgaris, which may indicate a prolonged course and severe disease and poorer therapeutic outcome. Positive family history may be an indicator of severe acne. Similarly, seborrhea, early-onset lesions, and prepubertal midfacial comedones may all give a clue to severe disease. Prolonged disease course points to poor therapeutic response and intense seborrhea relates to reduced response to antibiotic therapy. Truncal acne has a poor prognosis when compared to facial acne as the therapeutic response is much lesser when compared to the latter. Acne vulgaris when shows signs of insulin resistance is difficult to treat and has a poorer prognosis as against acne vulgaris without insulin resistance, even if the presentation is severe. In these patients, the disease runs a prolonged course and the lesions tend to be resistant to therapy. In many patients, the psychological impact also plays a major role in the treatment outcome and prognosis. These patients need extra attention through both counseling and drugs and procedures.

SEQUELAE AND COMPLICATIONS OF ACNE (FIGS. 21 TO 50)

Though acne is a self-healing disease without any sequelae and complications, majority of patients experience complications either due to disease or treatment. All types of acne lesions resolve with varying degrees of sequelae.

The most frequent disease-oriented complications are related to psychosocial disturbance and scarring. Albeit some complications are immediate and some are delayed in presentation. The important aspect of acne management is to prevent or minimize complications in patients which determine treatment success. The various complications encountered in acne patients are depicted in **Flowchart 1**.

Disease-induced Complications

Almost all patients with acne end up with dilated pores. In patients with minimal disease and effective treatment, the dilatation is not significant enough to go for further therapy.

BOX 1 | **Poor prognostic signs in acne vulgaris.**

- Positive family history
- Early onset
- Seborrhea
- Prepubertal midfacial inflammatory lesions
- More number of lesions
- Frequent relapses
- Truncal acne
- Longer duration

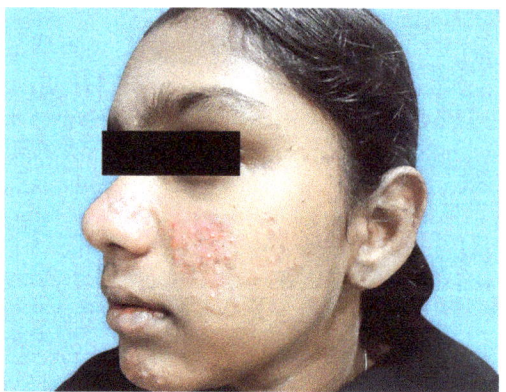

FIG. 21: Erythema is a frequent complication seen in acne patients.

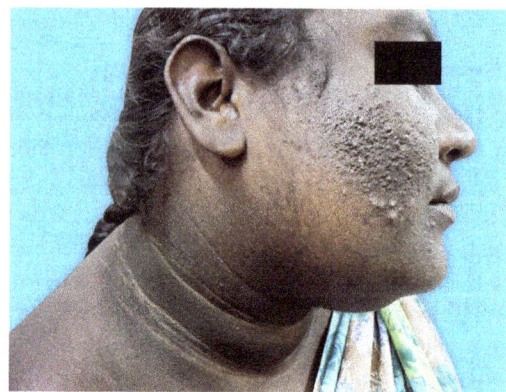

FIG. 22: Minocycline-induced pigmentation.

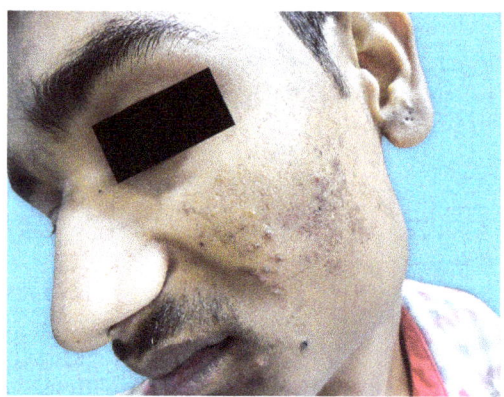

FIG. 23: Adolescent with pigmentation over scar after minocycline therapy.

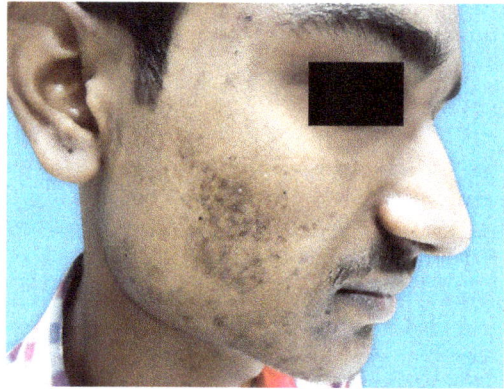

FIG. 24: Adolescent with pigmentation over scar after minocycline therapy. Same patient as in Figure 23.

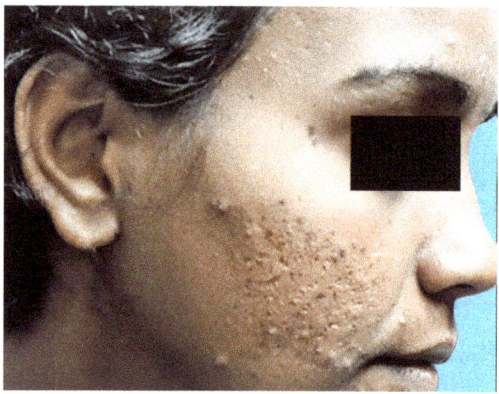

FIG. 25: Acne scar.

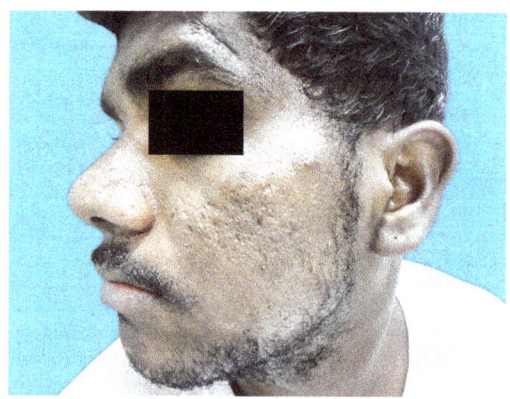

FIG. 26: Superficial scars post acne.

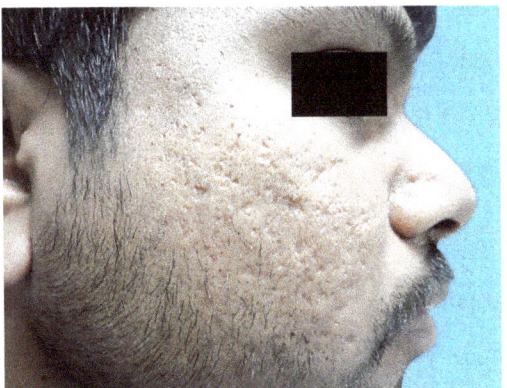

FIG. 27: Icepick scars of grade-III acne.

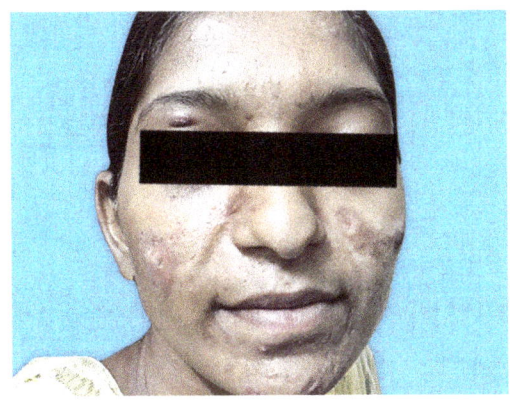

FIG. 28: Keloidal scars in acne.

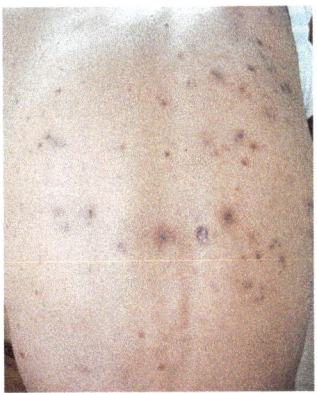

FIG. 29: Varioliform scars in a patient who had nodulocystic acne.

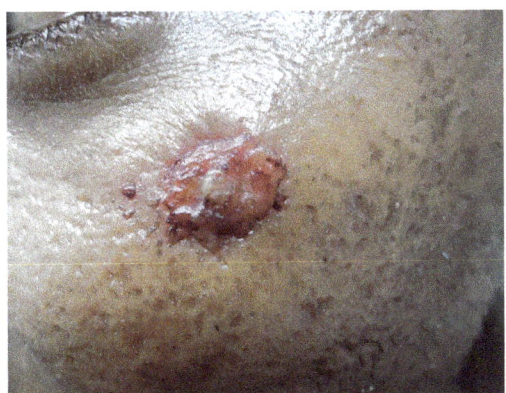

FIG. 30: Severe self-induced trauma leading to superficial ulcer in an acne patient.

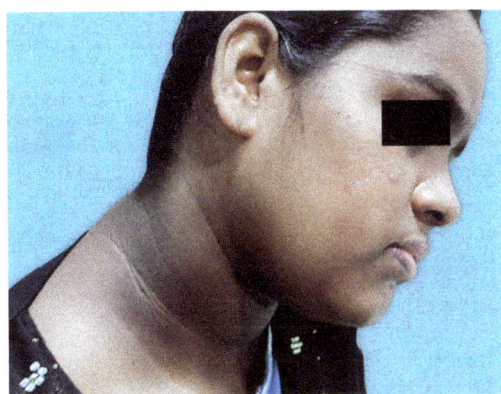

FIG. 31: Acanthosis nigricans in an obese girl with few acne papules with elevated testosterone level.

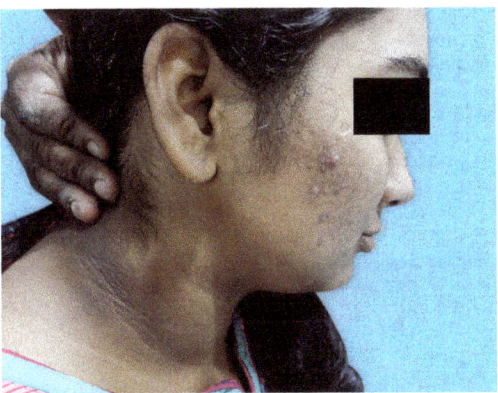

FIG. 32: Acanthosis nigricans in an acne patient showing normal endocrine work-up.

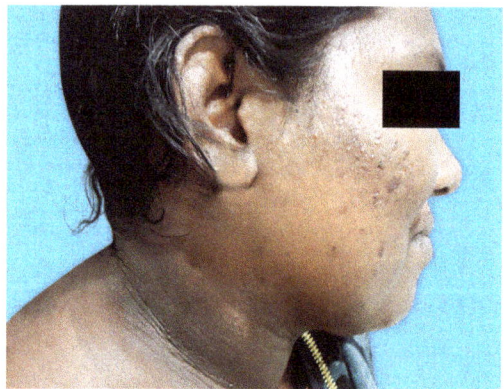

FIG. 33: Acne, acanthosis nigricans, seborrhea, and infertility need endocrine evaluation.

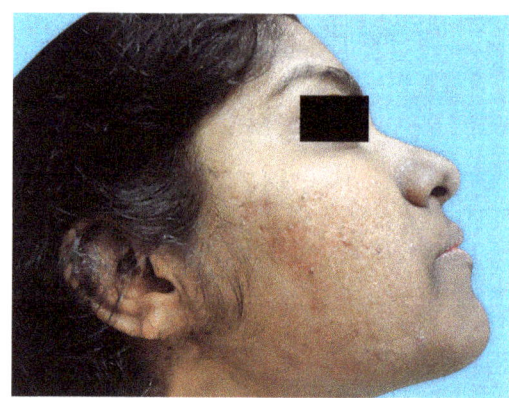

FIG. 34: Acne with hirsutism without other features of hyperandrogenism. Not necessary to subject for endocrine work-up.

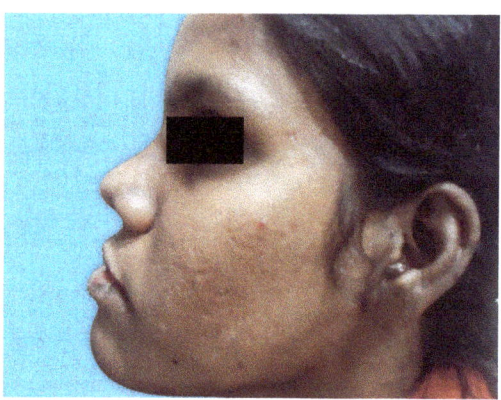

FIG. 35: Acne with menstrual irregularity showed normal endocrine profile.

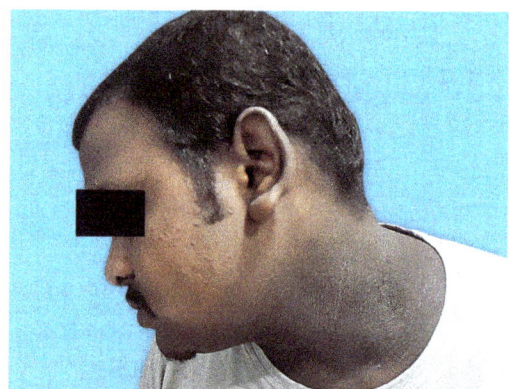

FIG. 36: APAAN (acne, patterned alopecia, and acanthosis nigricans) syndrome with abnormal glucose tolerance test (GTT).

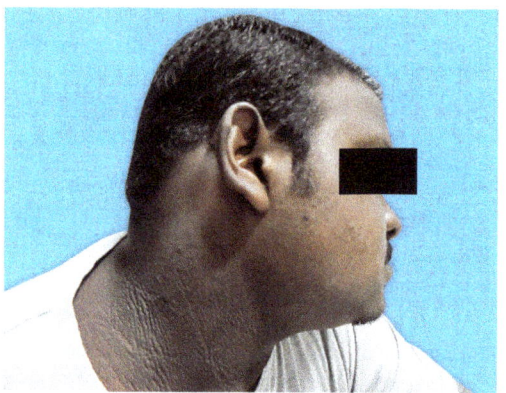

FIG. 37: APAAN (acne, patterned alopecia, and acanthosis nigricans) syndrome with abnormal glucose tolerance test (GTT). Same patient as in Figure 36.

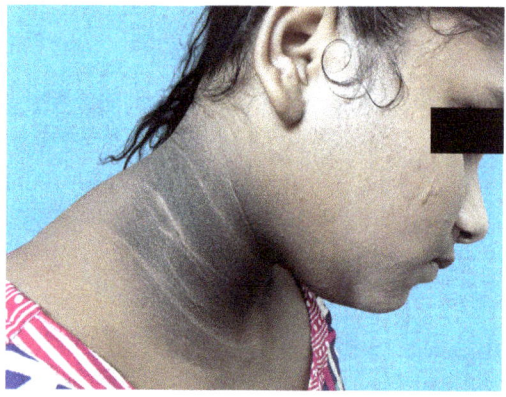

FIG. 38: APAAN (acne, patterned alopecia, and acanthosis nigricans) syndrome with diabetes.

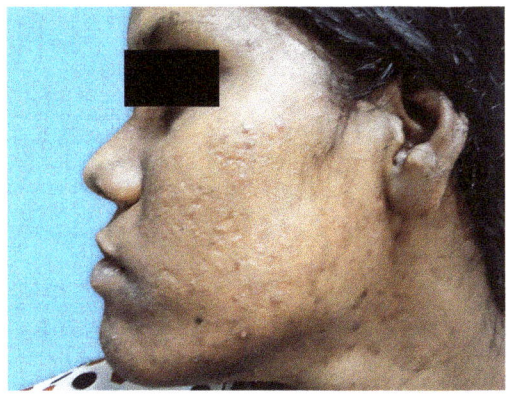

FIG. 39: Facial and truncal acne with oligomenorrhea in a girl with polycystic ovary syndrome (PCOS). Note the involvement of neck.

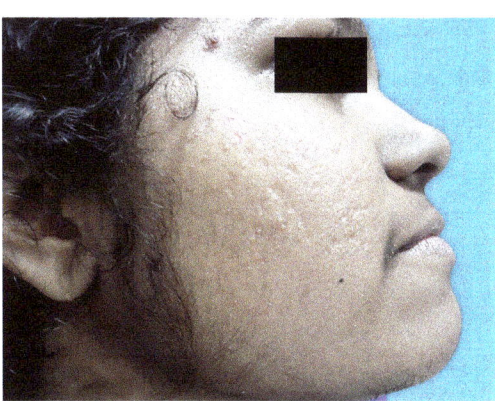

FIG. 40: Inflammatory acne in a girl with menstrual irregularity with abnormal scarring hormone profile.

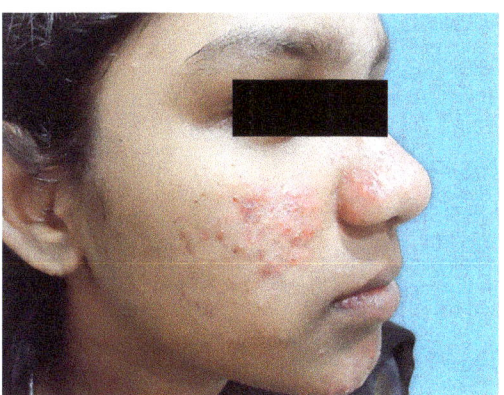

FIG. 41: Inflammatory acne in a girl with menstrual irregularity with abnormal hormone profile.

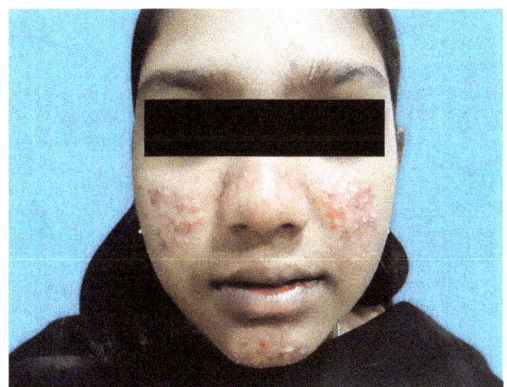

FIG. 42: Inflammatory acne in a girl with menstrual irregularity with abnormal hormone profile. Same patient as in Figure 41.

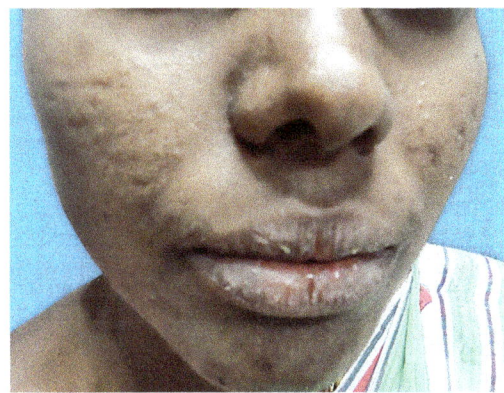

FIG. 43: Acne in a woman with altered glucose tolerance test (GTT). Note cheilitis following oral retinoids.

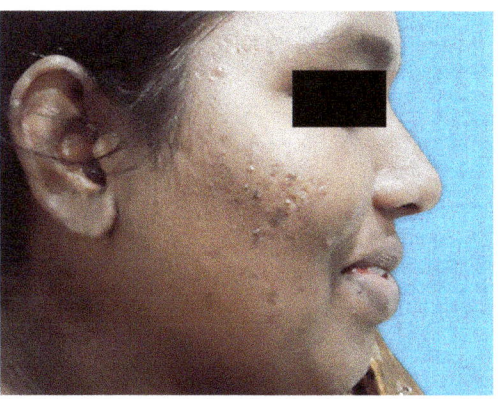

FIG. 44: Acne with abnormal glucose tolerance test (GTT) in a girl.

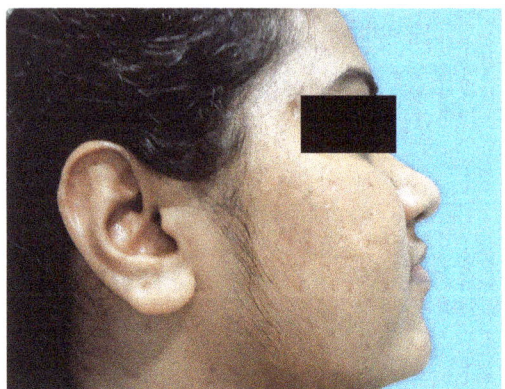

FIG. 45: Obesity and hirsutism in a girl with altered follicle-stimulating hormone:luteinizing hormone (FSH/LH) ratio.

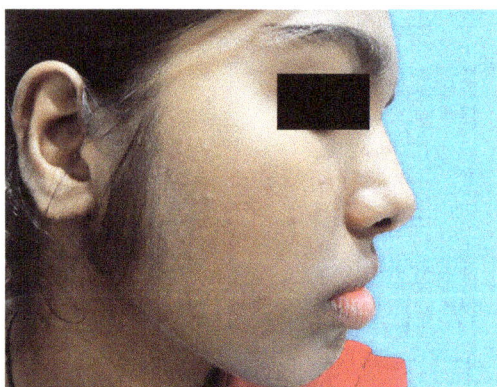

FIG. 46: A preadolescent girl with few acne papules and hirsutism needs follow-up and endocrine work-up.

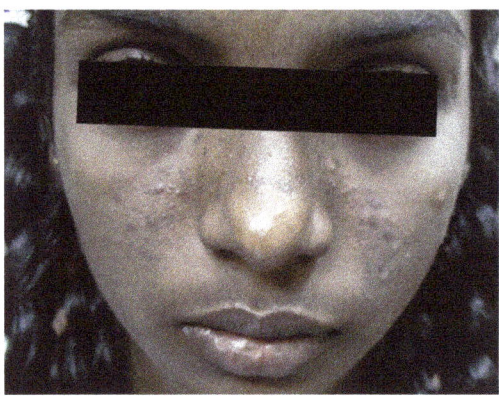

FIG. 47: Resistant acne in adolescents with polycystic ovaries.

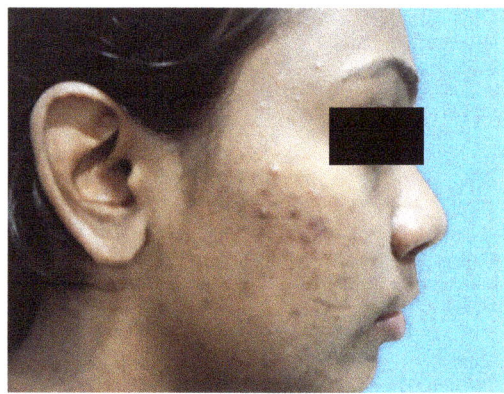

FIG. 48: SAHA (seborrhea, acne, hirsutism, and alopecia) syndrome with polycystic ovary syndrome (PCOS).

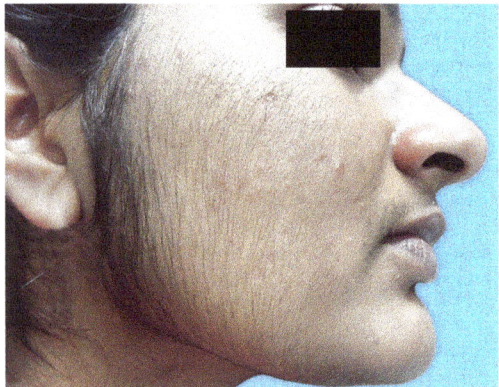

FIG. 49: SAHA (seborrhea, acne, hirsutism, and alopecia) syndrome in a girl who was detected to have polycystic ovary syndrome (PCOS) with ultrasonogram.

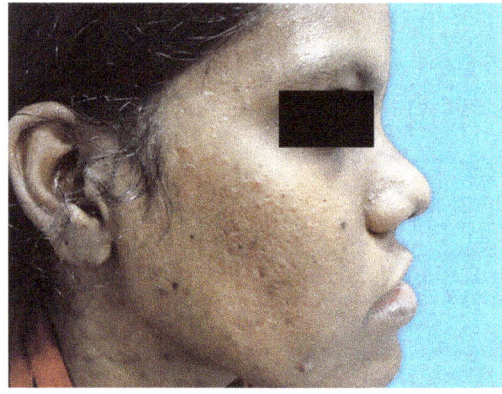

FIG. 50: Seborrhea and acne with persistent oligomenorrhea.

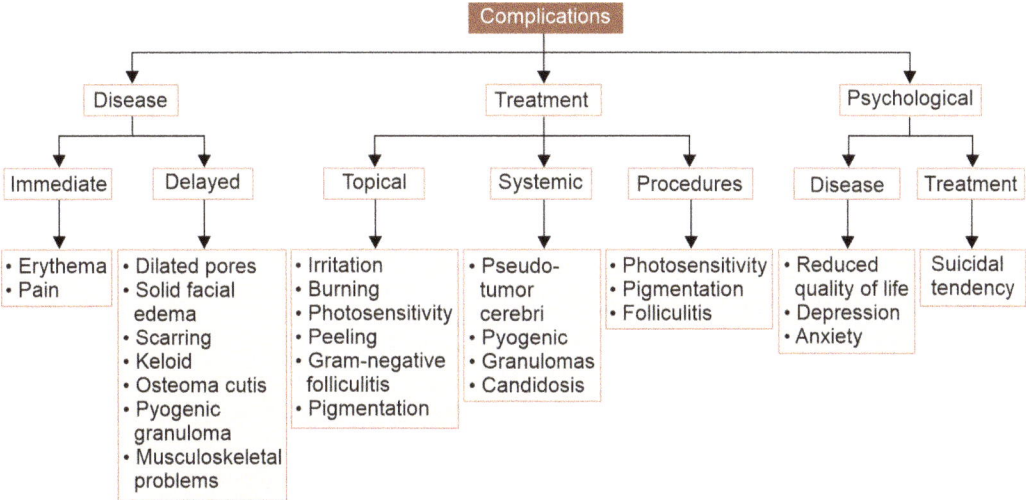

FLOWCHART 1: Complications of acne.

Erythema is a component of inflammatory lesions. This can be worsened with sun exposure or treatment. Transient macular erythema is a common sequela in almost all patients. Proper advice and effective measures can certainly minimize this problem.

Pain is usually not a feature of acne lesions. But some patients with inflammatory lesions complain of pain, which is commonly observed in those with severe forms of acne-like nodular acne, acne conglobata, and acne fulminans. Pigmentation is seen in a significant number of patients, especially dark-skinned individuals. In some, especially the dark-skinned individuals, this type of postinflammatory pigmentation may persist for many months after resolution of acne lesions. Pigmentation is also a sequela of treatment with drugs, such as minocycline.

Scarring

Scarring is a very common consequence of acne seen in as high as 90% of patients; however mild the disease be, indicating that a delay or incomplete treatment can lead to severe scar formation. Inflammatory acne lesions result in permanent scars. Delay in treatment is likely to worsen the severity of scars. Severe scarring leads to substantial physical and psychological stress, particularly in adolescents, in addition to reducing the job opportunities in a significant number of adults.

There are two different pathogenic mechanisms that determine the scar formation in an individual with scarring.

Genetic factors and the capacity to respond to trauma are considered the main factors influencing scar formation. The second important factor being the type, depth, and extent of inflammation.

It was found that in those patients not prone (genetically) for scar formation, the course was typical of delayed hypersensitivity response. In these people, both the innate and adaptive mechanisms led to effective resolution of inflammation without scarring, whereas in lesions of scar-prone patients, persistent adaptive immune response was acting, which was even upregulated in resolving lesions. These observations clearly suggest that effective treatment and management of inflammation will prevent scar formation, reducing the need for scar revision.

Hypertrophic scars are relatively less common in acne patients. Hypertrophic scars are seen more commonly in men and are usually seen over the back.

Solid facial edema, osteoma cutis, and pyogenic granuloma are very rarely reported complications of acne.

Solid Facial Edema of Rosacea

This is a rare disfiguring complication of acne and rosacea. There is progressive soft tissue swelling with thickened, woody facial edema, leading to midline distortion. This may be a result of preexisting hypoplastic lymphatics. If left untreated, it may end up in permanent swelling, which may not respond to medical treatment at a later date.

Osteoma Cutis

Osteoma cutis develops in long-standing disease, where the calcification manifests as firm persistent papules of 2–4 mm size. The histology shows calcified trabecular bone formation surrounded by perivascular proliferation and laying of fibrous tissue.

Pyogenic Granuloma

Pyogenic granuloma is a very rare complication of severe acne seen on the trunk. Such lesions may be a manifestation of acne fulminans. Some cases of pyogenic granuloma are precipitated by treatment with systemic isotretinoin.

Musculoskeletal Problems

Mild musculoskeletal discomfort seems to persist even after clearance of skin lesions in acne fulminans as has been documented. Radiographic changes such as hyperostosis and sclerosis persist in some patients even after treatment. These, however, are not symptomatic in many.

Complications due to treatment are discussed in Chapter 7.

PSYCHOLOGICAL EFFECTS OF ACNE

It will be alarming to know that as high as half of the adolescents suffering from acne experience psychiatric disturbances due to the disease. Certain studies have shown that the psychological disturbance due to acne is equal to that observed in chronic debilitating systemic diseases, such as diabetes, asthma, and epilepsy. The quality of life (QOL) shows a significant drop in patients with acne, more so in those with severe scars. When comparing with skin diseases, acne patients having depression have a severity same as seen in hospitalized patients of psoriasis. It is also very important to be aware that acne scars have been quoted as reason for unemployment, adding to the psychological problem in young adults. Therefore, it is better to obtain psychiatrist's assistance to counsel such patients with psychiatric disturbance. Nearly 70% of patients with acne experience shame. The different psychological disturbances observed among acne patients include depression, embarrassment, anxiety, lack of confidence, impaired social contact, and increased anger. There are reports on suicide due to acne and acne-related issues. Therefore, any acne patient showing signs of depression should be assessed for suicide risk.

CHAPTER 6

Assessment and Investigation

ASSESSMENT OF ACNE PATIENT

Patient assessment varies from disease to disease. In acne, the same protocol cannot be applied to all with a diagnosis of acne. Especially, with relation to psychological impact, the assessment varies between children, adolescents, and adults.

Acne is one disease for which most of the patients will require medical, psychological, and surgical assessment.

The following should be included under medical assessment:
- *History should include*:
  - Personal
  - Menstrual
  - Family
  - Treatment
  - Lifestyle
- *Physical examination will include assessment of*:
  - Extent
  - Severity
  - Grading
  - Associations

There are various methods adopted to assess the severity of acne. The evaluation can be either overall or global assessment, separate evaluations of individual lesions, or evaluation that is based according to predominant lesion type. In the recent days, patient-reported outcomes are given importance in the assessment methods.

According to LEEDS photometric grading scale, acne is graded in different locations, namely the face, back, and front of the chest. The grading is done on a scale of 0–10. The drawback with this system is that there is no definite differentiation between mild, moderate, or severe disease. The comprehensive acne severity system (CASS) applies six different gradings based on the severity of acne and the readings are done for the face, back, and chest separately. The CASS grading is briefly given in **Table 1**.

Psychological Assessment

Generic measures, generic health questionnaire, dermatology-specific measures such as dermatology life quality index (DLQI), and acne-specific quality of life (QOL) questionnaire instruments such as acne [quality of life inventory (QOLI)] are available to assess the psychosocial impact in acne patients.

It is difficult to apply the adult methods for adolescents to assess QOL—Skindex-Teen and teenagers' quality of life index (T-QOLI).

Similarly, the assessment of QOL in children is challenging due to difficulty in communication and the varying levels of maturity within children of the same age due to different lifestyle and exposure. For children, Children's Dermatology Quality of Life Index (CDQLI) can be used and assistance can be sought from parents.

TABLE 1: Grading by comprehensive acne severity system.

Grade	Description		
	Visibility	Number	Type of lesion
Clear	No to barely noticeable lesions	Few scattered	Comedones and papules
Almost clear	Hardly visible from 2.5 meter away	Few scattered	Comedones, small papules, and pustules
Mild	Easily recognizable	Many, <50% of affected area	Comedones, papules, and pustules
Moderate	Easily recognizable	Many, >50% of affected area	Comedones, papules, and pustules
Severe	Easily recognizable	Entire area affected	Comedones, papules, and pustules. Few nodules and cysts
Very severe	Easily recognizable	Entire area affected	Highly inflammatory, many nodules and cysts

INVESTIGATIONS IN PATIENTS WITH ACNE (FIGS. 1 TO 10)

The diagnosis of acne is clinical. In general, laboratory tests are not suggested for patients with acne, except during the following situations:
- Rule out mimickers
- Rule out or rule in associations
- Rule out hyperandrogenism
- Before starting therapy with certain drugs
- Follow-up
- Academic purpose

Microbiologic Tests

Microbiologic tests are, at times, carried out in patients with or suspected to have acne. Basically, culture and colony count testing of pustules of acne is needless as successful antibiotic therapy not always corresponds to reduction in bacterial numbers. However, patients with gram-negative folliculitis will benefit from microbiological testing who may show. Similarly, acute eruptions of staphylococcal folliculitis of face closely mimicking acne will grow *Staphylococcus aureus* in culture and antibiogram may help in deciding on the appropriate antibiotic. Gram-negative bacteria such as *Klebsiella* and *Serratia* can cause folliculitis in patients on prolonged treatment with antibiotics. In some patients having bacterial resistance, investigations for antibiotic-resistant *Cutibacterium acnes* (*C. acnes*) will help change the treatment, as it has been demonstrated that poor clinical response to antibiotics in some patients has been proved to be due to presence of resistant strains of *C. acnes*.

It was documented that blood culture yielded *C. acnes* in a patient with acne fulminans, the finding was not consistent though.

Biopsy and Histologic Examination

Biopsy is seldom indicated or done in patients with acne.

The classical lesions of acne, namely the comedone, whether open or closed, are histologically seen as cyst-like cavities lined by thin epithelium and filled with follicular keratotic material. The sebaceous acini may look atrophic. In case of open comedones, 10–15 hair structures can be seen in the lumen, whereas single or two such hair structures are seen in the lumen of closed comedones.

The inflammatory lesions show collection of neutrophils and fibrin within the infundibulum. There will be perifollicular inflammatory infiltrate composed of mononuclear cells and plasma cells.

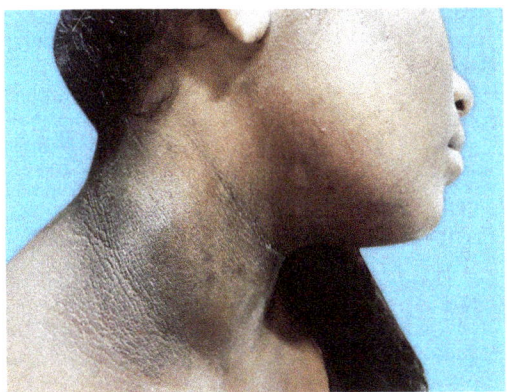

FIG. 1: Seborrhea, acne acanthosis nigricans, oligomenorrhea, and polycystic ovary syndrome (PCOS) to be excluded.

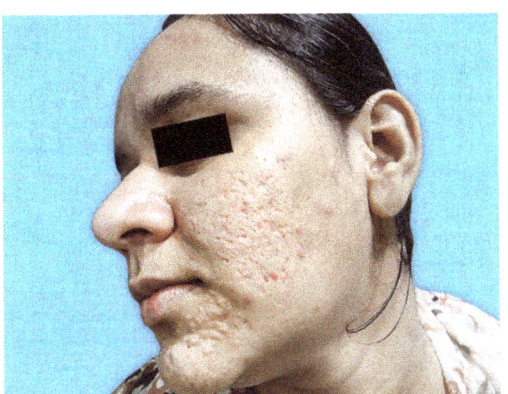

FIG. 2: Severe acne with altered hormone profile.

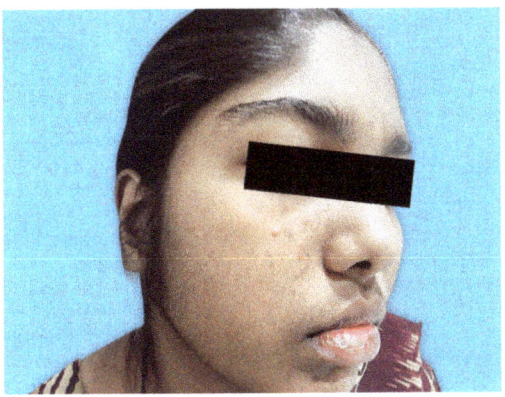

FIG. 3: Teenager with acne and polycystic ovary syndrome (PCOS).

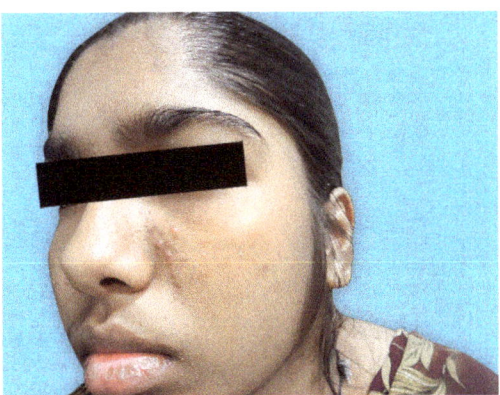

FIG. 4: Teenager with acne and polycystic ovary syndrome (PCOS). Same patient as in Figure 3.

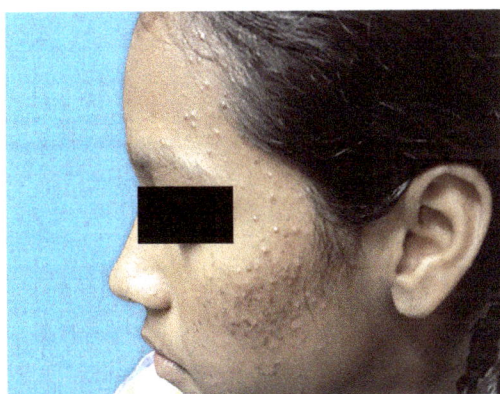

FIG. 5: Teenager with altered luteinizing hormone:follicle-stimulating hormone ratio.

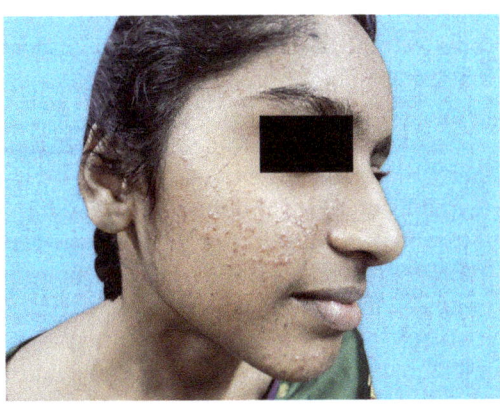

FIG. 6: Patient with abnormal prolactin levels.

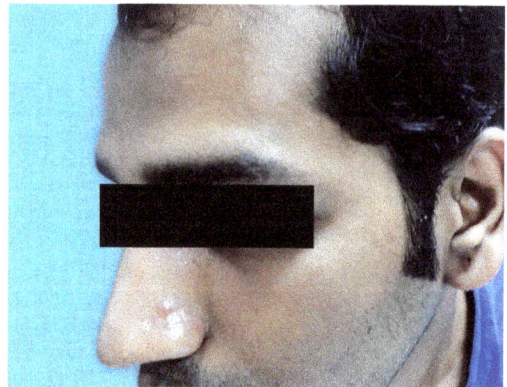

FIG. 7: Truncal acne and patterned alopecia in a man with abnormal lipid profile.

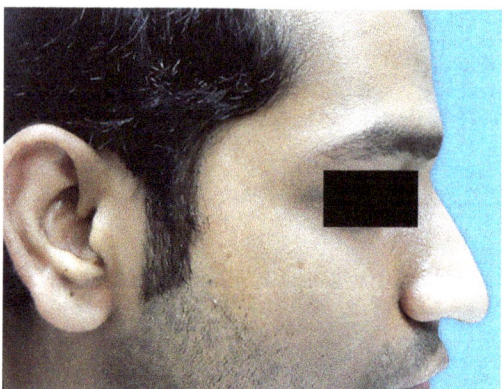

FIG. 8: Truncal acne and patterned alopecia in a man with abnormal lipid profiles. Same patient as in Figure 7.

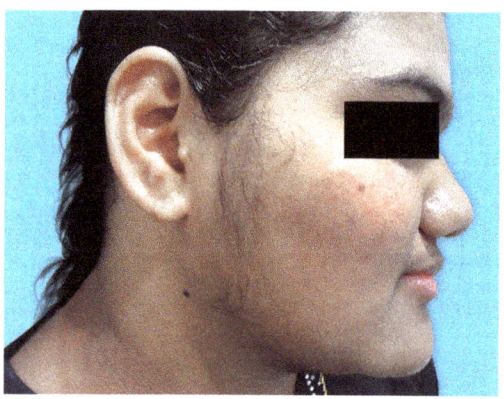

FIG. 9: Hirsutism acanthosis nigricans with truncal acne in a girl with oligomenorrhea.

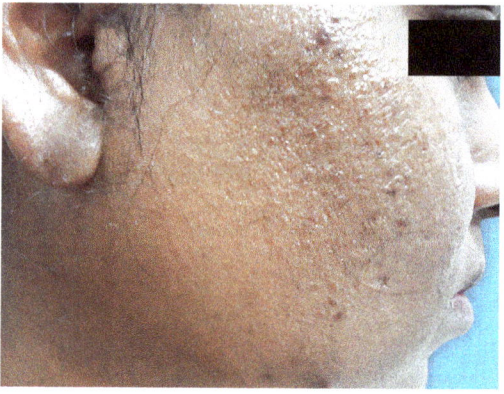

FIG. 10: Woman with persistent acne beyond adulthood with elevated testosterone.

When the follicle ruptures, the inflammatory infiltrate becomes intense to be followed by fibrous tissue replacement as the papule heals.

In case of deep nodulocystic lesions, there is formation of focal abscess containing remnants of follicular epithelium in addition to the neutrophils and other inflammatory infiltrate. It is documented that the clinically normal-looking skin also demonstrated features of inflammation, stating that inflammation starts much earlier than clinical manifestation of comedones.

Chloracne sometimes needs skin biopsy for confirmation. The histology of chloracne reveals acanthosis, follicular keratotic plugging, and loss of sebaceous gland structure, which are replaced by keratinizing epidermal cells.

In SAPHO (synovitis, acne, pustulosis, hyperostosis, and osteitis) syndrome, skin biopsy of the affected site shows neutrophilic pseudoabscesses. Bone biopsy shows sterile inflammatory infiltrate, composed predominantly of polymorphs in the early stages, and replaced by mononuclear cells as the disease progresses. During the late stage, there is enlargement of bone trabeculae, and increase in the number of osteocytes still later, resulting in marrow fibrosis.

Inflammatory Markers, Blood Counts, and Biochemical Tests

Inflammatory markers and biochemical tests are of value in severe forms of acne such as acne conglobata, acne fulminans, and SAPHO syndrome. However, they are not done as a routine practice. Immunoglobulin A gammopathy has been reported in patients with acne conglobata.

Chloracne: Though it is known that dioxins are the major causative chemical in chloracne, in serum titers of dioxin are found to be within normal range in these patients, and hence are not of diagnostic significance.

SAPHO syndrome: Elevated inflammatory markers, such as erythrocyte sedimentation rate (ESR), C-reactive protein (CRP), and elevated levels of components of complements C3 and C4. Mild leukocytosis and mild anemia were observed as well. Compared to healthy controls, these patients have elevated levels of immunoglobulin A.

Acne fulminans: Patients with acne fulminans show elevated ESR and CRP. Some patients may also demonstrate normocytic normochromic anemia and thrombocytosis. Leukocytosis and leukemoid reactions are reported in patients with acne fulminans. There are also reports documenting presence of myeloblasts, promyelocytes, and myelocytes in peripheral smear of patients.

Other laboratory findings include elevated liver enzymes, microscopic hematuria, proteinuria, and abnormal renal functions. Those patients who present with erythema nodosum also showed circulating immune complex in addition. Patients with bone involvement have elevated serum alkaline phosphatase levels.

Endocrine Tests

Endocrine evaluation is indicated in both adults and children where hormonal acne is suspected. In these patients, acne tends to be of sudden onset, very severe, rapidly relapsing, and resistant to therapy. The following features of cutaneous hyperandrogenism will help in selecting patients for evaluation:
- Androgenetic alopecia
- Marked seborrhea
- Hirsutism
- Acanthosis nigricans
- Cushingoid features
- Clitoromegaly
- Deepening of voice
- Increased libido

Box 1 gives indications for endocrine work-up in the following circumstances.

The hormone screening panel will include a long list of tests. The hormone and other blood tests done on patients with hormonal

---

BOX 1 | **Indications for endocrine work-up in female acne patients.**

- *Prepubertal children*:
  - Presence of acne between 7 and 12 years by itself
  - Early onset of body odor
  - Early development of axillary and pubic hair
  - Accelerated growth
  - Advanced bone age
  - Advanced genital maturation
- *Postpubertal girls and women*:
  - Recalcitrant acne
  - Irregular menstrual cycles
  - Polycystic ovary syndrome:
    - Adolescent girls:
      - Androgen excess (clinical or biochemical)
      - Persistent oligomenorrhea
    - Adult females—two of the following:
      - Androgen excess (clinical or biochemical)
      - Ovulatory dysfunction (oligo or anovulation)
      - Polycystic ovary (based on ultrasonographic findings)
  - Hirsutism
  - Androgenetic alopecia
  - Clitoromegaly
  - Truncal obesity
  - Infertility

> **BOX 2** | **Endocrine work-up.**
>
> - *Endocrine work-up in an adult*:
>   - 17α-hydroxyprogesterone
>   - Androstenedione
>   - Cortisol
>   - Dehydroepiandrosterone
>   - Estrogen
>   - Follicle-stimulating hormone
>   - Free 17β-hydroxysteroid
>   - Growth hormone
>   - Insulin
>   - Insulin-like growth factor
>   - Lipid levels
>   - Luteinizing hormone
>   - Progesterone
>   - Prolactin
>   - Sex hormone-binding globulin
>   - Dehydroepiandrosterone sulfate
>   - Total/free testosterone
> - *Endocrine work-up in a child*:
>   - Total/free testosterone
>   - Dehydroepiandrosterone sulfate
>   - Luteinizing hormone
>   - Follicle-stimulating hormone
>   - Prolactin
>   - 17α-hydroxyprogesterone

acne are given in **Box 2**. Before asking for hormonal testing, one must be aware of the interpretation of the testing.

If any of the values are found abnormal, it is better to get assistance from an endocrinologist for further evaluation before planning for the treatment.

Though there are several hormones in the panel, not all need to be tested in all patients. Each suspected disease association will have to be studied well and the list of hormones to be tested is selected appropriately. In addition to the hormones in many instances, other biochemical tests will be required to rule out insulin resistance or metabolic syndrome associated with endocrine acne.

Essential clinical and laboratory profile of the following five important endocrine associations, namely polycystic ovarian disease (PCOD), congenital adrenal hyperplasia (CAH), nonclassical congenital adrenal hyperplasia (NCAH), Cushing's syndrome (CS), and androgen-secreting tumors will help the reader to plan for the investigation to be ordered for different set of patients.

Polycystic Ovarian Disease

Clinical features:
- Positive family history of polycystic ovary syndrome (PCOS)/acne
- Hirsutism
- Infertility
- Obesity
- Menstrual abnormality
- Acanthosis nigricans
- Insulin resistance

Hormone profile: Luteinizing hormone (LH) and follicle-stimulating hormone (FSH) >2:1, T >150 ng/dL, and prolactin +/−.

Other investigations: Blood sugar, serum lipid, and serum insulin.

Congenital Adrenal Hyperplasia

Clinical features:
- Early onset of acne
- Hirsutism
- Accelerated growth
- Ambiguous genitalia
- Hypertension
- Infertility

Hormone profile: Dehydroepiandrosterone sulfate (DHEAS) >4,000–8,000 ng/dL, T >100–200 ng/dL, prolactin ±, 17-hydroxyprogesterone (17-OHP) normal/increased.

Other investigations: Blood pressure, blood sugar, sodium, and potassium.

Nonclassical Congenital Adrenal Hyperplasia

Clinical features:
- Decreased fertility anovulation
- Dysmenorrhea

- Acne
- Hirsutism
- Alopecia

Hormone profile: Adrenocorticotropic hormone (ACTH) stimulation test and 17-OHP >200 ng/mL.

Other investigations: Blood sugar, serum lipid, and serum insulin.

Cushing's Syndrome

Clinical features:
- Menstrual abnormality (oligomenorrhea)
- Central obesity
- Acne
- Hirsutism
- Acanthosis nigricans
- Insulin resistance
- Striae

Hormone profile: ACTH stimulation test, dexamethasone suppression test, serum, and urine cortisol level.

Other investigations: Blood sugar, serum lipid, and serum insulin.

Androgen-secreting Tumors

Clinical features:
- Fever
- Weight loss
- Abdominal pain
- Oligomenorrhea/amenorrhea
- Acne
- Features of CS
- Virilizing syndrome
- Hirsutism

Hormone profile: DHEAS >8,000 ng/dL (adrenal tumor) and testosterone 200 ng/dL (ovarian tumor).

Other investigations: Blood sugar and serum insulin.

Important instructions to be followed while suggesting endocrine work-up:
- Patients on oral contraceptive pills should be advised to discontinue hormones 4–6 weeks prior to hormone evaluation.
- Hormone profile is ideally performed in 1–3 days of menstrual cycle.
- In patients with amenorrhea, it is better that fasting samples are taken.

IMAGING STUDIES

In patients with acne fulminans, radiologic changes will include hyperostosis and sclerosis. These may persist even after treatment. Additional investigations such as ultrasonographic findings will add to the confirmation of the diagnosis in PCOD, whereas computed tomography (CT) and magnetic resonance imaging (MRI) will help in diagnosing CS and androgen-secreting tumors. Bone scan for determining bone age will be helpful in CAH.

In patients with insulin resistance, glucose, insulin levels, and glycosylated hemoglobin levels will aid the diagnosis. Thyroid profile will help in patients with hypothyroidism and metabolic syndrome.

Imaging studies are, at times, required in syndromes associated with acne and to assess the associations as in SAPHO syndrome and endocrine acne.

CHAPTER 7

Treatment

INTRODUCTION (FIGS. 1 TO 10)

Acne being a prolonged condition, the approach should be that of a chronic disease with psychosocial impact and warrants early and aggressive management. Maintenance therapy should be continued for better treatment outcome. Appropriate surgical assistance should be given wherever required. Nevertheless, timely and appropriate treatment, in majority of patients, will avoid complications and the need for surgery. With adequate and updated knowledge of disease pathogenesis and pharmacology of available drugs, the treatment outcome should be good in a compliant patient.

The treatment of acne should aim at:
- Alleviation of symptoms
- Clearance of lesions
- Halting occurrence of new lesions
- Avoiding or minimizing complications such as pigmentation and scarring
- Removal of negative impact on quality of life (QOL) and improvement of QOL
- Providing the benefit of procedural or surgical options wherever needed

The available treatment modalities for acne are shown in **Flowchart 1**. In this chapter, medical treatment will be discussed elaborately in order to enable the reader to get a clear picture about the drugs used in acne and their effectiveness.

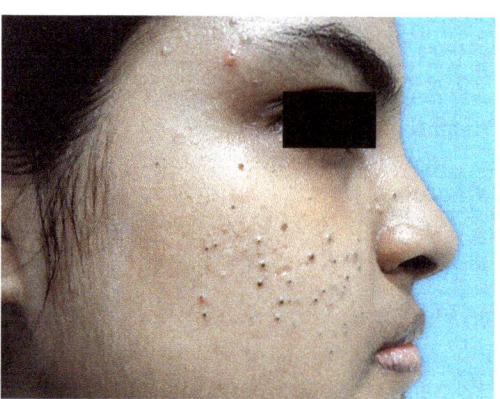

FIG. 1: Grade I acne ideal candidate for topical therapy.

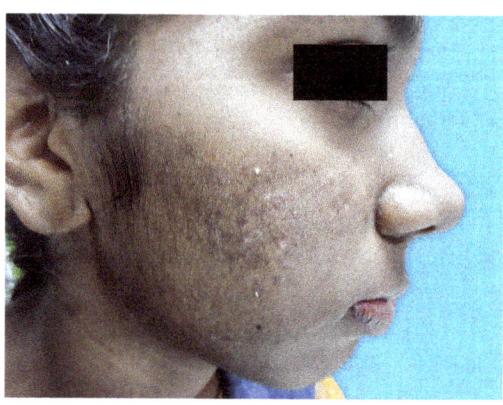

FIG. 2: Grade I and II acne ideal for topical retinoic acid.

CHAPTER 7: Treatment

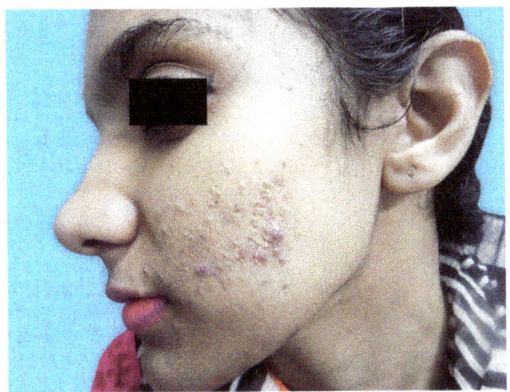

FIG. 3: Grade II acne to be treated with topical and systemic therapy.

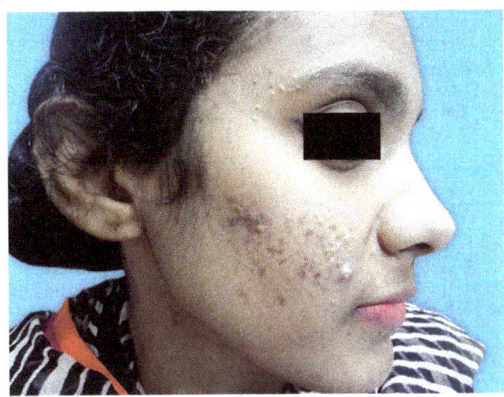

FIG. 4: Same patient as in Figure 3.

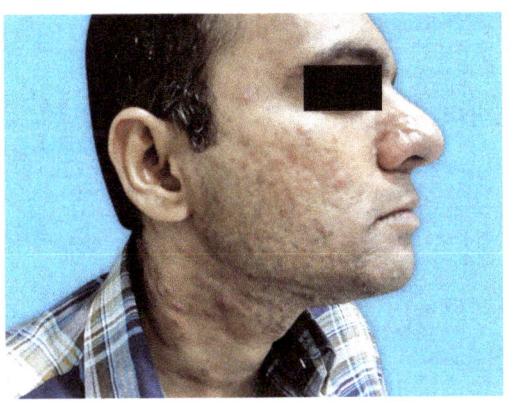

FIG. 5: Combination therapy should be tried with topical and systemic retinoids with proper monitoring.

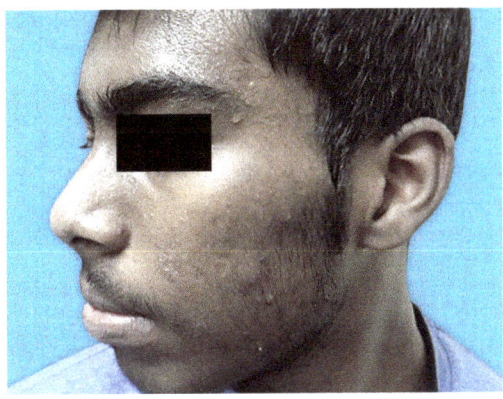

FIG. 6: Seborrhea will benefit from benzoyl peroxide face wash.

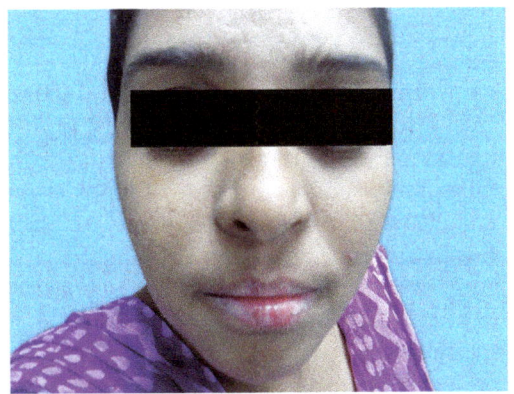

FIG. 7: Cheilitis following retinoid therapy.

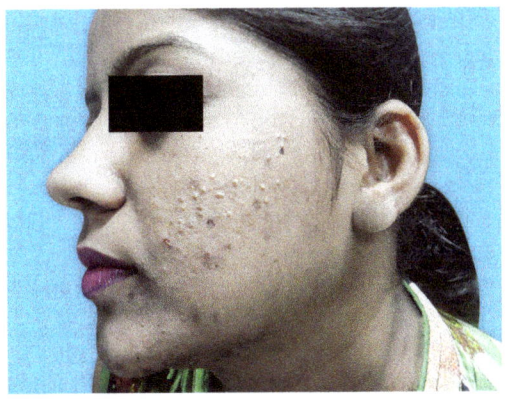

FIG. 8: Hormonal therapy can help this young patient opting for contraception.

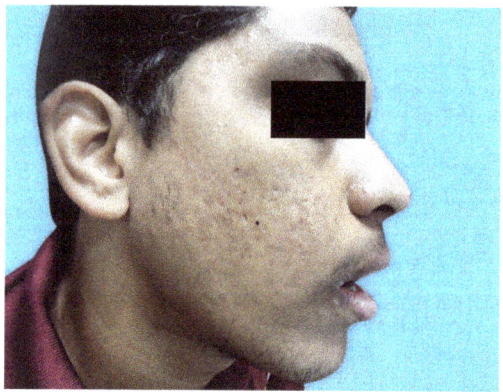

FIG. 9: Superficial scar will need procedural therapy.

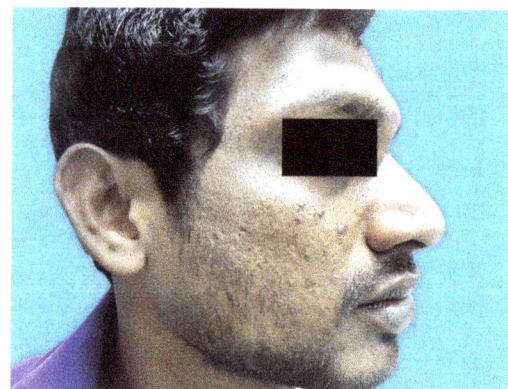

FIG. 10: Pitted scars of acne can be assisted by procedures.

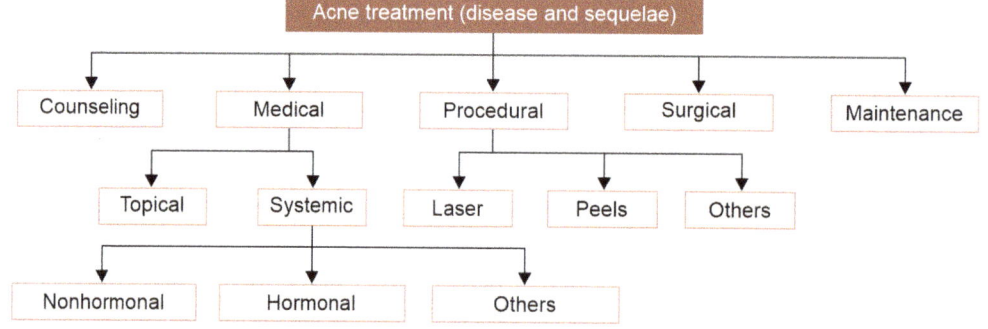

FLOWCHART 1: Options available for the treatment of acne.

DRUGS USED IN ACNE

Acne is a very common disorder seen in any age group starting from birth to almost the fifth decade. However, it affects predominantly the adolescent population, affecting up to 95% teens. Acne irrespective of severity can cause considerable scarring. The more severe the disease, the worse will be the scarring, both physically and psychologically. Correct choice of drug at the appropriate time will reduce the sequelae to a great extent. The drugs used in acne are targeted against the four pathogenic factors, namely:
1. Follicular epidermal hyperproliferation
2. Increased sebum production
3. Inflammation
4. *Cutibacterium acnes (C. acnes)*

Figure 11 gives a bird's-eye view of various drugs used in the treatment of acne and their level of action.

TREATMENT PROTOCOL

Very mild forms of acne in some patients may resolve spontaneously or with topical treatment alone. In a significant number of them, the disease evolves into a more severe manifestation. All forms of severe acne will require systemic treatment. With the available long list of drugs in the market, it will be easy to follow some guidelines or protocol while treating acne patients. The guidelines and protocol though are applicable to vast majority of patients, modifications should be considered to suit the individual patient, their lifestyle,

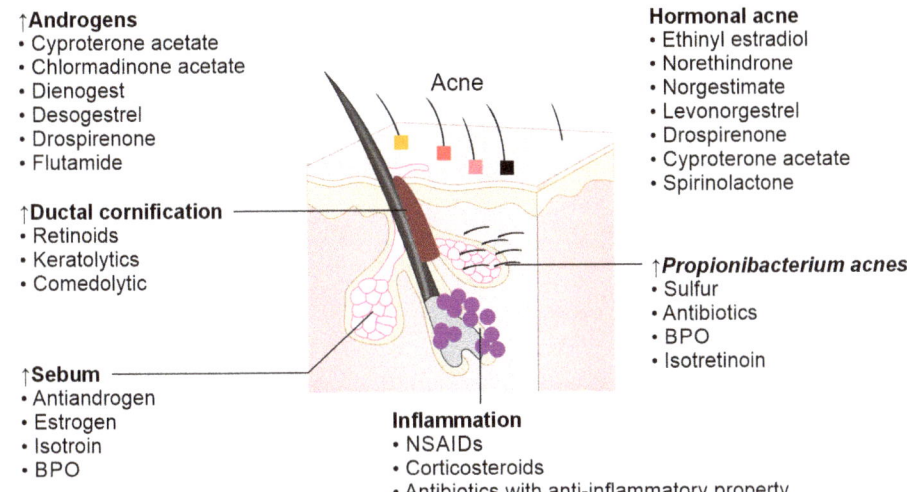

FIG. 11: Level of action of drugs used in the treatment of acne.
(BPO: benzoyl peroxide; NSAIDs: nonsteroidal anti-inflammatory drugs)

and other disease associations. A simple algorithmic approach to acne management is given in **Flowchart 2** and based on severity, the suggested treatment protocol is depicted in **Table 1**.

Of all the available drugs, oral isotretinoin is capable of acting at all four levels of the pathogenic mechanism involved in acne. However, due to the side effects, it is not used as first-line drug in mild and moderate acne. However, appropriate usage of isotretinoin with proper monitoring will certainly yield good results in majority of acne patients. In the current era of antibiotic resistance, newer anti-inflammatory drugs like 5-lipoxygenase inhibitors, such as zileuton, may find greater role in acne management in future.

A combination of topical retinoid and systemic antibacterial agent can be used as first-line therapy in all grades of acne. The complementary mechanisms of action will be working on all four major pathogenic factors of acne. While retinoids take care of the hypercornification and sebum production, antibiotics will exert antibacterial and anti-inflammatory effects. Retinoids, in addition, have anti-inflammatory effect and indirect antibacterial effect by bringing down the C. acnes colony count, thus minimizing the need for oral antibiotic therapy.

TREATMENT OF ACNE VARIANTS

There are very few literature data available on treatment of *childhood acne*. A fixed combination of benzoyl peroxide (BPO) 2.5% and adapalene 1% gel is approved by the Food and Drug Administration (FDA) for children above 9 years of age and 0.05% tretinoin for children above 10 years of age. All other retinoids are approved only for children above 12 years of age. Topical BPO and dapsone are safe in children.

Neonatal acne needs no treatment. Ketoconazole cream seems to be effective in treating neonatal acne, whereas topical retinoid in low concentration and BPO have been beneficial in *infantile acne*. Oral drugs such as erythromycin and trimethoprim can be used in refractory cases.

A simple algorithmic approach to the management of childhood acne is given in **Flowchart 3**.

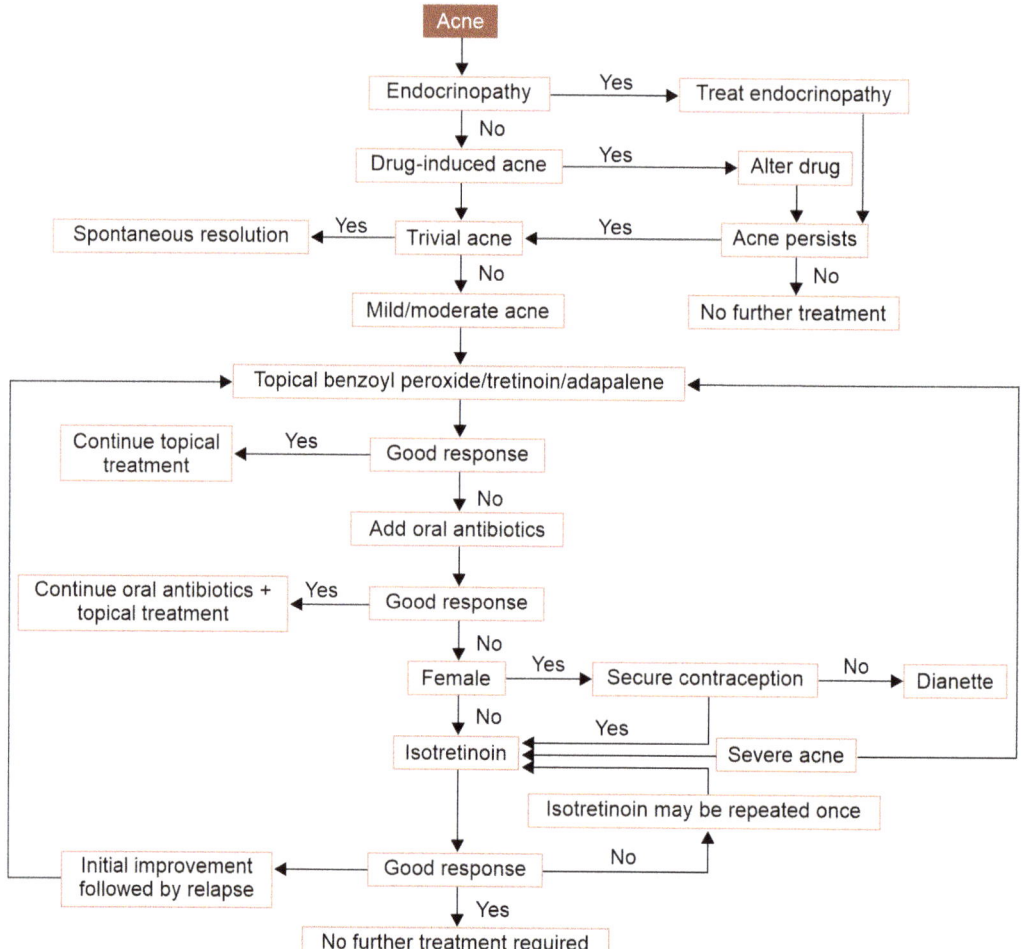

FLOWCHART 2: Algorithmic approach to treatment of acne.

TABLE 1: Acne treatment based on severity.			
	Mild—comedonal	**Moderate—papulopustular**	**Severe—nodulocystic**
First line	• Topical retinoid • BPO • BPO + Clindamycin • BPO + Adapalene • Clindamycin + Tretinoin	• BPO + Clindamycin • BPO + Adapalene	• Systemic antibiotics + BPO ± Topical retinoid • Oral isotretinoin monotherapy
Second line	• Azelaic acid • Combined OCP	• BPO • Topical retinoid • Topical retinoid ± Systemic antibiotics • Combined OCP	• BPO + Systemic antibiotics • BPO + Systemic antibiotics ± Topical retinoid

Continued

Continued

	Mild—comedonal	Moderate—papulopustular	Severe—nodulocystic
Additional recommendation		• Blue light • Oral zinc • Topical clindamycin/erythromycin + Isotretinoin/tretinoin • Systemic antibiotics + Azelaic acid • Systemic antibiotics + Adapalene + BPO • Zileuton	• Systemic antibiotics + BPO • Combined OCP (if not contraindicated)
Maintenance	Topical retinoid	Topical retinoid ± BPO	Topical retinoid ± BPO

(BPO: benzoyl peroxide; OCP: oral contraceptive pill)

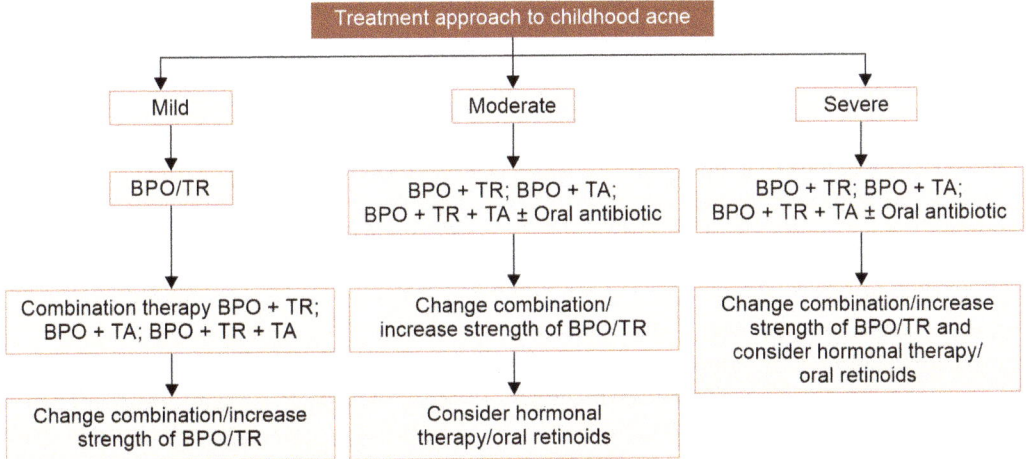

FLOWCHART 3: Algorithmic approach to treatment of acne in children.
(BPO: benzoyl peroxide; TR: topical retinoid; TA: topical antibiotic)

Acne conglobata can be best treated with oral isotretinoin. The dose can be 5 mg/kg to begin with and escalated to as high as 2 mg/kg and continued for a long period up to nearly 5 months. Intensive high-dose oral antibiotics, systemic glucocorticoids, and intralesional triamcinolone are also helpful in patients with acne conglobata. Some authors advise to start systemic corticosteroid before initiating isotretinoin therapy in order to combat the inflammation caused by isotretinoin.

Acne fulminans is a difficult condition to treat. Systemic glucocorticoid therapy along with oral antibiotics is the treatment of choice in acne fulminans. Isotretinoin, though is beneficial, should not be started before initiating steroid therapy to prevent explosive flares. Even after induction of isotretinoin, systemic steroid should be continued and tapered over a period of 2–3 weeks. Dapsone was found to be very useful, especially in patients who present with erythema nodosum. Dapsone is effective as both anti-inflammatory and steroid-sparing agent. History of known allergy to sulfa group of drugs and glucose-6-phosphate dehydrogenase (G6PD) deficiency are definite contraindications for dapsone therapy.

Chloracne lesions may clear in 2 years' time on stopping exposure to the chemical. These lesions do not respond to routine anti-acne measures and topical or systemic antibiotics are not very effective as they do so in acne vulgaris (AV). However, tetracycline (TC) with short course of prednisolone may be useful if the disease is severe. This is probably due to the anti-inflammatory property of both the drugs. Topical retinoic acid in higher concentration up to 0.3% can help control comedones. Early administration of oral isotretinoin may help in the prevention of cystic lesions. Procedures like dermabrasion will be beneficial and should be advised to patients who are concerned about the scar. Nonabsorbable, nondigestible, lipophilic dietary fat substitute has been reported to accelerate intestinal excretion of tetrachlorodibenzodioxin (TCDD) by up to 10 times, which will reduce elimination half-life.

Oil acne responds to routine anti-acne regimens. But unless future avoidance of contact with oil and grease is strictly adhered to, the treatment outcome will not be as expected. In those who continue to be exposed to oil, practicing good personal hygiene, periodic regular changing of work clothes, and frequent cleansing of skin with nonallergenic, noncomedogenic soaps are the key factors to prevent or reduce recurrence of oil acne.

Pitch acne can be prevented by providing proper ventilation and exhaust systems. Proper clothing and cleansing will further help in the prevention of pitch acne. These lesions respond to standard acne therapy.

Mechanical acne will improve on removal of causative mechanical and physical factors. Gentle skin washing with mild cleansing agent may reduce the risk of acne mechanica.

Once a diagnosis of *gram-negative folliculitis* has been made, the causative antibiotics should be stopped and replaced by antimicrobial agent with adequate gram-negative coverage. Topical retinoids should replace antibiotics, which have the added advantage of drying the skin. This drying effect of topical retinoids will help in the elimination of gram-negative organisms, which require a moist environment for survival. Oral isotretinoin is beneficial in recalcitrant cases.

Radiation acne is best treated with topical or oral retinoids. In patients who do not respond to medical treatment, surgical extraction will help.

Tropical acne can never be treated if the patient continues to work in the same atmosphere. Removal to cool place and administration of systemic antibiotics will be useful in the management of tropical acne. In addition to topical anti-acne medications, such as BPO and retinoids, systemic antibiotics should be given in order to treat the secondary infection caused by coagulase-positive *Staphylococci*.

Ultraviolet protection is the best way to prevent *acne aestivalis*. Topical BPO and retinoids are effective in the management of acne aestivalis, whereas oral antibiotics are not. Patients should be adequately warned about flare-up of disease on re-exposure to ultraviolet (UV) light and advised to avoid exposure to UV light.

Acne excoriée needs extra care and attention. An expert assistance from psychiatrist wherever required will change the treatment outcome in a big way. Antidepressants and psychotherapy can be helpful in selected patients.

Granulomatous acne or *acne agminata* responds better to steroids and sometimes to oral contraceptives, in addition to doxycycline, dapsone, and retinoids.

Drug-induced acneiform lesions normally resolve spontaneously on withdrawal of the offending agent. Topical BPO and retinoids are used to give faster clearance of lesions.

Epidermal growth factor receptor (EGFR)-induced papulopustular eruptions can be prevented by avoiding excessive sun exposure and use of adequate and frequent sunscreen formulations. It has also been recommended to use topical moisturizers and sunscreens along with topical 1% hydrocortisone and systemic doxycycline in a dose of 100 mg twice a day or minocycline 100 mg, 24 hours prior to initiating EGFR through 6 weeks in those under preemptive treatment. Once skin lesions are established as papulopustular eruptions, potent topical steroids and oral TCs should be advised. It is suggested that for severe reactions, isotretinoin in the dose of 20-30 mg/day should be used.

Syndromes associated with acne are rare. Knowledge and awareness aid in correct diagnosis and appropriate treatment. In Apert syndrome, the skin lesions respond well to anti-acne treatment. Severe cases may be treated with isotretinoin with proper advice to the patient and regular monitoring. Nonsteroidal anti-inflammatory drugs (NSAIDs), sulfasalazine, and infliximab have been reported to be successful in the treatment of *SAPHO* (synovitis, acne, pustulosis, hyperostosis, and osteitis) syndrome. The associated bone pain can be benefitted by bisphosphonates. Similarly, anakinra, an IL-receptor antagonist, and infliximab have been tried with success in the management of *PAPA* (pyogenic arthritis, pyoderma gangrenosum, and acne) syndrome.

Solid facial edema is best treated with oral isotretinoin (0.2-0.5% mg/kg/day) either alone or in combination with clofazimine or ketotifen for a period of 4-5 months. Some authors advise short intermittent course of oral glucocorticoids to combat the inflammatory component. Morbihan's disease, the solid facial edema, is highly resistant to oral antibiotics but responds well to isotretinoin and glucocorticoids. Some feel that it is a complication of rosacea and some feel it is a separate entity.

Acne keloidalis nuchae can be a marker of diabetes, and hence metabolic screening is important. Intralesional steroids are the best way to treat the keloidal lesions. Topical antibiotics such as clindamycin and oral TC are preferred during the papulopustular stage. Resistant cases can be treated with cryotherapy or laser therapy. Surgical excision is the last option in recalcitrant cases.

Acne varioliformis responds to oral antibiotics and topical and intralesional steroids. Surgical treatment of larger scar is advised for better results.

The treatment options available for the rare complication *osteoma cutis* are limited. The best method would be surgical ablation and laser therapy. However, in small lesions, topical tretinoin can be used to induce transepidermal elimination of the content.

Potent topical steroid for over a period not exceeding 2-3 weeks is effective in managing *pyogenic granuloma* consequent to severe acne.

TOPICAL AGENTS USED IN THE TREATMENT OF ACNE

Topical agents are used in the treatment of acne in almost all patients with acne. Some of the topical agents are easily available over the counter without prescription. This makes self-medication in most of the patients a failure, which brings them to the physicians. Hence, it is important to get the correct information about all the previous topical treatment used by the patient in detail. It is only wise to avoid those drugs to which the patient reacted adversely. A list of topical agents used in acne is given in **Box 1**. These agents can be used as monotherapy or in combination with other

---

BOX 1 | **Topical agents used in acne.**

- Antibiotics
- Dapsone
- Retinoids
- Benzoyl peroxide
- Azelaic acid
- Salicylic acid
- Zinc
- Sulfur and sodium sulfacetamide
- Resorcinol
- Combinations

topical or systemic agents, depending on the severity of the disease.

The appropriate topical agent/s should be selected taking into consideration the following factors:
- Age of patient
- Skin type
- Site of involvement
- Grade of acne
- Nature of outdoor activities and light exposure
- Response to medication used earlier
- Patient preference

The topical preparations commonly preferred include cream, lotion, gel, ointment, pledget, and wash-off lotion or foam.

Topical Antibiotics

Topical antibiotics once applied accumulate in the hair follicle and exert an anti-inflammatory effect as well. They are superior to placebo but inferior to BPO and retinoids. Monotherapy with topical antibiotics is not recommended for fear of development of antibiotic resistance, which can be avoided by combining with BPO and retinoids.

Topical antimicrobials used in acne are listed in **Box 2**.

Topical antibiotics are usually well tolerated. The side effects of topical antibiotics include irritation and gram-negative folliculitis. Very rarely diarrhea and colitis due to *Clostridium* have been reported as side effects of systemic absorption of topical minocycline.

Erythromycin is a safe topical antibiotic. It binds to the bacterial ribosome and blocks transfer ribonucleic acid (RNA) interfering with the polypeptide chain formation and inhibits protein synthesis. It is both antibacterial and anti-inflammatory. Clindamycin, similar to erythromycin, suppresses bacterial protein synthesis by binding to the bacterial 50S ribosome. Though they are well tolerated, rare instances of pseudomembranous enterocolitis have been reported following topical clindamycin therapy. *Nadifloxacin*, a fluoroquinolone derivative, has been approved by some European countries for the treatment of AV. However, because of the fear of development of quinolone resistance, this molecule is not used as the other two molecules, namely erythromycin and clindamycin. It has been observed that topical nadifloxacin can result in a plasma concentration of 3 ng/mL, which can lead to development of quinolone resistance.

Topical *metronidazole* is commonly used in the management of gram-negative folliculitis and rosacea. It has a broad spectrum of activity against anaerobes and protozoal organisms.

Resorcinol, a keratolytic agent, was used in acne for its antibacterial effect, either alone or in combination with sulfur. It is also an antifungal agent.

Topical *dapsone* 5% has both anti-inflammatory and antimicrobial properties. As an anti-inflammatory agent, diaminodiphenyl sulfone inhibits neutrophil myeloperoxidase and eosinophil peroxidase activity. It also suppresses hypochlorous acid production and scavenges reactive oxygen species. As an anti-microbial, dapsone inhibits bacterial dihydropteroate synthase in the folic acid metabolic pathway. This combined effect seems to be beneficial in the management of acne. Topical dapsone was found to be safe in patients with G6PD deficiency unlike oral dapsone.

Topical Retinoids

Retinoid is a wonder drug in the management of acne. The binding of retinoid molecule

---

BOX 2 | **Topical antimicrobials in acne.**
- Clindamycin
- Erythromycin
- Minocycline
- Nadifloxacin
- Dapsone
- Metronidazole

to nuclear retinoic acid receptor affects the genes involved in keratinocyte proliferation and differentiation, melanogenesis, and inflammation. The end result being altered corneocyte cohesion and accumulation. Retinoids are thus potent comedolytics and anti-inflammatory agents. Topical retinoids, apart from altering the follicular keratinization, also enhance the penetration of other topical medications used. Tretinoin, isotretinoin, adapalene, and tazarotene are the first-, second-, third-, and fourth-generation molecules of topical retinoids, respectively. Molecules bind to different receptors, thereby conferring different degrees of activity, tolerability, and efficacy. Of all the topical agents used in acne management, retinoids are the best performers not only because of their action at different levels of pathogenesis, but also because they can enhance other topical regimens and can be used as maintenance therapy. They are ideal for inflammatory and non-inflammatory lesions and can be used alone or in combination with other drugs, both topical and systemic. However, the common side effects of retinoids should be kept in mind before giving it as a prescription.

Tretinoin is not a photostable molecule and hence should be avoided during daytime and advised to be used in the evening. Similarly, BPO can inactivate tretinoin and hence such a combination or coadministration should be avoided, but can be applied at different parts of the day. All prescriptions with retinoids should include a topical sunscreen. Retinoids should be avoided during pregnancy and in women planning for pregnancy.

All forms of topical retinoids can induce an irritant reaction and alcohol-based preparations have greater irritancy potential. The newer microsponge or polymer technology, wherein the drug is incorporated within a polyol prepolymer helps reduce the irritancy potential of the molecule at the same time, increasing the concentration. Because of the irritant nature of the drug, treatment should be initiated with a lower concentration for a short contact time before using the required concentration, depending on the tolerability of the patient. While tretinoin is photolabile, adapalene, a synthetic retinoid, is photostable, specifically targeting retinoid-related orphan receptor. The advantage of adapalene is that it can be combined to BPO without degradation of the drug. Adapalene is more efficacious and better tolerated than tretinoin. Tazarotene, another synthetic retinoid, exerts its action through its metabolite tazarotenic acid. Tazarotene is more efficacious than tretinoin. Like other topical retinoids, tazarotene also has irritant properties, which can be minimized by reducing the contact time. It is very important to know that retinoids are pregnancy category X drugs and hence should be avoided during pregnancy. Counseling is important while prescribing topical retinoids for women in the childbearing age group.

Topical sulfur is both comedolytic as well as comedogenic. Sulfonamides are antibacterial agents. They inhibit para-aminobenzoic acid (PABA), an important substance for the growth of *C. acnes*. Sulfur can inhibit formation of free fatty acid and also has mild keratolytic effect, which is considered important in acne management. In the keratinocyte, sulfur interacts with cysteine, releasing hydrogen sulfide, which through its keratolytic property subsequently ruptures disulfide bond in cysteine, and consequently exerts an inhibitory effect on *C. acnes*. When used with BPO or sodium sulfacetamide, sulfur shows better results in the management of acne. Sulfur is used in strengths up to 10% as creams, ointments, lotions, foams, and soaps. Sulfur is well tolerated, except for mild irritation. The comedogenic potential should be kept in mind, which can lead to exacerbation of lesions.

Salicylic acid is a lipid soluble O-hydroxybenzoic acid with a comedolytic and keratolytic property. The anti-inflammatory effect exerted by salicylic acid is due to its ability to affect arachidonic acid cascade. Salicylic acid decreases corneocyte cohesion and aids exfoliation by breaking down the follicular keratotic plug through dissolving the intercellular cement and promotes desquamation of follicular epithelium. The concentration of salicylic acid used in acne varies from 0.5 to 3% in topical preparations. It is available as creams, ointments, lotions, and washes and in a higher concentration as high as 30% in chemical peels. Salicylic acid can be used in both inflammatory and noninflammatory lesions. Mild irritation is a common side effect of topical salicylic acid.

Azelaic acid (AA) is a dicarboxylic acid having antimicrobial as well as comedolytic property. AA competitively antagonizes and inhibits the activity of mitochondrial oxyreductase and 5α-reductase. AA inhibits the DNA synthesis and has an antibacterial action against *C. acnes* by inhibiting protein synthesis. AA also has a modest comedolytic activity by controlling the proliferation and differentiation of keratinocytes. The anti-inflammatory action of AA is due to its ability to inhibit generation of proinflammatory oxygen derivatives in neutrophils. The added advantage of AA is its ability to decrease postinflammatory pigmentation by competitively inhibiting tyrosinase. Apart from a transient burning or stinging sensation, the drug is well tolerated.

Benzoyl peroxide is the most commonly used anti-acne preparation and is easily available over the counter. BPO is an antimicrobial, keratolytic, and comedolytic agent. The whitening effect of BPO is advantageous while using it in patients with postinflammatory pigmentation. The absence of drug resistance makes it superior to all topical antibiotics.

Topical Zinc

Zinc has a beneficial role in the management of acne due to its anti-inflammatory activity and its ability to reduce *C. acnes* count by inhibiting *C. acnes* lipase and free fatty acid levels in the skin. Zinc is capable of reducing sebum production, which is an important factor in the pathogenesis of acne. Zinc is safe and devoid of irritant potential. It is nonallergenic and noncomedogenic. Zinc is also being used in combination with antibiotics and nicotinic acid in the management of acne with good results. However, used alone, topical zinc may not yield the expected result.

Topical Nicotinamide

Nicotinamide is a pyridine-3-carboxylic acid amide of nicotinic acid. It is a potent anti-inflammatory and sebostatic agent. The anti-inflammatory effect is through the inhibition of *C. acnes*-induced interleukin 8 production in keratinocytes through interference with nuclear factor (NF) kappa B by inhibiting poly-adenosine diphosphate (ADP)-ribose polymerase-1 (PARP-1) and mitogen-activated protein kinases (MAPKs) pathways. It is noncomedogenic and can cause mild irritation.

Table 2 gives the effect of different topical agents used in acne.

Combination therapy in acne is superior to monodrug therapy.

In general, topical application of medications is rather tedious, more so if multiple formulations have to be applied, leading to poor medication adherence. Combining monotherapies may add undue cost to the patient. Therefore, especially formulated combination therapies have been developed.

Since acne has more than one pathogenic mechanism, the goal of combination therapy is to target multiple areas of acne pathogenesis to get the best therapeutic outcome. There are many such combinations available in the market. The following combinations have been studied and found useful in the treatment of acne:
- Adapalene + BPO
- Adapalene + Clindamycin

TABLE 2: Effect of different topical medications used in acne.

	Sebum	Comedones	Cutibacterium acnes	Inflammation
Benzoyl peroxide	—	↓	↓↓	↓↓
Topical retinoids	—	↓↓↓	—	↓↓
Topical antibiotics	—	↓	↓↓	↓↓
Oral isotretinoin	↓↓↓	↓	↓↓↓	↓↓↓
Oral tetracyclines	—	↓	↓↓↓	↓↓↓
Cyproterone acetate	↓↓	—	↓	↓↓
Spironolactone and combined oral contraceptive pills	↓↓	—	—	↓↓
Azelaic acid	—	↓	↓	↓

- Adapalene + Nadifloxacin
- BPO + Hydrating gel
- BPO + Clindamycin
- BPO + Erythromycin
- BPO + Sulfur
- Clindamycin + AA
- Clindamycin + BPO
- Clindamycin + Nicotinamide + Tea tree oil
- Clindamycin + Nicotinamide + Allantoin
- Clindamycin + Tretinoin
- Erythromycin + Zinc
- Erythromycin + Tretinoin
- Erythromycin + Isotretinoin
- Dapsone + Tazarotene

Synergistic effect means that the effect of combination of the two drugs used will be greater than the sum of the benefit of the two drugs when used as monotherapy.

Side Effects of Topical Treatment in Acne

The most common side effects of topical preparation used in acne include erythema, dryness, scaling, and irritation. Burning or stinging sensation and tightness are usually the result of overuse of medication with higher concentration, more quantity, or prolonged contact time. Bleaching of skin and hair is frequently observed with BPO and AA. The comedogenic property of sulfur is a therapeutic paradox, which has to be considered whenever there is an exacerbation of comedonal acne while treating acne patient with sulfur creams. Gram-negative folliculitis presenting as sudden eruption of pustular lesions or worsening of existing lesions following prolonged therapy with antibiotics is not infrequent. Postinflammatory pigmentation and tanning is a disturbing side effect seen with topical agents such as retinoids and salicylic acid preparations, which can be prevented by appropriate use of topical sunscreen.

The common side effects encountered with frequently used topical anti-acne medications are given in **Table 3**.

The clinical manifestations of side effects are variable depending on the strength used, amount applied, condition of skin prior to application, type of soap and cosmetics used, sun exposure, and skin type. Almost all patients will need topical sunscreen to avoid or minimize the side effects from topical application.

SYSTEMIC AGENTS USED IN ACNE

Majority of acne patients will require systemic drugs. The systemic medications used in acne can be divided into nonhormonal agents and hormonal agents.

The list of systemic drugs used in acne is given in **Flowchart 4**.

TABLE 3: Side effects of topical anti-acne medications.

Topical agent	Dryness	Erythema	Stinging/Burning	Scaling	Bacterial resistance
Tretinoin 0.05%	++	+++	++	++	–
Tretinoin 0.025%	+	++	++	+	–
Isotretinoin 0.05%	+	+	+	+	–
Adapalene 0.1%	+	+	+	+	–
Azelaic acid 20%	+	++	++	–	–
Benzoyl peroxide 5%	++	++	++	+	–
Erythromycin	–	–	–	–	++
Clindamycin	–	–	–	–	++
Sulfur precipitate 10%	–	–	–	–	–
Dapsone	+	+	–	–	–

Systemic antibiotics were the mainstay of acne management till recently. The use of systemic antibiotics is indicated in moderate-to-severe forms of acne along with topical agents. When antibiotics are derived from other organisms, antibacterial agents such as sulfur are useful in treating acne. The following antimicrobial agents were found to be efficacious in the management of acne:
- Tetracycline
- Oxytetracycline
- Doxycycline
- Lymecycline
- Minocycline
- Erythromycin
- Azithromycin
- Amoxicillin
- Cephalexin
- Trimethoprim + Sulfamethoxazole
- Trimethoprim
- Dapsone

The TC group of antibiotics are considered the first-line treatment in moderate-to-severe forms of AV unless otherwise contraindicated. The TC group of drugs inhibit protein synthesis by binding to the 30S subunit of bacterial ribosome. By inhibiting metalloproteinase activity and chemotaxis, they act as good anti-inflammatory agents as well.

Various molecules of the TC group are different in their potency, tolerability, and exerting side effects. Doxycycline and minocycline are considered superior to TC. Doxycycline is less nephrotoxic and therefore can be used in patient with renal disease where TC cannot be used.

The macrolide antibiotics, namely erythromycin and azithromycin, like the TC group of drugs inhibit protein synthesis by binding to the 30S subunit of bacterial ribosome with anti-inflammatory property. Penicillin and cephalosporin can be used where erythromycin is not tolerated well. However, the usage of these alternative drugs is not much practiced.

Trimethoprim + Sulfamethoxazole combination is not infrequently used in the management of acne, especially in situations where cost is a major constraint. Sulfamethoxazole is a bacteriostatic drug. It acts by blocking bacterial synthesis of folic acid necessary for cell division, while trimethoprim is a folic acid analog that inhibits the enzyme dihydrofolate reductase. These two agents work synergistically to block bacterial nucleotide and amino acid synthesis. All antibiotics have cutaneous and systemic side effects, which have to be borne in mind

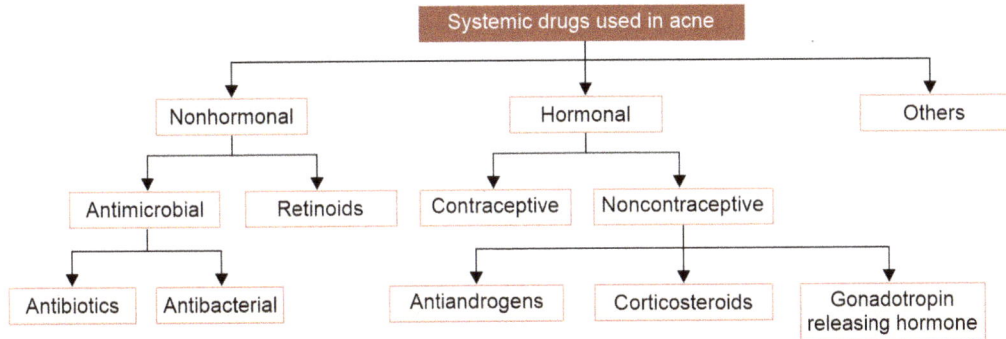

FLOWCHART 4: Systemic drugs used in acne.

and should be looked for during follow-up and detected early.

The dosage and side effects of common antibacterial agents used in acne are listed in **Table 4**.

Azithromycin is being used as pulse therapy in the management of acne. Different dosing schedules are being followed. A commonly followed schedule is:

Azithromycin 500 mg once a day, 3 days a week for 8–12 weeks.

Prolonged use of any antibiotic can give rise to vaginal candidiasis. With each class, the manifestation is variable. For instance, photosensitivity is more with doxycycline than minocycline, while hyperpigmentation occurs the other way round. Similarly, doxycycline causes more gastrointestinal (GI) symptoms, while minocycline causes tinnitus and dizziness. Fulminant hepatic necrosis and blood dyscrasias like agranulocytosis are more common with trimethoprim + sulfamethoxazole. Severe forms of drug reactions to antibiotics used in acne are rare. However, one has to remember that serious conditions such as Stevens–Johnson syndrome are seen more frequently in patients with human immunodeficiency virus (HIV) infection.

With frequent inappropriate use of antibiotics, bacterial resistance remains a major concern.

This issue can be effectively tackled by promoting correct use of them adopting the following norms:

- Antibiotic use should be limited to less than 3 months.
- Continue antibiotic only if there is clinical improvement.
- Use the same antibiotic that gave good clinical response earlier for the same patient.
- Monotherapy using antibiotics should be avoided.
- Standard dosing regimens should be followed.
- Encourage the use of combination regimens.
- Add topical agents such as retinoids or BPO.
- Advice BPO for a week between two courses of oral antibiotics.
- Avoid two different molecules for topical and systemic use concomitantly.
- As far as possible, systemic antibiotics other than TC and macrolides should be discouraged.

Poor or inadequate response should be spotted and appropriate alternate drug should be prescribed. However, before declaring poor response, patient compliance and proper adherence to therapy should be ascertained.

TABLE 4: Side effects of common antibacterial agents used in acne.

Side effects	TC	Doxycycline	Minocycline	LC	Erythromycin	TMP + SMZ
	500 BD*	100–200 OD*	100–200 OD*	300–600 OD*	500 BD*	200–300 BD*
Pigmentation	–	–	+	–	–	–
Phototoxicity	+	+	–	+	–	+/–
Drug-induced LE	–	–	+	–	–	–
Exanthem	+	+	+	+	+	+
TEN/SJS/Skin rash	+	+	+	+	+	+
(Photo) Onycholysis	+	+	+	+	–	–
Vaginal candidiasis	+	+	+	+	+	–
Headache	+	–	+	+	–	–
Benign ICT	+	–	+	+	–	–
Esophagitis	+	+	–	+	–	–
Gastrointestinal symptoms	+	+	+	+	+	–
Hepatitis	+	+	+	+	+	+
Fulminant hepatic necrosis	–	–	–	–	–	+
Pancreatitis	+	–	–	+	–	+
Respiratory hypersensitivity	–	–	–	–	–	+
Blood dyscrasias	–	–	–	–	–	+
Renal toxicity	–	–	–	–	–	+
Weight gain	–	–	–	+	–	–

*All doses in milligram (mg).
(ICT: intracranial hypertension; LC: lymecycline; LE: lupus erythematosus; SJS: Stevens–Johnson syndrome; TC: tetracycline; TEN: toxic epidermal necrolysis; TMP + SMZ: trimethoprim + sulfamethoxazole)

RETINOIDS

The advent and use of oral retinoids have revolutionized the management of acne.

Oral retinoids have been used with success in acne patients above the age of 18 years. Oral isotretinoin, an isomer of retinoic acid, has been approved by the FDA for the use of nodulocystic acne in 1982. Its use has proven successful in patients with severe acne. The early response in the reduction of seborrhea and prevention of scarring has led to its frequent usage in acne patients. Oral retinoids can be used even in moderate acne or patients with resistant acne. The indications of oral retinoids in acne are given in **Box 3**.

The mechanism of action of isotretinoin is not completely evaluated. However, the profound inhibition of sebaceous gland activity produced by the drug seems to be the most important factor in lesion clearance and patient compliance. In some patients, the sebaceous gland inhibition continues for over a period of 1 year, while in vast majority of patients, sebum production returns to normal after 2–4 months of stopping the drug. Retinoid is supposed to exert its effect through the following mechanisms, the schematic representation of which is given in **Figure 12**.

BOX 3: Indications for oral retinoid in acne.

- Nodulocystic acne—first-line therapy
- As first-line therapy in any other forms of severe acne
- Moderate acne—failure of 3 months of conventional treatment
- Acne rosacea
- Hidradenitis suppurativa
- Apert syndrome
- Acne fulminans
- Acne variants

Mode of Action of Retinoids

- Reduce abnormal keratinocyte proliferation within pilosebaceous duct
- Causes reversal of hypercornification within follicular canal
- Induction of follicular epithelium leads to unplugging of follicle
- Inhibit development of comedone formation
- Reduce rupture of the comedone into surrounding
- Reduce *Pityrosporum acnes* population
- Downregulate toll-like receptor 2 (TLR2) expression and function
- Reduce inflammation

Being a drug with a wide profile of local and systemic side effects, the dosing should be carefully planned and monitored. Isotretinoin is commonly initiated at a starting dose of 0.5 mg/kg body weight/day. Some authors recommend concomitant use of systemic corticosteroids to prevent the side effects in the early period of the course. The dose of isotretinoin advised is in the range of 0.1–1 mg/kg body weight. Patients treated with higher doses exhibited lower relapses when compared to those treated with lower dose regimens. Because of the local side effects, it is suggested to start with lower dose, escalate the dose, and treat with higher dose. According to some studies, low-dose treatment yielded similar treatment outcome as high-dose therapy but with lesser side effects. Intermittent dose is not recommended as it is not so effective and is associated with higher relapse rates. Being a lipophilic molecule, isotretinoin should be taken with meals. Isotretinoin formulations encased in lipid agents can be taken without food. Normally, procedures should be delayed for 6–12 months of retinoid therapy. However, reports endorse the safety of laser procedures like those using pulsed dye and CO_2 lasers even while on treatment with isotretinoin. However, treatment with oral retinoids is not without adverse reactions. The most common side effects of oral retinoids met within daily practice include mucosal erosion and symptoms of hypervitaminosis A. Almost all patients treated with high-dose isotretinoin develop cheilitis, which can be treated with topical corticosteroid cream application.

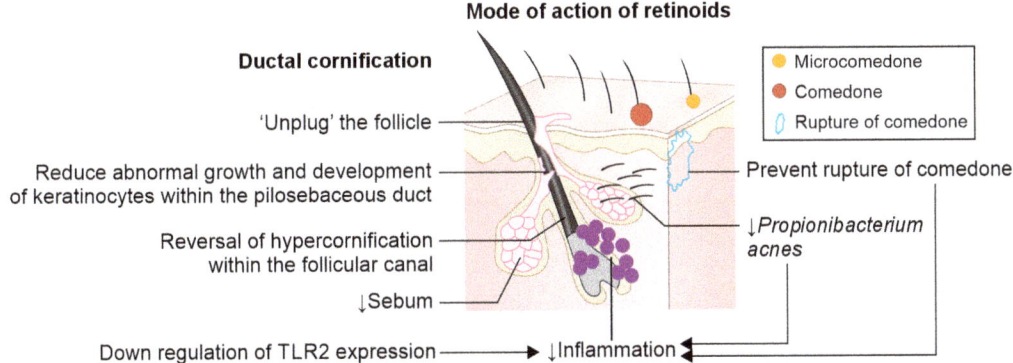

FIG. 12: Mechanism of action of oral isotretinoin in acne.

Sometimes, the secondary bacterial infection with *Staphylococcus aureus* requires flucloxacillin and/or topical antibiotic such as mupirocin.

Due to its proven teratogenicity, all patients, especially women in the childbearing age group, should be carefully counseled regarding contraception during the course of treatment and for a minimum of 1 month after the last dose of isotretinoin treatment. It has been estimated that while on oral isotretinoin, 50% of pregnancies spontaneously abort and half of the children born suffer cardiovascular or skeletal deformity. Females in the childbearing age should be strictly advised on contraception. Pregnancy prevention programs include advice on education and treatment schedule and most importantly to prevent pregnancy during treatment with oral isotretinoin. In the United States as mandated by the FDA, all patients receiving isotretinoin, both men and women, should enroll in and adhere to the iPLEDGE risk management program, which is executed to prevent isotretinoin exposure during pregnancy.

Relapse of skin lesions is a very common phenomenon with oral isotretinoin and special mention about this during counseling is important. Studies document that the younger the patient, the more the relapse rate. Drug interactions with systemic isotretinoin are not uncommon, which should be appropriately handled. Important information about oral isotretinoin treatment is given in **Box 4**.

The side effects of isotretinoin can be classified as very common, common, and significant but rare which are listed as follows:

Very common side effects:
- *Mucocutaneous*:
    - Cheilitis
    - Pruritus
    - Dry skin
    - Localized exfoliation
- *Hematological*:
    - Increased erythrocyte sedimentation rate

> **BOX 4** **Important facts about oral isotretinoin in acne.**
>
> - Recommended as first-line drug for severe nodulocystic acne
> - Can be used in moderate acne resistant to basic therapy
> - Reduces scarring
> - Low but not intermittent dose is effective
> - Routine monitoring of liver, renal functions, and lipid profile are important but not the blood count
> - All patients in the childbearing age must follow contraceptive measure(s)
> - All patients should be explained adequately about the side effects of the drug
> - All patients should be monitored for all the documented side effects

- Thrombocytopenia
- Thrombocytosis
- *Ocular*:
    - Conjunctivitis
    - Dry eyes
    - Eye irritation
- *Hepatic*:
    - Elevated transaminase
- *Musculoskeletal*:
    - Arthralgia
    - Myalgia
    - Back pain
- *Lipid profile*:
    - Increased triglyceride
    - Decreased high-density lipoprotein

Common side effects:
- *Hematological*:
    - Neutropenia
- *Nervous system*:
    - Headache
- *Respiratory system*:
    - Epistaxis
    - Nasal dryness
    - Nasopharyngitis
- *Renal*:
    - Hematuria
    - Proteinuria

- *Biochemical profile*:
  - Increased blood cholesterol
  - Increased blood glucose

Rare side effects:
- *Immune system*:
  - Anaphylactic reaction
  - Hypersensitivity reaction
- *Psychiatric*:
  - Depression
  - Anxiety
  - Aggressive tendency
  - Mood alterations
- *Cutaneous*:
  - Alopecia

Very rarely reported side effects:
- Infections (gram-positive organisms)
- *Cutaneous*:
  - Acne flare
  - Acne fulminans
  - Facial erythema
  - Exanthem
  - Hirsutism
  - Nail dystrophy
  - Paronychia
  - Photosensitive reaction
  - Pyogenic granuloma
  - Pigmentation
- *Lymphatic system*:
  - Lymphadenopathy
- *Metabolic*:
  - Hyperuricemia
- *Psychiatric*:
  - Suicidal ideation
  - Suicidal attempts
  - Suicide
- *Neurological*:
  - Drowsiness
  - Dizziness
  - Convulsions
- *Ocular*:
  - Blurred vision
  - Cataract
  - Color blindness
  - Photophobia
  - Decreased night vision
  - Contact lens intolerance
  - Corneal opacity
  - Keratitis
  - Papilledema
- *Otic*:
  - Impaired hearing
- *Vascular*:
  - Vasculitis
- *GI*:
  - Nausea
  - Ileitis
  - GI hemorrhage
  - Inflammatory bowel disease
  - Hepatitis
  - Pancreatitis
- *Musculoskeletal*:
  - Arthritis
  - Calcinosis
  - Premature epiphyseal fusion
  - Exostosis
  - Hyperostosis
  - Osteopenia
  - Tendinitis
- *Renal*:
  - Glomerulonephritis
- *Biochemical*:
  - Increased creatine phosphokinase

Of the several complications, the important complications to be kept in mind while treating different groups of patients are given in **Table 5**.

A common drug interaction of oral isotretinoin observed by dermatologists is with ketoconazole, which increases the levels of isotretinoin. Vitamin A in other forms should

TABLE 5: Most important complications of oral retinoids.

Complications	Groups affected
Irreversible bone damage	Children
Teratogenicity	Pregnant woman
Abnormal lipid profile and risk of heart disease	Young and middle aged
Hepatotoxicity	Excess alcohol intake
Hypervitaminosis A	All

be avoided in patients on oral isotretinoin to prevent additive toxic effects.

Baseline investigations before starting and during therapy are mandatory as is exclusion of pregnancy in females. Baseline lipid profile, complete blood count, renal function test, and liver function test are to be done. Renal and liver function tests are repeated after 1 month after reaching the maximum dose, and every 3 months thereafter throughout the course of treatment. Special attention has to be paid while monitoring the lipid profile. Serum triglycerides should be repeated every month. If values are normal after 2 months of therapy, there is no need to repeat every month. If there is an elevation of triglyceride level (TGL) above 500 mg/dL, the test has to be repeated monthly. If there is elevation of serum TGL beyond 700 mg/dL, the drug has to be stopped or lipid lowering drugs have to be supplemented. If left untreated, further elevation of TGL may lead to pancreatitis. Another important reason to stop oral isotretinoin is the development of bowel symptoms.

HORMONAL THERAPY

One of the major etiological factors involved in acne is androgen excess. The source may be either from one or more of the following:
- Increased production
- Increased circulating free testosterone [that is not bound to sex hormone-binding globulin (SHBG)]
- Peripheral conversion
- Increased receptor response

The main goal of hormonal therapy is to counteract the effect of androgen on the sebaceous gland inducing increased sebum production. This can be accomplished with drugs having antiandrogen property, namely the oral contraceptive pills, antiandrogens, glucocorticoids, or gonadotropin-releasing hormone agonists.

Hormonal therapy in acne is of two kinds. One kind uses hormonal contraceptives, the combination oral contraceptive (COC) pills and the other uses a group of noncontraceptive hormonal therapies that include spironolactone, cyproterone acetate, and flutamide. Apart from these, corticosteroids and gonadotropin-releasing hormone agonists are also being used.

Oral Contraceptives

Combined oral contraceptive pills have been widely used in the management of acne of all degrees of severity. They exhibit their anti-acne action by the following mechanisms, effectively tackling androgen excess.
- Suppress luteinizing hormone production, thereby decrease in gonadal androgen production
- Increase SHBG, thereby decrease in amount of free testosterone
- Inhibit activity of 5α-reductase, thereby prevent conversion of testosterone to more potent dihydrotestosterone
- Block the androgen receptors of keratinocytes

Combination oral contraceptive pills contain both estrogen and progestin components. There are currently four COCs approved by the FDA for the treatment of acne, which is given in **Box 5**.

Norgestimate, gestodene, and desogestrel are third-generation progestins and are less selective for the androgens and more selective for progesterone receptors. Drospirenone, a novel progestin, is derived from 17α-spironolactone with an antiandrogenic activity. According to some authors, the

---

BOX 5 | **Food and Drug Administration-approved combination oral contraceptive pills in acne.**

- Ethinyl estradiol/norgestimate
- Ethinyl estradiol/norethindrone acetate/ferrous fumarate
- Ethinyl estradiol/drospirenone
- Ethinyl estradiol/drospirenone/levomefolate

proven efficacy and the long-term safety profile of these drugs have placed them into the first-line treatment for all severity grades of acne. In mild acne in female patients who do not want to get pregnant, COCs are used as an adjuvant to topical treatments. In moderate and severe acne, COCs are used as first-line therapy in those who are not planning for pregnancy. Here, the contraceptive effect of COC is advantageous to the patient.

By and large, the recommendations for hormone therapy in acne are indicated in females in the following situations:
- Not responding to conventional therapies
- Significant premenstrual flare-up
- Clinical findings of hyperandrogenism [androgenetic alopecia, hirsutism, and SAHA (seborrhea, acne, hirsutism, and alopecia) syndrome]
- Proven ovarian hyperandrogenism
- Not suitable for other therapy
- Late-onset acne
- Polycystic ovarian syndrome
- As an alternative in women who require repeated course of isotretinoin
- Those who require contraception (as desired by patient and while on isotretinoin)

Before prescribing COC, it is mandatory to identify every risk factor and contraindication for hormonal treatment. The following should be ruled out:
- Genetic clotting factors
- Prolonged immobilization
- History of venous thromboembolism (VTE)
- Heart disease
- Hypertension
- Obesity
- Smoking
- Diabetes
- Liver disease
- Migraine and headache
- History of estrogen-dependent malignancies (breast, endometrial, and hepatic)

Based on analysis, it has been concluded that all COC users have an increased risk of developing VTE, myocardial infarction (MI), hemorrhagic stroke, and breast cancer compared to nonusers. The risk of developing MI increases in the presence of other factors such as cigarette smoking, diabetes, and hypertension.

Albeit the noncontraceptive benefits of COC include regulation of menstruation and correction of menorrhagia and associated anemia, there is a reduction in the formation of benign ovarian tumors and colorectal, ovarian, and endometrial cancers. COC can also be given in combination with other medications such as oral antibiotics and spironolactone.

Spironolactone

Spironolactone is an aldosterone-receptor antagonist, exhibiting potent antiandrogen activity. It decreases testosterone production, inhibits 5α-reductase, increase SHBG, and completely impedes binding of testosterone and dihydrotestosterone to androgen receptors in the skin. However, the FDA has not approved spironolactone as an antiandrogen for the treatment of acne. Despite lack of evidence to prove its effect in acne, many experts support the use of this drug in acne. The side effects of spironolactone are mostly dose dependent and include diuresis, menstrual irregularities, breast enlargement, hyperkalemia and tenderness, fatigue, headache, and dizziness. Being a pregnancy category C drug, concomitant COC is advised in female patients of childbearing age, and hence, it is better to avoid this drug on a routine basis.

Flutamide

Flutamide is a nonsteroidal selective androgen receptor-blocking agent and is not approved by the FDA for the treatment of acne. The common side effects encountered with use of flutamide include headache, GI distress, breast tenderness, hot flushes, xerosis, and decreased libido. Fatal hepatotoxicity, a dose and age-related idiosyncratic reaction, has been documented with flutamide.

Cyproterone Acetate

Androgen-receptor blockers, such as cyproterone acetate, directly inhibit the androgen receptors and suppress sebum production. It has been used in the management of acne with relative success. Cyproterone acetate is licensed for acne treatment in most European countries but not in the United States.

The various levels of action of hormonal and antiandrogen therapy in acne are depicted in **Figure 13**.

The dose, mechanism of action, contraindications, side effects, monitoring tests, advantages, and disadvantages of hormonal therapy in acne are given in **Table 6**.

The management of *hormonal acne* in adult female is difficult as more often than not they are resistant to conventional acne regimens.

Flowchart 5 gives the treatment of adult woman with hormonal acne.

Corticosteroids

The use of systemic steroid in patients with acne is a therapeutic paradox as prolonged use of corticosteroid by itself can lead to acneiform eruptions. While combining with estrogen, there is greater reduction of plasma androgen levels than when using either drug alone. Owing to their anti-inflammatory action, low-dose prednisone in a dose of 5–15 mg/day used along with COC has proven efficacious in treating acne and seborrhea. Prednisone in dose of 0.5–1 mg/kg/day is effective in the treatment of acne fulminans as well as prevention of isotretinoin-induced acne fulminans-like eruptions. The drug has to be tapered and stopped. Sometimes high-dose glucocorticoids are used in severe forms of acne.

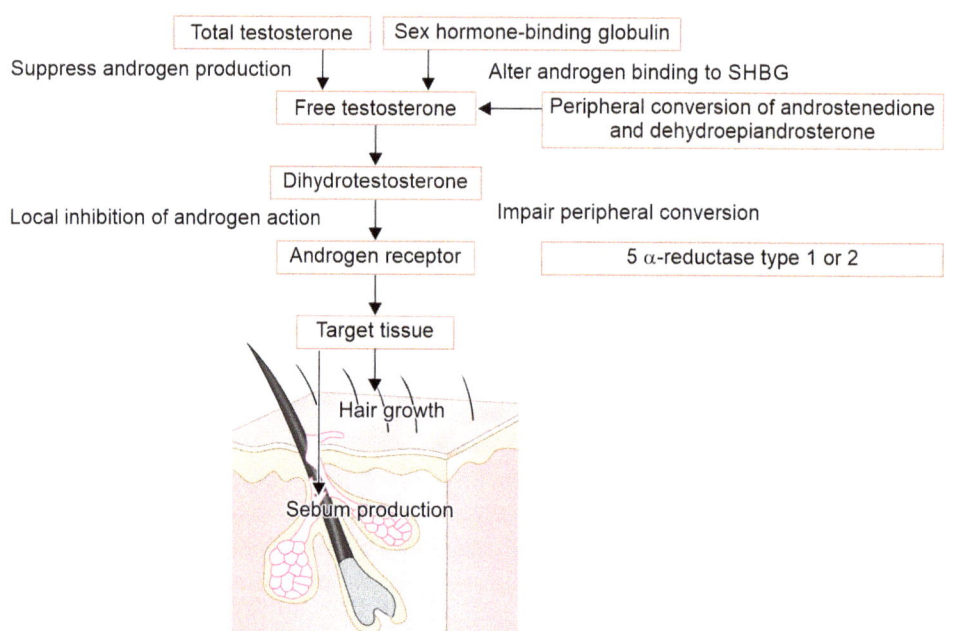

FIG. 13: Levels of action of hormonal and antiandrogen therapy in acne.

TABLE 6: Hormonal therapy in acne.

	COCs	Spironolactone	Flutamide	Cyproterone acetate
Dose		25–100 mg once or twice daily taken with meals	Initial dose of 62.5 mg of flutamide was given, which was increased to 125 mg after 1 month	50–100 mg/day when used alone. Should be initiated from first day to 14th day of menstrual cycle. If added to COC 12.5–50 mg/day
Mechanism of action	• Reduction in 5α-reductase activity • Level of free testosterone • Sebaceous gland activity • Size of the gland	• Reduction in 5α-reductase activity • Level of free testosterone • Testosterone and dihydrotestosterone binding • Sebaceous gland activity • Size of the gland	Blocks nuclear binding of androgens	• Blocks testosterone • Reduces secretion of gonadotropins
Contraindications	• Smoking in patients >35 years of age • Cardiovascular disease • Hematological disorders • BMI >35 kg/m² • Migraine • Estrogen-dependent malignancy	Estrogen-dependent malignancy	Liver disease	• History of meningioma • Liver disease • Malignancy other than prostatic cancer • Hematological disorder • Severe diabetes • Sickle-cell anemia • Chronic severe depression
Side effects	GI disorders, spotting, headache, breast tenderness, fluid retention, and depression	Hyperkalemia, hypercalcemia, breast tenderness, menstrual irregularities, hypotension, and reduced libido	• GI disorders • Hematological disorders • Muscle cramps • Gynecomastia • Acute liver failure	• GI disorders • Headache, breast tenderness, menstrual irregularities, fluid retention, liver dysfunction, and clotting disorders
Monitoring tests	Not needed unless in the presence of risk factors	Serum potassium levels, blood pressure, and electrocardiogram	Liver function tests	Liver function test and clotting factors

Continued

Continued

	COCs	Spironolactone	Flutamide	Cyproterone acetate
Advantages	• Good clinical efficacy • Contraceptive effect	• Good clinical efficacy and tolerability at regular dose • Good alternate when COC cannot be used	Good antiandrogen effect	Increased efficacy of COC containing cyproterone acetate
Disadvantages	• Delayed onset of clinical efficacy • Severe side effects (rare)	Dose-related side effects	Dose-related liver toxicity	Dose-related side effects

(BMI: body mass index; COCs: combined oral contraceptives; CPA: cyproterone acetate; EE: ethinyl estradiol; GI: gastrointestinal)

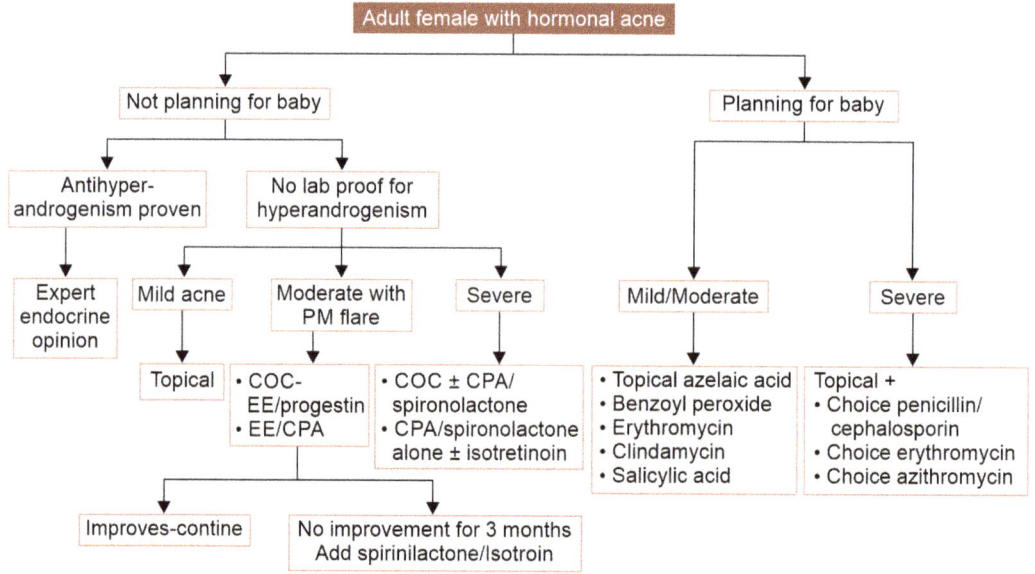

FLOWCHART 5: Treatment of an adult woman for hormonal acne.
(COC: combined oral contraceptive; CPA: cyproterone acetate; EE: ethinyl estradiol)

Gonadotropin-releasing Hormone Agonists

Gonadotropin-releasing hormone agonists such as leuprolide act on the pituitary gland, disrupting the cyclical release of gonadotropin, leading to a fall in the ovarian production of steroids. These are exclusively used where ovaries are the source of increased androgen production. Menopausal symptoms and loss of bone restrict their use in acne.

ROLE OF SKIN CARE AS AN INTEGRAL COMPONENT IN THE MANAGEMENT OF ACNE: IMPORTANCE OF CLEANSERS AND MOISTURIZERS

Representative global data has established that acne is one among the foremost causes of patient visits to the dermatologist. Surprisingly, self-diagnosis and diagnosis made by contemporaries have deemed to be the cause of nonphysician-directed and over-the-counter options. Furthermore, the availability of products that are retailed for AV sold over-the-counter at pharmacies, stores, and skin care centers as well as over the internet has led to a number of people settling for self-treatment. These skin care centers are devised in such a way as to attract people with skin care needs, in particular AV. Numerous pharmaceutical and cosmetic companies have separate departments for the purpose of developing and marketing over-the-counter products for AV. In short, people with acne have a wide variety of choices when it comes to receiving advice and treatment from sources other than the dermatologist, and this proves demanding for the dermatologist and his/her team while dealing with such patients. It is essential for the dermatologist and his/her team to administer a high level of integrated and inclusive care to patients who can otherwise seek treatment for AV from nondermatological sources. The long-term success of management of AV depends on educating the patient on AV, the available treatment options and their side effects, the expected outcome, response time, as well as the significance of proper use of medications, patient adherence, and regular follow-up. The relevance of proper skin care and choice of products in the management of AV has long since been forgotten, but they are essential as AV on its own and the various treatment options such as BPO, topical retinoids, and oral isotretinoin can cause impaired permeability of the stratum corneum (SC), leading to increased transepidermal water loss (TEWL), xerosis, increased sensitivity of the skin, and inflammatory skin changes.

Epidermal Barrier Dysfunctions in Acne Vulgaris

The approach to acne calls for a reasonable choice of therapeutic agents and other modalities equivalent to the severity of AV as well as other factors pertaining to the patient, their adherence, and follow-up. Nonetheless, proper skin care adds an additional value to the medical regimen and can decrease topical medication-associated local tolerability reactions.

Epidermal Barrier Impairments Innate to Acne

There is some data regarding the SC permeability impairment characteristic of AV despite the requirement of more research on the structural and functional integrity of the epidermal barrier and SC functions fundamental for acne-prone and acne-affected skin. There is impaired SC permeability barrier as evidenced by high levels of TEWL and sebum loss as well as reduced SC conductance (determined by corneometry), demonstrated in patients with AV. These patients also revealed reduced levels of free sphingosine and total ceramides in the SC, supporting a deficiency of the intercellular membrane, providing a limited explanation for decreased TEWL as well as corresponding directly with the SC permeability barrier dysfunction. In addition, the increase in TEWL and the decrease in the SC hydration were of greater consequence in people with moderate AV severity as compared to people with mild AV severity and in normal controls, suggesting that the significance of SC permeability barrier impairment corresponds directly with the severity of AV. It is unknown whether the qualitative or quantitative changes in SC structure and/or function recognized with AV develop only in combination with the inflammation present in active AV or if they are also present in the epidermis of unaffected facial skin of AV patients where AV lesions are not seen at the time of SC testing. However, untreated skin in people with AV reveals impaired SC permeability barrier that is essential to correct as part of the management of AV in order to decrease signs and symptoms of facial irritation, dryness like peeling due to faulty desquamation, and skin sensitivity.

Medication-induced Epidermal Changes

Some topical medications and/or vehicle formulations and oral medications such as BPO, topical retinoids, and oral isotretinoin employed to treat AV can cause alterations within the epidermis that result in modified barrier functions, especially the SC permeability barrier.

Skin Care Formulations for Acne-prone and Acne-affected Skin

There is good pragmatic and scientific rationale for the regular use of proper skin care in patients with AV, especially those subjected to professionally approved therapy. The application of proper skin care for facial skin is beneficial when AV is actively present (acne-affected skin) and also during periods of quiescence when facial acne is substantially clear and well controlled (acne-prone skin). In addition, both groups (acne-affected skin and acne-prone skin) are frequently using over-the-counter or prescription therapies for acne that can induce SC permeability barrier damage, which can be subclinical or conspicuous with signs of dermatitis. In both cases, proper skin care is advantageous for these patients.

Various alternatives are available for selection of a gentle cleanser and moisturizer as well as photoprotectant formulations. Unfortunately, there is an apparent lack of many studies assessing specific skin care products (specifically cleansers, moisturizers, and photoprotectants) in patients with AV, both with and without adjuvant treatments, especially well-designed studies that analyze the advantages and disadvantages of specific formulations and ingredients.

A complete analysis of the formulation of cleansers, moisturizers, and photoprotectants for use in patients with AV and acne-prone skin is far beyond the extent of this book. Nevertheless, a few general remarks will aid the reader in discerning what the added ingredients are designed to provide, specifically for patients with acne-prone and acne-affected skin, and what potential advantages may be extended for many of the patients with AV, with additional information on preparation and study data accessible through direct contact with the manufacturer or in the literature.

Cleansers

- *Surfactant*: The foam wash employs a unique surfactant (zinc coceth sulfate), which aids to balance tolerability, enhances the ability to lather, adequately cleans skin and removes surface debris such as dirt and sebum, and preserves its potency at a low pH.
- *Skin type*: The foam wash can be utilized in patients with oily, normal, dry, or combination skin ("T zone").
- *Clinical use*: The foam wash is used as a constituent of the skin care regimen (along with moisturizer SPF 30) in patients subjected to treatment for AV with an array of topical medications, such as retinoids and BPO-containing formulations. A greater number of subjects are satisfied with the cosmetic acceptability and absence of irritation connected with use of the foam wash.

Moisturizers

- *Barrier protection/repair*: Moisturizers have been shown to bring down TEWL and increase skin hydration, even when used in patients under active treatment with an array of topical medications for AV, such as topical retinoids and BPO-containing formulations.

- Ceramide-containing formulations are shown to reconstruct human skin model and to boost (epidermal) cutaneous levels of endogenous ceramides.
- As ceramides are the predominant constituent of the intercellular lipid membrane of the SC, which serves to regulate TEWL, the addition of pseudo-ceramide 5 (a ceramide precursor), along with other ingredients made to bring down cutaneous irritation and inflammation, such as allantoin and glycyrrhetinic acid, is scientifically reasonable.

Photoprotection

- An SPF 30 is optimal and can also be used in combination with a moisturizer.
- The moisturizer SPF 30 inherently provides photoprotection as is commonly sought in a daily moisturizer product that is also produced to protect against concomitant UV exposure. This is beneficial in patients with AV as they are frequently on medications where photoprotection is expressly recommended.
    - The addition of SPF 30 averts the need to purchase an additional sunscreen product that may not get used regularly, adds an additional topical application step reducing patient compliance, can independently cause skin irritation that baffles clinical assessment, and stacks on an added expense to the management program.

Therefore, the importance of integrating dermatologist-selected skin care into the long-term management plan for AV for both the patient and the clinician needs no elaboration.

DRUGS THAT CAN BE USED FOR ACNE IN PREGNANCY

While treating acne in pregnant women, it is better to limit to topical agents as far as possible. **Tables 7 and 8** give the pregnancy category of drugs used in acne.

Oral retinoids and topical tazarotene belong to pregnancy category X.

OTHER THERAPIES AND DIET IN ACNE

Dapsone

Oral dapsone in the dose of 25-200 mg/day was used in severe nodulocystic acne with good results. With the advent of retinoids and because of the side effects induced by dapsone, the drug is not so frequently used as before. However, in the author's point of view, dapsone is a cost-effective drug for those who cannot afford expensive drugs, such as hormones and retinoids. One should always keep in mind the side effects of dapsone before prescribing.

Zinc

Topical zinc exerts effective antioxidant property. Zinc was found to be more effective when combined with other topical medicines such as erythromycin. Some authors, however, feel that oral zinc has been used in acne for its

TABLE 7: Pregnancy category of systemic anti-acne drugs.

Drugs	Pregnancy category
Tetracycline	D
Oxytetracycline	D
Doxycycline	D
Lymecycline	D
Minocycline	D
Erythromycin	B
Azithromycin	B
Amoxicillin	B
Cephalexin	B
Trimethoprim + Sulfamethoxazole	C
Trimethoprim	C
Prednisolone	C

TABLE 8: Pregnancy category of topical anti-acne drugs.

Drugs	Pregnancy category
Erythromycin	B
Clindamycin	B
Dapsone	C
Tretinoin	C
Adapalene	C
Benzoyl peroxide	C
Azelaic acid	B
Salicylic acid	C
Zinc	C
Sulfur and sodium sulfacetamide	C
Resorcinol	C

antioxidant effect. Apart from being an antioxidant, the proposed mechanism of action of zinc in acne includes suppression of sebum production and through its antiandrogenic property.

Nonsteroidal Anti-inflammatory Agents

Nonsteroidal anti-inflammatory agents such as ibuprofen have been recommended for the treatment of SAPHO syndrome. In the authors' experience, early administration of NSAIDs in selected patients on oral retinoids has yielded good results.

Biologics

Infliximab, a monoclonal antibody against tumor necrosis factor alpha (TNF-α), has been used with success in SAPHO syndrome.

Topical Nicotinamide

Topical nicotinamide is an anti-inflammatory agent. The advantage of using topical nicotinamide is the absence of development of resistance. Some authors even showed that the efficacy of topical nicotinamide in a strength of 4% gel was similar to that of topical 1% clindamycin gel.

Salicylic Acid

Salicylic acid was used as a keratolytic agent in acne. It can be used in both inflammatory and noninflammatory lesions. However, because of the irritation caused by salicylic acid, it is not frequently used nowadays when newer, more cosmetically, more suitable preparations are available.

Sulfur

Sulfur can be used as a safe agent even in children. However, prolonged use of sulfur can lead to systemic absorption. Being a comedogenic agent itself, it can exacerbate the acne lesions in some patients. Owing to the unacceptable smell, the use of topical sulfur has come down in the recent days.

Other Modalities

Thyroid replacement, hypoglycemic agents to handle insulin resistance by administering thyroxine and metformin, will help in those patients who show signs and features of metabolic syndrome. In future, inhibition of androgen-metabolizing enzymes in the skin and usage of such drugs will be the main line of management in the armamentarium of acne therapies.

Complementary Therapy

Research done on the traditional herbs shows the usefulness of certain herbal medicines in the management of acne. These include topical tea tree oil and consumption of green tea, barberry extract, and gluconolactone solution. However, there is no consistent evidence to show their usefulness in managing acne.

Diet in Acne

The role of diet in acne has been a long-debated topic. Based on research, diets with high glycemic index are to be avoided in patients with acne as they have been shown to exacerbate the lesions. Diets with low glycemic index are to be advised, especially in those who show features of insulin resistance. Limited data indicate the adverse effects of dairy products in flare-up of acne lesions. Antioxidants such as zinc, probiotics, and fish oil in few selected studies have proved beneficial in acne patients.

PROCEDURAL MANAGEMENT IN ACNE

Beyond the medical drugs and prescriptions, diet, and alternate medicine, the therapy of sequelae of acne continues. Despite the best of treatment and patient compliance, sequelae-like pigmentation and scarring are inevitable in acne. The trend of nonmedical management of acne has been the recent developing field in acne management. However, it has to be emphasized that early appropriate treatment of acne for adequate period of time with proper maintenance therapy will certainly prevent most of the sequelae seen in acne patients who had medical line of treatment.

Procedural treatment, however, hastens the process of acne resolution. Of the post-acne sequelae, pigmentation does resolve completely over a period of time with treatment. 100% resolution of acne scars is not possible with any procedure. Procedures reduce the visibility of acne scars to a considerable extent and prevent visibility of the scars at a social distance (considered to be 25 cm). This in turn emphasizes the need for early treatment, control, and prevention of acne to prevent post-acne scarring, which is expensive to treat, needs multiple sittings, and also cannot be completely treated.

Therefore, the patients must be counseled to not pick their acne lesions to prevent post-acne scars and advised regarding the necessity of prevention and early treatment of acne if a breakout occurs. Also, if scarring has taken place, the patient must be counseled regarding the limitations of acne scar treatment procedures so that they do not have unrealistic expectations.

The following are the procedures commonly employed to manage acne and acne scars beyond medical treatment:
- Comedone extraction
- Peels (salicylic, acetic, mandelic, and retinoic acid peels)
- Blue light therapy
- Evacuation surgery
- Light electrodessication
- Microdermabrasion
- Subcision
- Trichloroacetic acid (TCA)–chemical reconstruction of skin scars (CROSS) cautery
- Cryoslush
- Intralesional steroid
- Platelet-rich plasma (PRP)
- Dermaroller
- Microneedle fractional radiofrequency
- Fillers
- Lasers (Q-switched, pixel, and fractional CO_2 laser)

Generally, a combination of procedures according to the need of the patient works better than a single line of treatment alone. Medical and procedural treatments yield better results when combined.

For acne patients who present with pigmentation or unacceptable scars following treatment, various procedures and their application are given in **Table 9**.

Comedone Extraction

This is a simple in-office method by which mechanical pressure is applied by means of a comedone extractor, and it helps in expressing

TABLE 9: Various procedures and their application in acne and acne sequelae, such as pigmentation and scars.

Procedure	Application or lesion
Extraction	Comedones
Drainage	Pustules and cysts
Excision	Sinus tracts and cysts
Blue light therapy	Acne
Peeling	Acne, post-acne pigmentation, and superficial scars
Intralesional steroid injection	Large cysts and nodules
Cryotherapy	Chronic cysts and superficial scars
Q-switched laser	Acne (when used with carbon) and post-acne pigmentation
Subcision	Post-acne scars
Dermaroller	Acne scars
Platelet-rich plasma	Acne, acne scars, and open pores
Microneedle fractional radiofrequency	Pigmentation, post-acne scars, and open pores
Punch excision and punch elevation	Acne scars
Erbium-doped yttrium–aluminum–garnet (Er:YAG) pixel and fractional CO_2 lasers	Post-acne pigmentation and scars
Restylane vital	Post-acne scars
Juvederm ultra plus XC	Very deep, rolling post-acne scars

the contents of the blocked pilosebaceous follicle.

The area is cleaned with alcohol swabs or spirit and the comedone extractor is centered over the comedone. Downward firm pressure is applied in the direction of the hair follicle to express the contents. Excessive force must be avoided since it will lead to inflammation and thus potential scarring.

In case of closed comedones, the top of the lesion can be pierced with a 26G needle for easier extraction. Mild radiofrequency energy with an epilating needle (after topical anesthesia) can be used to make a tiny puncture to facilitate easier and less traumatic extrusion of closed comedones.

Comedone extraction helps prevent the progression of acne into the inflammatory stage. It is helpful to treat recalcitrant macrocomedones. It can be done with treatment with isotretinoin to treat comedones, which are slow to resolve.

The timing of the extraction plays a role in preventing premenstrual acne. When comedones are removed at the time of ovulation prior to the sebaceous orifice size reduction, this prevents blockage of the pores and thus prevents bacterial colonization and inflammation and thus prevents inflammatory acne, which might lead to potential scarring.

Cryotherapy

This is done by using cryoslush, which is a paste prepared from acetone and crushed solid carbon dioxide. This is applied to the nodulocystic lesions and papules in acne and kept for around 2–10 seconds. Alternatively, a metal cryoroller can also be dipped in liquid nitrogen and rolled over the acne lesions for 2–10 seconds. It is done every week to 2 weeks and repeated two to three times.

Mechanism of Action

Cryofreezing the tissue, which leads to desquamation of comedones, epidermal necrosis, and resolution of the inflammatory acne lesions.

The complications include pigmentation, scarring, and persistent erythema. The complications are more common in dark-skinned individuals.

Intralesional Corticosteroids

These are used to treat cystic and nodular acne lesions. It helps in rapid resolution of larger lesions, reduces pain and post-acne scarring.

Procedure

Triamcinolone acetonide is used in a concentration of 2.5–5 mg/mL (10 mg/mL vial diluted with xylocaine of normal saline).
- After cleaning the area with alcohol swab or spirit, around 2–3 units are injected into the base of each lesion with the help of an insulin syringe.
- The cyst usually resolves in around 2–3 days.
- Repeat injection is advised after a month in case of incomplete resolution.

Complications include atrophy, hypopigmentation, infections, and hematoma formation.

The most common complications are hypopigmentation and atrophy, which are due to injection of higher concentrations or larger doses of the medication. These can be prevented by using only 2.5 mg/dL concentration or less and not injecting in the dermis or subcutaneous tissue. This side effect is reversible; however, it takes around a few months to a year to resolve depending on the severity.

Aspiration of the Cysts

Aspiration of the cyst is done for nodulocystic acne to reduce scarring and inflammation. The cyst is aspirated with the help of a wide-bore needle. This can be followed by intralesional steroid injection to reduce fibrosis and scarring in and around the lesion.

Incision and Drainage of the Cysts

Incision and drainage is also done for nodulocystic acne. A nick is made with a No. 15 surgical blade under aseptic precautions and the cystic is drained by manual pressure. Following this, to prevent recurrence, the walls of the cyst may be cauterized with 88% phenol using a cotton swab.

Blue-, Red-, and Green-light Therapy

Blue light (407–420 nm) targets the endogenous porphyrins. Free radicals are produced by this photoexcitation reaction, which destroys *C. acnes*.

Red light has anti-inflammatory properties and penetrates deeper than blue light.

Potassium-titanyl phosphate (KTP) or 532 nm green light laser also targets porphyrin.

Postinflammatory Pigmentation

The common peels used in the management of postinflammatory pigmentation include alpha hydroxy acids or beta hydroxy acids. TCA (10–35%), glycolic acid (20–70%), and salicylic acid (20–30%) are commonly used as office procedures.

Salicylic Acid

Salicylic acid is a beta hydroxy acid with a phenolic ring. It is lipophilic and hence penetrates into the pilosebaceous unit and thus has comedolytic effect. It has anti-inflammatory activity and hence reduces erythema and controls inflammatory lesions in acne. It has keratolytic action and dissolves intercellular cement and reduces corneocyte adhesion. It also reduces postinflammatory hyperpigmentation of acne. It is economical, easy to apply, and the side effects are minimal.

Glycolic Acid

Glycolic acid is an alpha hydroxy acid that has exfoliative properties. It reduces corneocyte adhesion, decreases keratinocyte plugging, corrects abnormal keratinization and thus reduces follicular occlusion. It also had bactericidal action on *C. acnes* and thus has anti-inflammatory action.

Trichloroacetic Acid

Depending on the concentration, it can be a deep, medium depth, or superficial peel. Higher concentrations are used in the TCA-CROSS method for treatment of acne scars. The TCA peels cause dermal and epidermal protein coagulation and also leads to collagen necrosis up to the upper portion of the reticular dermis. The skin appendages and the islets of keratinocytes lead to reepithelialization. It also increases the volume of collagen, elastin, and glycosaminoglycans. The TCA is a self-neutralizing peel and therefore is not absorbed systemically even in high concentration usage.

Phenol peels are not commonly used in Asians due to hypopigmentation and hyperpigmentation following the usage of the peel.

Newer peels containing AA, mandelic acid, pyruvic acid, retinoic acid, and lactic acid are available.

Scars

Scars are of different types and depth. The procedures adopted to correct them include:
- Dermabrasion
- Microdermabrasion
- *Surgical repair*:
  - Subcision
  - Punch excision
  - Punch elevation
  - Grafting
- Microneedling or dermaroller
- Fillers
- *Lasers include ablative/nonablative/ fractional types*:
  - Pulsed dye
  - CO_2
  - Erbium-doped yttrium–aluminum–garnet (Er:YAG) (Pixel)
  - Diode
  - Combination of CO_2 or Er:YAG.

No single procedure can give the desirable effect for any patient. Therefore, proper patient selection, counseling, and planning are essential before contemplating procedural management in acne.

Dermabrasion

Dermabrasion is a sequential planning of the skin with the help of a manual or electrical dermabrader to the required level. Usually, a manual dermabrader is used for spot lesions.

Mechanism of Action

After dermabrasion, re-epithelialization occurs from the wound margin and also from the remnants of appendages, i.e., sweat glands, hair follicles, and sebaceous glands. Since the face has more density of these appendages, healing is faster over the face as compared to other body areas.

Procedure

Spot dermabrasion can be done under local anesthesia, whereas whole-face dermabrasion requires an operation theater with the availability of emergency resuscitation.

After cleaning the area and marking the scars, the skin is stretched and the base of the scars is dermabraded. The maximum level of dermabrasion should be the junction of the mid-reticular and the upper dermis. This end point is seen as a firmer surface, large bleeding points, and breaks in the skin.

Even if an electrical dermabrader is used, a manual dermabrader can be used to correct the edges and uneven areas. Following the procedure, pressure and ice-cold saline compresses are used to achieve hemostasis. Dressings, which are nonadherent, are used for a week. Crusting usually takes about a week or two to subside, depending on the depth of the dermabrasion.

Complications include persistent hyper- or hypopigmentation, erythema, infections, and scarring.

Microdermabrasion

Microdermabrasion is a superficial, minimally invasive, mechanical abrasion of the skin. It is done by using a pressurized stream of abrasive materials, such as aluminum oxide crystals. Alternatively, it can be done using a diamond tip. It is useful for very superficial scars, and it is not much useful for deeper acne scars. Multiple sittings are needed.

It is contraindicated in the presence of concurrent dermatoses or active infection or acne over the face.

Mechanism of Action

Superficial wounding of the skin leads to stimulation of epidermal cell turnover and stimulation of dermal collagen.

Procedure

- The skin is cleaned and degreased.
- Contact lenses are to be removed and eye protection must be given to prevent crystals from entering the eyes.
- Pressure is kept from 10 to 30 mm Hg. The pressure depends on the depth required, the number of passes planned, and the epidermal thickness.
- The hand piece is moved over the area to be treated in an outward direction. Second passes are usually done in a perpendicular direction to the first pass. The end point is erythema.
- The skin is stretched under tension and a vacuum is created to aspirate the used crystals and epidermal debris.
- The treated area is wiped with moist gauze to remove crystals and moisturizers can be applied.
- Sittings can be done once a week.

The complications include edema, erythema, infection, pigmentary changes, purpura, and scarring. In case the crystals enter the eye, crystal adherence to the cornea, superficial punctate keratopathy, and conjunctival congestion can occur.

Subcision

Introduction

Subcision is also known as subcutaneous incision surgery. It is a method to treat acne scars. It is especially useful for rolling scars in acne.

Mechanism of Action

Subcision releases the subcutaneous fibrotic bands, which pull the overlying epidermis down and thus helps to elevate the scar. There is formation of hematoma in the dermis beneath the scar, which helps to elevate the scar. Connective tissue forms in the area as a process of wound healing.

Procedure

- The area is cleansed with alcohol swabs or spirit.
- The scar margins can be defined with surgical markers.
- Local anesthesia can be given if needed.
- 25–27-gauge needles can be inserted at an acute angle nearby the scar. The bevel should face up and should be parallel to the skin surface.
- The needle is moved through the dermis in a fan-like motion. Fibrous bands are transected and a snapping sound is heard.
- The needle is removed and pressure and ice are applied on the wound for a few minutes.
- Topical antibiotics can be applied for a few days after the procedure.

Complications of the procedure include hematoma, tenderness and pain, infection, injury to nerve or blood vessel, keloids, or hypertrophic scars.

TCA CROSS

Introduction

TCA CROSS is the process of chemical reconstruction of skin scars (CROSS) by the means of trichloroacetic acid (TCA). In this, high concentrations (70–100%) of TCA are placed on the base of the atrophic scar. It is mainly useful in rolling, boxcar, and ice-pick type of acne scars.

Mechanism of Action

Trichloroacetic acid leads to a local inflammatory reaction, which leads to the formation of new collagen fibers. This helps decrease the depth of the scar and also reduces the shadow effect.

Procedure

- The skin is cleansed with saline or chlorhexidine.
- A blunt end instrument such as a toothpick is dipped into the TCA solution and the excess solution is wiped off. Dripping should be avoided.
- The TCA is then applied to the base of the atrophic scars.
- Once frosting occurs, TCA is removed.
- Eyes and mucosal surfaces must be avoided.
- Frosting will be visible for 12 hours.
- Redness and soreness in and around the area may be seen for 1–2 days.
- Strict sun protection must be used for a few days following the procedure.
- The treatment is repeated at intervals of 4–8 weeks.

The complications include damage to mucosal surfaces, leading to ulceration and scarring, postinflammatory hyper- and hypopigmentation, formation of larger scars, and continuous irritation and erythema.

Dermaroller

Introduction

Dermaroller is a drum-shaped device having 192 microneedles in 8 rows. The dermaroller used for acne scars ranges in length from 0.5 to 1.5 mm and has a diameter of 0.1 mm. They are made by ion etching on medical grade stainless steel or silicon and gamma irradiation is used to presterilize them. The dermaroller is meant for single use only.

Mechanism of Action

The dermaroller pierces the SC during treatment and causes microholes without damaging the epidermis. This microtrauma leads to the release of growth factors, which result in the formation of new collagen, elastin, and also neovascularization in the papillary dermis. This formation of regular collagen (percutaneous collagen induction theory) and release of fibrous bands leads to scar reduction.

Procedure and Postcare Instructions

- It is an outpatient department (OPD) procedure.
- Topical anesthesia is applied for a period of 45 minutes to 1 hour over the area to be treated. A block can also be given if the patient has very low pain tolerance.
- The area is sterilized with alcohol swabs and betadine and with saline at the end.
- Rolling is done with the dermaroller in three different directions (horizontal, vertical, and diagonal) for 15–20 times till pinpoint bleeding occurs.
- The area is covered with cold saline pads following the treatment for around 5 minutes.
- The area is cleaned and topical antibiotics are applied.
- The patient is instructed to apply topical antibiotics twice a day for around 3 days.
- Photoprotection is advised for a week.
- Topical steroids and anti-inflammatory agents are to be avoided as inflammation is necessary for collagen induction.
- The erythema and swelling lasts for a period of 1–3 days.
- A gap of 4–6 weeks is recommended in between two treatments as this is the time taken for new collagen formation.
- Multiple treatments (4–8) are necessary depending on the severity of the scarring.
- It can be combined with PRP injection (after dermaroller) or application prior to the dermaroller for better results.
- Dermastamps have also been developed and are useful for localized scars.

Exclusion criteria for procedures like dermaroller, microneedle radiofrequency, ablative lasers, and subcision include active acne, keloidal tendency, pregnancy, immunosuppression, active skin disease interfering in wound healing, local or systemic active infection, connective tissue disorders, active vitiligo or psoriasis, body dysmorphic disorder, unrealistic expectations, and patients on isotretinoin. A course of oral acyclovir is needed for individuals with history of recurrent herpes simplex.

Microneedle Fractional Radiofrequency

Introduction

Microneedle fractional radiofrequency is a treatment by which controlled radiofrequency energy is introduced into prefixed depths in the skin by minimally invasive microneedles. It is done by means of a probe, which has 25 gold-coated (conductor) needles. The depth of the needles can be adjusted from 0.5 to 3.5 mm depending on the target area. The tip is for single use only and each tip delivers 1,000 shots.

The needles are insulated except for the distal 0.3 mm. This helps in precise treatment of the affected area and prevents damage to the surrounding tissue. It has lesser downtime than Er:YAG laser and fractional CO_2 laser.

Mechanism of Action

The electrical energy is transformed into thermal energy, which leads to a uniform, deep tissue warming, which initiates a wound healing process within the affected area, causing regeneration of collagen and elastin and thus reduces the depth of scars. Radiofrequency thermal zones are created in the reticular dermis, which lead to neocollagenogenesis, neoelastogenesis, long-term dermal remodeling and thus dermal thickening.

Since the needles are insulated except for the tips, the microholes created on the epidermis are not subject to thermal damage, and thus the side effects of pigmentation and damage to the epidermis seen with ablative lasers are absent. The authors actually observed a reduction of pigmentation, which could possibly be due to creation of microchannels for passage of the pigment.

Procedure and Postcare Instructions

- Topical anesthesia is used for around 45 minutes to 1 hour prior to the procedure. Nerve blocks can also be given if necessary.
- The area is cleansed with alcohol swabs or spirit.
- Shots are given with the tip touching the skin in horizontal, vertical, and diagonal directions.
- A medial-to-lateral direction is preferred as it helps in tightening of the skin.
- Three to four passes can be given. The needle depth can be kept at 3.3–3.5 mm for the first pass, 2.5 mm for the second pass, and 1.5 mm for the third pass.
- A depth of 1–1.3 mm is used over the forehead, nose, and upper lip for all passes.
- For the eyelids, a depth of 0.5–0.6 mm can be used after pulling it up or down.
- Extra passes with higher energy can be given on the affected areas.
- By reducing the exposure time, higher energies can be given; however, in acne scars, a low energy for a longer duration of time gives better results compared to a high energy for shorter duration.
- Lower energy is used at lower depths to prevent epidermal damage.
- Patient is instructed to use topical antibiotics with re-epithelializing agents containing sodium hyaluronate, cyclohexasiloxane, and cyclopentasiloxane for around 7 days.
- Thermal water can be sprayed over the area to retain moisture.
- Patient is advised strict sun protection for 7 days following the procedure.
- Anti-inflammatory agents are to be avoided.

- Erythema and edema are seen for the first 1 or 2 days, following which the skin becomes dry and flaking is seen. By 7 days, the skin becomes normal.
- This procedure can also be combined with PRP and subcision for better results.
- The patient may need around 3–6 sessions, depending on the severity of the scars.
- The procedure is done once in 4–6 weeks.

Platelet-rich Plasma

Introduction

Platelet-rich plasma is an autologous concentration of plasma with more count of platelets than of whole blood. Growth factors are released from platelets, which help in wound healing, release of fibrous bands, new regular collagen formation and thus reduce acne scars. Patients on aspirin and other NSAIDs should discontinue treatment 7 days before treatment.

Mechanism of Action

Platelets are a natural source of growth factors. Growth factors stored within platelet α-granules include insulin-like growth factor (IGF), platelet-derived growth factor (PDGF), platelet-derived angiogenic factor (PDAF), epithelial growth factor (EGF), vascular endothelial growth factor (VEGF), and transforming growth factor-beta (TGF-β).

Platelets also release other substances such as vitronectin, sphingosine 2-phosphate, and fibronectin that help in wound healing. PRP regenerates and rejuvenates soft tissue, thus helping in acne scar healing. It also stimulates growth of new capillaries and thus helps to improve the texture of the skin.

When done in combination with laser, it helps in healing laser-damaged skin and reduces the downtime of laser such as erythema and edema by release of growth factors, especially PDGF, which stimulates the production of other growth factors, upregulates protein and collagen synthesis and thus helps in connective tissue healing and collagen remodeling.

Insulin-like growth factor helps in the proliferation and migration of fibroblasts and thus increases collagen production. EGF effects are limited to the lower layers of the epidermis. It promotes cell re-epithelialization and differentiation. TGF-β hastens tissue recovery by upregulation of cell proliferation and migration and also directly by stimulating fibronectin-binding interactions and stimulating cell replication.

Procedure

- Local anesthesia can be applied for around 30–45 minutes prior to the procedure. A block can also be given if necessary.
- Around 8–10 mL of blood is collected from the antecubital vein of the patient and transferred to ethylenediaminetetraacetic acid (EDTA) or sodium citrate-containing tube. Regen tubes containing a thixotropic gel for separation of plasma and red blood cells and sodium citrate solution can also be used.
- It is centrifuged at 1,500 g for around 5 minutes in case of Regen tubes. In case of EDTA tubes, double centrifugation initially for 12 minutes and the removal of plasma and recentrifugation for 12 minutes is done.
- The supernatant PRP is loaded into insulin syringes and injected into the affected areas. Alternatively, it can be applied on the skin and dermaroller can be done.
- The activation of plasma occurs during the process of injection.
- The treatment is usually repeated every 4–6 weeks.
- Erythema and edema may be there for 1–3 days following the procedure.
- There is slight brightness of skin when injected superficially after around 2–3 days.

The advantage of PRP is that it can be combined with all the other procedures such as dermaroller, fractional CO_2 laser, Er:YAG laser, and microneedling radiofrequency, and it gives better results when combined than when the above are done as a stand-alone treatment.

Fractional Lasers

Initially, CO_2 laser was used for acne scars, traumatic scars, and treatment of facial lines. This laser removed the epidermis and a part of the dermis by a continuous beam mode. Healing occurred by neocollagenesis and fibroplasia. The downtime was for a week or even more. Many side effects such as edema, pain and persistent erythema, and postinflammatory hyper- and hypopigmentation were seen. The hypopigmentation was seen even 2 years after the procedure. The side effects are more in Indian skin.

The nonablative near-infrared lasers [KTP laser and pulsed dye lasers (PDL)] and intense pulse light devices were then introduced. But even though the side effects and downtime were minimal with these procedures, the effects were also less. They were more useful for vascular lesions but had less effect on collagen and elastin and thus were not much useful for scars.

The fractional lasers came into the picture, which minimized the side effects and downtime of ablative nonfractional lasers and at the same time provided results closer to ablative laser resurfacing. It was first described in 2003 by Huzaira.

The fractional lasers produce injury to the skin with skip areas instead of ablating the whole skin. These produce small columns of thermal injury also known as microthermal zones (MTZ). The depth and diameter of the injury varies with the laser. Once these zones develop, the repair process of the skin begins. The depth of the laser should have a nonlinear correlation with the energy and the density of shots.

The repair is by transepidermal delivery of the treated necrotic skin into the SC, also known as microscopic epidermal necrotic debris (MENDs). The healing process is possible due to the presence of the surrounding normal or untreated skin.

The fractional lasers can be further divided into ablative and nonablative lasers. Ablative lasers can be CO_2, Er:YAG, or yttrium–scandium–gallium–garnet (YSGG). The ablative lasers can also be microablative, which produces epidermal and dermal damage to depth <750 microns and deep dermal ablative lasers, which produce damage of >750 microns in the skin.

The CO_2 laser has carbon dioxide gas as its medium and emits energy at 10,600 nm. Er:YAG laser has a flash lamp-excited system, which emits light of wavelength 2,940 nm. This light is 16 times better absorbed by tissue water. It also causes tissue ablation with less of tissue desiccation and vaporization. The thermal damage caused by Er:YAG laser is less compared to CO_2 laser.

Procedure

- A topical anesthetic cream can be applied for around 1 hour on the treatment area.
- The area should be cleaned with betadine and saline. Alcohol or spirit should be avoided in case of CO_2 lasers.
- Ice cooling is given.
- Fractional laser is given on the affected areas. The energy can be kept from 30 to 40 Joules and the gap between each shot from 1 to 1.5 mm. Two passes can be given with an overlap of around 10%.
- The area is cooled with ice packs and a topical antibiotic is applied. Re-epithelializing agents can be used for around 7 days.
- Erythema and swelling persists for around 3 days. The crusts persist for 7–10 days.
- The patient is instructed to maintain strict sun protection for a week following the procedure and a broad-spectrum sunscreen is advised.

Punch Techniques for Acne Scarring

This is useful for deep scars of acne, especially of the boxcar type.

Punch Excision and Closure

Punch excision and closure technique is useful in ice-pick and boxcar scars. This is the least invasive among the punch techniques and is useful for scars <3.5 mm in size.

The area is marked out and local anesthesia is infiltrated. A surgical biopsy punch of diameter according to the diameter of the scar is used to punch out the scar after undermining in a direction parallel to the relaxed skin tension lines up to the subcutaneous layer. The wound then becomes elliptical and is then sutured. A linear scar along the relaxed skin tension lines is present, which fades over a period of time.

Punch Excision and Grafting

Punch excision and grafting technique is used for deep ice-pick scars. It is useful for scars up to 4 mm in size. In this, instead of suturing the wound after excision of the punch, a full thickness skin punch graft taken from the retroauricular area or the gluteal region is placed over the area.

Punch-floatation Technique (Punch Incision and Elevation)

Punch floatation technique is done for depressed scars in which the skin texture is normal. The scars are marked and the area is infiltrated with 2% xylocaine. The size of the punch depends on the diameter of the scar. The scar is incised with the punch up to the subcutaneous layer. Lateral and upward pressure is given so that the punch moves up. The punch is fixed parallel to the level of the skin surface with the help of surgical glue. The advantage of punch elevation is that the skin has the same color as the surrounding skin.

Fillers for Acne Scars

Fillers for acne scars are most useful in the case of broad-rolling scars. Tiny scars do not respond much to fillers. It is important to remove fibrous bands under the scar to prevent uneven distribution of the filler and extrusion into normal skin.

- Hyaluronic acid fillers can either be directly injected underneath the scar or can be injection with a cross-hatching technique.
- The effect is temporary and generally lasts for a couple of months.
- Juvederm Ultra and Juvederm Ultra Plus can be used for deeper scars caused by severe nodulocystic acne.

Undercorrection is preferred as fillers tend to absorb water and touch-up treatments if needed can be done later.

CHAPTER 8

What is New in Acne Vulgaris—from Recent Literature

CORRELATION IDENTIFIED BETWEEN ABO BLOOD TYPES AND ACNE SEVERITY

As per late discoveries, the ABO antigenic framework, alongside tumor necrosis factor alpha (TNF-α) and different sorts of supportive fiery particles, is generally accepted to assume a part in sickness pathogenesis. Additionally, certain conditions may be influenced by the transmission of blood group genes.

Increased TNF-α levels have been linked to inflammation, which is thought to be an etiopathogenic factor in the development of acne vulgaris. Some studies have looked at the relationship between blood group and acne vulgaris. However, the findings of previous studies have been inconsistent, which is why this study was conducted. Neşe Göçer Gürok, MD, of Fethi Sekin City Hospital in Turkey authored the study.

"Possible correlations were investigated in diseases such as rosacea, lichen planus, skin cancer, vitiligo, pemphigus, and psoriasis in dermatology," Gürok and colleagues wrote. "Also recently, the correlation between acne vulgaris and blood group was investigated but contradictory findings were reported. In This study aimed to investigate the correlation between acne vulgaris severity and somewhere in the range of 2019 and 2022, the specialists led their concentrate on 380 members matured 18 to 65 who had gone through a clinical assessment and been determined to have skin breakout vulgaris at the Dermatology Center at Wellbeing Sciences College, Elazig Fethi Sekin City Clinic. Also used by the researchers was a healthy control group of 1,000 people in the same age range who had been to the hospital for checkups or health reports.

263 out of 380 people in the first group said that they had mild acne vulgaris, while 117 said that they had more severe acne vulgaris. There were no dermatological comorbidities, systemic diseases like cardiovascular disease, drug abuse, or cancers among the included participants.

The examiners likewise dissected seriousness of skin breakout vulgaris through the worldwide skin inflammation evaluating framework [Global Acne Grading System (GAGS)]—a device utilized regularly in this specific center—estimating seriousness in light of both the blood gathering and Rh factor values noticeable through tolerant records.

Overall, the team came to the conclusion that the acne vulgaris arm had a lower mean age and a higher proportion of females than the control arm. The data also showed that participants with severe acne were typically younger than those with mild acne.

The specialists noticed that among members with blood classification A, extreme skin breakout occurrence was viewed as higher in contrast with both those with gentle skin inflammation and those in the benchmark group. Having said that, mild acne was found to be more prevalent in the other blood type groups than in the control arm.

Finally, they came to the conclusion that participants with either type of acne or those in the control arm did not have significantly different Rh blood groups.

"The expression of A blood type antigens, which was reported to be significantly higher in the present study, especially in severe acne patients, could contribute to the etiopathogenesis of acne vulgaris and alleviate acne severity via follicular hyperkeratinization," they wrote. "Further studies that would be conducted with larger samples in different centers could confirm the current study findings."

TRIPLE-COMBINATION TOPICAL TREATMENT EFFECTIVE FOR ACNE IN PEDIATRIC PARTICIPANTS

A new, fixed-portion skin treatment made of a blend of clindamycin phosphate 1.2%, benzoyl peroxide (BPO) 3.1%, and adapalene 0.15% treatment—given the title of IDP-126—saw positive outcomes in patients as long as 17 years old with moderate-to-serious skin inflammation, as per late findings.

This post hoc examination was directed to analyze potential enhancements made in skin breakout medicines for pediatric members, with the upgrades having involved a few consolidated skin medicines that designated various pathogenic elements.

This expansion in intricacy of treatment and ensuing potential for additional unfriendly occasions was recognized by the review's examiners. Lawrence F Eichenfield, MD, from the School of Medicine at the University of California, San Diego's Departments of Dermatology and Pediatrics, led their study.

"Topical clindamycin phosphate 1.2%/BPO 3.1%/adapalene 0.15% gel (IDP-126) is the first fixed-dose triple-combination formulation in development for acne," Eichenfield and colleagues wrote. "This post hoc analysis investigated efficacy and safety of IDP-126 in children and adolescents with moderate-to-severe acne."

Background and Findings

A post hoc analysis of the data from a phase 2 study evaluating the efficacy of IDP-126 treatment for moderate-to-severe acne in individuals was carried out by the researchers. As part of the randomization process, 394 individuals were randomly assigned to one of three other dyad combination gel treatments and a vehicle gel.

The first review inspected the outcome of the medicines, incendiary and non-fiery sore counts, the Skin Break Out Unambiguous Personal Satisfaction Poll [skin break out quality of life (QoL)], treatment-developing unfriendly occasions, and cutaneous security as well as bearableness.

The post hoc analysis by the research team looked at patients between the ages of 10 and 17 years, with the intent-to-treat (ITT) population consisting of all randomized participants who received the study drug and the safety population consisting of patients who received the study drug at least once with a one post-baseline safety evaluation.

IDP-126 had a significantly higher treatment success rate of 55.8% after 12 weeks of treatment than the vehicle, according to the post hoc analysis of these pediatric participants.

This pace of achievement was likewise higher than that of the other dyad blends (range: 30.8–33.9%). In addition, the researchers noted that, in comparison to the vehicle and the other dyad combinations, the study drug led to greater reductions in both inflammatory (78.3% vs. 45.1%) and noninflammatory lesions (70.0% vs. 37.6%).

In addition, the team discovered that the IDP-126 study arm had generally higher improvements in acne-specific quality of life (Acne-QoL) domain scores compared to the other treatment arms. Finally, they mentioned that mild-to-moderate application site dryness and pain were the most common treatment-related side effects in all of the study's arms.

"The efficacy and safety profile of IDP-126—the only fixed-combination acne medication in development containing three recommended treatments for once-daily use—demonstrates its potential as an effective acne treatment option," they wrote.

TNF INHIBITORS SHOWN TO BE EFFECTIVE FOR REFRACTORY ACNE TREATMENT, MAY ALSO INDUCE ACNE

Growth putrefaction factor-alpha inhibitors [TNF inhibitors (TNFis)] were viewed as compelling in recalcitrant skin breakout treatment, despite the fact that they can be related to skin inflammation event in certain occurrences, as suggested by a new efficient survey.

Tumor necrosis factor alpha inhibitors—prescriptions supported for treating provocative infections—are infrequently involved off-name for serious skin breakout that does not respond to customary medicines. Notwithstanding this, their utilization can advance the improvement of skin breakout, demonstrating a potential connection between TNFis and skin inflammation.

The specialists decided to look at this association further, as a significant part of the accessible writing regarding this matter comprises unreviewed case reports. The survey was created by Aaron Gabriel W Sandoval, MPhil, MSc, from Harvard Clinical School.

"Given the elevation of cytokines, such as TNF-α, interleukin (IL)-17, and IL-1β in acne, TNFis have been considered as a potential treatment option for severe, recalcitrant acne or in the setting of inflammatory syndromes," Sandoval and colleagues wrote. "However, acne occurrence following TNFi use for other conditions has also been reported."

The research that has been done on the use of TNFi to treat acne as well as the occurrence of acne is detailed in the literature review conducted by the researchers.

Background and Findings

Using PubMed and Web of Science searches for articles published between the beginning of these databases and October 2022, the researchers carried out a methodical review of the available literature.

They remembered investigations for their audit that had covered patients of all ages or orientation who had been given TNFis and created or settled their skin breakout. The group additionally utilized two analysts to freely survey the examinations, remove information from each, and break them down quantitatively.

The researchers discovered that 64 patients from the 53 studies included had received TNFis to treat acne or had developed acne after receiving TNFi treatment for another condition. 8.8% of the patients were female, with a mean age of 28.7 years.

The researchers came to the conclusion that 53.2% and 40.4%, respectively, of patients who received the TNFi etanercept, adalimumab, or infliximab had experienced either partial improvement or acne clearing up.

They discovered that just 6.4% of these patients reported experiencing any side effects. Additionally, the researchers found that acne was present in 63.8% of the patients evaluated as part of an inflammatory syndrome.

"Further studies elucidating the role that TNF plays in treating and inducing acne could yield insight into off-label TNFi use and acne pathogenesis, potentially guiding clinical care of patients with acne treated or induced by TNFis," they wrote.

ROLE OF TUMOR NECROSIS FACTOR-ALPHA INHIBITORS IN THE TREATMENT AND OCCURRENCE OF ACNE

Important Uses

Off-label uses of TNFis, which are approved to treat a number of inflammatory diseases, can occasionally be used to treat severe forms of acne that do not respond to conventional treatments. However, acne can also occur after TNFis use, indicating a connection between TNFis and acne. The majority of the literature on the subject consists of case studies and series that have not been thoroughly examined.

Objective

The objective is to describe the segment attributes, clinical introductions, medicines, and results of patients getting TNFis to treat skin breakout and patients who foster skin breakout following treatment of different circumstances with TNFis.

Proof Survey

As per the Favored Revealing Things for Orderly Audits and Meta-examinations Detailing Rules, a deliberate writing survey was done and detailed. PubMed and Web of Science were searched from the beginning to October 17, 2022. Patients of all sexes and ages who received TNFis and whose treatment was followed by a goal or event of skin breakout were the subject of included investigations, which provided details. Each study's data were quantitatively combined after being screened by two independent reviewers using predefined criteria.

Discoveries

A sum of 53 investigations providing details regarding 64 patients who got TNFis for the treatment of skin inflammation ($n = 47$) or who experienced skin breakout after treatment with TNFis for an alternate condition ($n = 17$), mean age 28.7 years; span of 12–64 years; six women, or 8.8% of the total, were included. Adalimumab, infliximab, and etanercept were the TNFis used. The majority of the 47 acne patients treated with TNFis had previously received antibiotics (31, or 66.0%) or isotretinoin (32, or 68.1%). The majority (44, or 93.6%) experienced partial improvement (25, or 53.2%), clearance (19, or 40.4%), and very few adverse effects (3, or 6.4%) were reported. 30 patients (63.8%) had acne as part of an inflammatory syndrome. Only 1 patient, or 5.9%, of the 17 patients who received TNFis for a different condition and then developed acne, reported having a history of acne. Due to the occurrence of acne, treatment with TNFis was either discontinued (8, or 47.1%) or modified (6, or 35.3%) in the majority of patients, typically with an improvement in symptoms.

Conclusions and Importance

The findings of this systematic review suggest that TNFis can be effective in treating acne that does not respond to other treatments, but that they can also be linked to the development of acne in some cases. Acne pathogenesis and off-label TNFi use could be better understood if more research is done on the role that TNF plays in treating and causing acne. This could help the clinicians in better treatment of patients with acne treated or induced by TNFis.

Only one of the 17 patients who developed acne following TNFi treatment for a different condition had a history of acne, according to the team. After the onset of acne, TNFis were typically stopped or adjusted, resulting in symptom relief.

CLASCOTERONE CREAM LINKED TO FACIAL ACNE CLEARANCE IN ADOLESCENTS AND ADULTS AT 12 WEEKS

According to new phase 3 results, a topical 1% clascoterone cream may treat adult and adolescent patients with facial acne vulgaris with significant efficacy and favorable safety.

This week, at the Society of Dermatology Physician Assistants (SDPA) 2022 Annual Meeting in Miami, Florida, a group of industry researchers presented brand-new data. After 12 weeks of treatment, the Food and Drug Administration (FDA)-approved topical androgen receptor inhibitor was associated with clear or nearly clear skin in about one in five patients under the age of 12 years with acne vulgaris, according to the findings. Clascoterone cream, a promising treatment for acne vulgaris with a novel mechanism of action, now has a new set of findings to add to its arsenal.

A new pooled study on the safety and viability of 1% clascoterone cream in a stage 3 preliminary program's subgroup of adolescents and adults with facial skin breakout vulgaris was conducted by specialists. The program consisted of two identical studies in which patients with moderate-to-severe disease and Investigator's Global Assessment (IGA) score of 3 or 4 were given the medication twice daily for 12 weeks. Essential viability results for the multicenter, randomized, twofold visually impaired, and vehicle-controlled preliminaries included extent of patients to accomplish IGA 0 or 1—demonstrating clear or practically clear skin—in addition to a ≥2-point decrease in IGA score from gauge as well as outright change from standard [count from baseline (CFB)] in noninflammatory sore counts (NILCs) and fiery injury counts (ILCs) at 12 weeks.

From the beginning to the end of week 12, the researchers also looked for safety results per local skin reaction every 4 weeks.

The trial's data included 1,421 patients under the age of 12 years who were randomly assigned to receive either vehicle ($n = 712$) or 1% clascoterone cream ($n = 709$). 90% of patients were white, approximately 60% were female, and the median age was 19 years old. A baseline IGA score of 3 was recorded by approximately 8 out of every 10 patients.

By week 12, the team found that 19.9% of patients who received clascoterone cream had IGA score of 0 or 1, compared to 7.7% of patients who received vehicle. At week 12, the absolute change in NILC from baseline was −11.9% in patients receiving vehicle and −20.8% in patients receiving therapy ($p = 0.0031$). At week 12, ILC's changes were −19.7% and −14.0%, respectively ($p = 0.0031$).

In terms of safety, the majority of patients did not experience any local skin reactions at week 12. The majority of the reactions that were reported were mild. More than 1.7% of patients who were treated had no reactions that were rated as moderate to severe.

The team came to the conclusion that topical 1% clascoterone cream has "favorable efficacy and safety" for treating facial acne vulgaris in patients under the age of 12 years and that the novel agent has a low risk of serious side effects.

"These phase 3 studies did not contemplate the concomitant use of 1% clascoterone cream with other anti-acne medications," they wrote. "Larger studies are necessary to investigate the long-term efficacy and safety of 1% clascoterone cream alone or in combination with other topical acne medications."

The study "Efficacy and safety of 1% clascoterone cream through 12 weeks in patients >12 years of age with facial acne vulgaris: pooled data analyses of two phase 3 randomized clinical trials" was presented at SDPA 2022.

Background

Following 12 weeks of treatment, two randomized stage 3 examinations analyzed the viability and well-being of 1% clascoterone cream, a skin androgen receptor inhibitor, in patients younger than 9 years with moderate-to-extreme facial skin inflammation vulgaris.

Objective

The objective was to present a pooled analysis of the two phase 3 trials' efficacy and safety of 1% clascoterone cream after 12 weeks of treatment for patients younger than 12 years.

Methods

Clascoterone or vehicle was administered twice daily to the entire face to patients in a 1:1 randomized fashion. The primary efficacy outcomes were the absolute change in noninflammatory lesion count and inflammatory lesion CFB. The percentage of patients who successfully completed their treatment [IGA score of "clear" (0) or "almost clear" (1) with a 2-point reduction from baseline] was the primary outcome. At week 12, absolute CFB in total lesion count was a secondary efficacy outcome. From treatment-related adverse events (AEs) and local skin reactions, safety was evaluated.

Results

709/712 patients under the age of 12 years were treated with clascoterone/vehicle. In view of the level of patients who made treatment progress (19.9% vs. 7.7%) and CFB as far as NILC (20.8 vs. 11.9), provocative injury count (19.7 vs. 14.0), and complete sore count (40.0 vs. 26.1; all $p < 0.0001$). There were no new well-being signals, and the frequency of nearby skin responses was low and comparable between the treatment arms.

Conclusions

Clascoterone is effective in patients under the age of 12 years with facial acne vulgaris, has a favorable safety profile, and has a low rate of local skin reactions.

MEDICAL FACE MASKS

Half of Romanian healthcare providers (HCPs) reported acne during the coronavirus disease 2019 (COVID-19) pandemic, according to a recent survey that detailed inadequate management of the condition that is associated with prolonged use of medical face masks.

An online cross-sectional survey of healthcare workers working in medical centers across Romania between December 17, 2020, and February 17, 2021, was part of the study.

About 50% of the 134 people who took the survey said they had acne lesions now, and 56.7% of them needed treatment. Only 34.2% sought medical advice, and 9% reported using antiacne medication despite identifying as not having acne. The majority of those (65.8%) self-medicated.

The authors of the review, led by Stefana Cretu, MD, of Hymn Davila College of Medicine and Drug Store in Bucharest, Romania, wrote, "Our results from a public overview recommend inadequate therapy of skin breakout corresponding to clinical facial covering use". Medical care suppliers ought to get clear preparation, sufficient screening, and therapy for unfriendly responses connected with personal protective equipment (PPE), in the same manner as all specialists get preparing and schooling in regard to other word-related perils and legitimate utilization of individual defensive gear (PPE).

Salicylic acid was used by 61.36% of those who received treatment. Next came topical retinoids (40.91%), BPO (20.45%), and azelaic acid (18.8%). Effective antimicrobials were utilized by four members (9.09%).

The most frequently linked treatments were azelaic acid and salicylic acid, retinoids and BPO (13.64%), salicylic acid and BPO (13.64%), and retinoids and salicylic acid (18.18%). Furthermore, just 14.2% of medical services suppliers were available to utilizing telemedicine as a patient, as indicated by the review.

Doctors (79.9%), millennials (74.62%), and women (86.6%) made up the majority of respondents. Acne sufferers reported black dots (59.7%), red papules (54.5%), erythema (41.8%), nodules (29.1%), itching (27.6%), and scales (26.9%).

"The members from our companion revealed a high profound effect of the injuries, and the people who were more impacted would in general look for help," examiners composed. Despite not identifying as having acne, few individuals reported receiving treatment for their acne; disagreements regarding the minimal diagnostic criteria for acne could be one explanation.

Patients were more likely to seek treatment if they reported a greater emotional impact from the acne lesions.

To account for any additional lifestyle factors that might influence acne, a multivariate analysis was used.

Because of friction, occlusion, moisture, an increase in temperature, and changes to the microbiota on the skin, using medical face masks for an extended period of time can exacerbate acne. According to the study's authors, the discomfort that results from using face masks improperly highlights the importance of treating skin conditions appropriately.

In addition to treatment, other possible measures that could lessen the effects of prolonged medical mask use include shorter shifts, frequent breaks, resting in areas that are not contaminated, and telemedicine. During the pandemic, dermatologists provided more virtual screening and treatment, and a 2020 study found that teledermatology was more cost-effective than traditional treatment.

"Reluctance regarding the use of telemedicine by the HCP from our cohort in their capacity as patients was surprising, considering that most of the cohort consisted of young individuals," investigators wrote. "Although not evaluated in our study, this hesitancy may also be due to a preference for a physical consultation."

The disadvantages of the review were its little size, absence of variety in orientation and age, and the shortfall of a clinical assessment of members. Additionally, the study did not investigate the kind of face masks used.

STUDY OBSERVES DIFFERENCES BETWEEN LATE-ONSET AND EARLY ONSET ACNE IN WOMEN

A new study suggests that women with late-onset and early onset acne have distinct clinical characteristics.

At Seoul National University College of Medicine, 89 female patients with a clinical diagnosis of acne vulgaris <5 years after onset were recruited for the observational study. "Although there have been some studies documenting the clinical characteristics of postadolescent acne, little is known about the clinical characteristics of acne based on the age of onset," the investigators wrote.

"Accordingly, this is the first study that investigates the clinical characteristics of acne based on the age of onset by using objective and quantitative evaluation methods and elucidates the relationship with topographical and etiological factors, such as the density of *Cutibacterium acnes* and the level of sebum secretion."

They performed a quantitative assessment of the prevalence of *C. acnes* by employing a stereotactic fluorescent photography unit.

The team used the student's t-test to compare the groups and Pearson's correlation test to see how clinical characteristics, onset age, sebum level, and *C. acnes* density were correlated.

Outcomes

The examiners found that patients with skin inflammation that erupted after the age of 21 years gave different clinical qualities in contrast to those with skin inflammation beginning at more youthful ages.

The late beginning gathering had essentially lower mean sore counts for comedones and all out skin breakout injuries in the T-zone than the beginning stage bunch did ($p = 0.001$ and $p = 0.001$, separately). Mean lesion counts for the entire face were also significantly lower in the late-onset group than in the early onset group ($p = 0.001$ and $p = 0.031$, respectively).

The late beginning gathering gave a fundamentally lower extent of comedones in the T-zone and whole face than the beginning stage bunch ($p = 0.021$ and $p = 0.013$, separately). However, the researchers found that neither group had significantly different mean lesion counts for the inflammatory lesions.

These findings were not considered statistically significant, even though the level of sebum secretion was generally higher across all regions in those with late-onset acne compared to those with early onset acne. Additionally, there was no statistically significant difference in the groups' *C. acnes* densities.

"The clinical characteristics of early onset acne and late onset acne may indicate a need for different treatment approaches," the investigators concluded. "Further studies are needed to investigate differences in men with regard to age of onset of acne," they wrote.

The study, "The clinical features of late-onset acne compared with early-onset acne in women," was published online in the *Journal of the European Academy of Dermatology and Venereology*.

ENCAPSULATED BENZOYL PEROXIDE CREAM AND TRETINOIN COMBINATION EFFECTIVELY AND SAFELY TREATS ACNE

Embodied BPO and tretinoin may give advantage to clinician scores to fiery and nonprovocative skin breakout sores in patients >12 weeks.

New information from a group of US-based specialists recommends that the typified mix of effective clean BPO and vitamin A subordinate tretinoin gives a successful, protected, and decent advantage as a fixed-portion routine for patients with moderate-to-serious skin inflammation.

Driven by James Q Del Rosso, DO, of JDR Exploration, specialists looked for viability and security results from a couple of stage 3 preliminaries including fixed-portion 3.0 mg BPO cream in addition to microencapsulated tretinoin 0.1%. They mentioned that, despite not utilizing silica microencapsulation, previous studies have demonstrated the effectiveness of this combination for treating acne vulgaris. "BPO degrades tretinoin through a process of oxidative decompensation," investigators wrote. "Treatment with BPO and tretinoin can also result in significant skin irritation, and there is evidence suggesting that their irritative effects may be additive."

The silica miniature epitome permits BPO from debasing the vitamin A subsidiary and permits a controlled arrival of both gainful specialists to patients' skin with further developed decency.

859 individuals with moderate-to-severe acne participated in their two multicenter, double-blind, parallel-group, vehicle-controlled assessments. For a period of 12 weeks, patients were assigned 2:1 to receive either vehicle cream or once-daily BPO with tretinoin.

Co-primary endpoints were sought by the researchers. The first was the percentage of participants with score of clear (0) or almost clear (1) on the IGA at week 12 from baseline and a grade reduction of <2. The second was outright change in provocative and nonfiery sore counts at week 12 to standard. They also used methods such as AE reporting, physical examination, and other approaches to find safety and tolerability outcomes.

In the primary outcomes of both trials, Del Rosso and colleagues found that microencapsulated BPO with tretinoin performed significantly better than vehicle cream. IGA success was achieved by nearly two out of five (39.9%) patients in the first study, compared to 14.3% in the vehicle arm. In the second trial, 26.8% of treated patients, compared to 15.1% of those in the vehicle arm, achieved this result.

In the first and second studies, patients who received BPO plus tretinoin had mean inflammatory lesion reductions of 21.6 and 16.2 from baseline, respectively, in comparison to reductions of 14.8 ($p = 0.001$) and 14.1 ($p = 0.018$) in the vehicle arms, respectively. Treated patients furthermore detailed 29.7 and 24.2 mean decreases in nonfiery sores from benchmark in the two preliminaries, versus 19.8 ($p < 0.001$) and 17.4 ($p < 0.001$) in the vehicle arms, separately.

In both studies, the combination therapy was tolerated well by the researchers, with application site pain (10.6%), dryness (4.9%), and exfoliation (4.1%) being the most frequently reported AEs.

They came to the conclusion that a fixed-dose regimen of encapsulated BPO and tretinoin was safe and effective for treating patients with moderate-to-severe acne.

The researchers wrote that treatment "reduced both inflammatory and noninflammatory lesions in subjects with moderate-to-severe acne and provided statistically significant improvements in IGA scores." The review met every essential endpoint and showed critical improvement over vehicle at 12 weeks, with no treatment-related serious unfriendly occasions.

INFLAMMATORY BOWEL DISEASE RISK IN ACNE MAY BE DUE TO "SHARED MECHANISTIC PATHWAYS"

While acne was associated with the incidence of inflammatory bowel disease (IBD), two drug classes used to treat acne had no such association, according to a study.

"There have been concerns about whether treatments for acne such as isotretinoin and oral antibiotics may be associated with inflammatory bowel disease," study author John S Barbieri, MD, MBA, of the department of dermatology at Brigham and Women's Hospital in Boston, told Healio. "However, an important consideration for studying these associations is whether acne itself may be associated with inflammatory bowel disease, as both processes share some of the same underlying inflammatory pathways." In the current propensity score matched cohort study, the researchers assessed whether exposure to isotretinoin, oral tetracycline-class antibiotics, and/or acne itself carry associations with IBD. Data were collected for the period between 2001 and 2022.

One-year incidence of IBD for patients with acne and/or treated with one of the two drug classes served as the outcome of interest.

"Our study design is unique in that we explored both the potential association between acne itself and inflammatory bowel disease as well as the potential association between acne treatments and inflammatory bowel disease," Barbieri said. "We also tried to take steps to reduce the potential for confounding, which can lead to identification of spurious associations."

Barbieri noted that previous research did not explore whether treatment with oral antibiotics before isotretinoin could lead to detection of those "spurious associations" between isotretinoin and IBD.

Results showed that acne itself had a statistically significant association with risk for incident IBD [odds ratio (OR) 1.42; 95% confidence interval (CI) 1.23–1.65]. However, no such association was observed for either drug class.

"We were surprised that we did not find an association between oral antibiotic exposure and risk of inflammatory bowel disease as one other study in acne and several other studies outside of acne have suggested that (this association may exist)," Barbieri said. "However, while we do not identify an association between oral antibiotic use in acne and inflammatory bowel disease, I would still encourage that oral antibiotics be prescribed thoughtfully given the risk of antibiotic resistance and other antibiotic associated complications."

Barbieri concluded that while the risk for IBD in acne is statistically significant, it is small. "The risk may reflect shared underlying mechanistic pathways," he said. "Our data also provide further reassurance that isotretinoin use for acne does not appear to be associated with a significant increased risk of inflammatory bowel disease."

ACNE INCIDENCE ASSOCIATED WITH AGE AND BODY MASS INDEX IN CHILDREN AND ADOLESCENTS

Among children and adolescents with acne, prescription systemic medications were more likely to be used by those with a higher body mass index (BMI) than those with a low or normal BMI, according to a study.

The population-based retrospective cohort study included 643 children and adolescents aged 7–12 years who had an initial acne diagnosis between 2010 and 2018.

For each case, the group also selected two age- and sex-matched controls. BMI was recorded for all participants.

In an analysis that adjusted for age and sex, the annual incidence rate of acne was 58 per 10,000 person-years.

According to the study, girls were more likely to experience acne than boys (89.2 vs. 28.2 per 10,000 person-years; $p < 0.001$).

Acne was also age-dependent. The incidence rate was 4.3 per 10,000 person-years for children aged 7–8 years compared with a 24.4 rate per 10,000 person-years for those aged 9–10 years and 144.3 per 10,000 person-years for those aged 11–12 years ($p < 0.001$).

Participants with acne had a median of 75% in BMI percentile, whereas the median BMI percentile among controls was 65% ($p < 0.001$). Moreover, 16.7% of participants with acne versus 12.2% of controls were in the 95th or greater percentile for BMI.

Further results showed that 99% of the acne group began some type of acne therapy, with 75.1% using prescription topical medications, 47.7% using over-the-counter (OTC) medications and 8.2% using prescription systemic medications.

As BMI increased, so did the likelihood of receiving systemic medication to treat acne (OR 1.43 per 5 kg/m^2 increase in BMI; 95% CI 1.07–1.92).

Rates of prescription systemic acne medication use were 5.4% among participants with underweight or normal weight, 8.1% among those with overweight, and 10.3% among those with obesity.

"Future studies investigating the effect of measures taken to improve BMI status on acne should be considered as appropriate," the researchers wrote. "Increasing understanding of preadolescent acne epidemiology and risk factors may allow earlier intervention and prevent undesirable sequelae."

ANTI-IL-17A BLOCKADE DID NOT SIGNIFICANTLY REDUCE INFLAMMATORY LESIONS IN A PLACEBO-CONTROLLED PILOT STUDY IN ADULT PATIENTS WITH MODERATE-TO-SEVERE ACNE

Abstract

Investigators randomly assigned patients aged 18–45 years with moderate-to-severe acne who had failed other systemic therapies to three treatment groups: CJM112 300 mg, 75 mg, or placebo via subcutaneous injection for three doses given 4 weeks apart. Treatment period 2 began at week 12, at which time patients receiving placebo were re-randomly assigned to receive monthly doses of either CJM112 300 or 75 mg from weeks 12 to 24 and the patients who received CJM112 300 or 75 mg in treatment period 1 continued to do so. All patients completed a 13-week safety follow-up after the last dose. The primary endpoint was to determine if CJM112 was significantly better than placebo in reducing total facial inflammatory lesions at week 12, defined as at least a 30% reduction. Investigators used a Bayesian model for repeated measurements to analyze the log-transformed inflammatory lesion count.

There were 52 patients included in the study: 21 randomly assigned to CJM112 300 mg, 13 to CJM112 75 mg, and 18 to placebo. The mean age was 24.3 years and 35% were male. There were 42 patients who continued to treatment period 2 (17 in CJM112 300 mg, 10 in CJM112 75 mg, and 6 in the placebo group). There were 11 patients who directly entered the follow-up period. Based on results from an interim analysis, the study was terminated early due to futility. 14 patients in the CJM112 300 mg, 3 in the CJM112 75 mg, 5 in the placebo/CJM112 300 mg, and 4 in the placebo/CJM112 75 mg group had completed week 24 at the time of the interim analysis.

At week 12, all groups saw a decrease in the total number of inflammatory lesions, but there was no significant difference between the groups. Dermatology Life Quality Index (DLQI) scores improved in all groups as well with no differences seen between CJM112 and placebo.

Overall, 71.2% of patients experienced at least one AE in treatment period 1 and no serious AEs. The incidence of AEs was higher in the pooled CJM112 groups compared with placebo, but there was no dose–response association. Infections were the most common AEs in patients treated with CJM112, with nasopharyngitis, upper respiratory tract infection, and urinary tract infection being the most frequently reported.

The study was limited by its small sample size and early termination.

Researchers noted that other study "Data indicates that anti-IL-17A therapy may be effective in a more inflamed acne phenotype." "Further clinical studies should be undertaken to delineate the underlying role of IL-17A in driving inflammation in acne, leading to the clinical applicability of anti-IL-17 agents in the treatment of this skin disorder," the study authors wrote.

A TOPICAL COMBINATION REGIMEN OF BENZOYL PEROXIDE AND RETINOL MOISTURIZER FOR MILD-TO-MODERATE ACNE

For mild-to-moderate acne, a topical regimen consisting of BPO, salicylic acid, and retinoids can be used in conjunction with a moisturizer containing retinol. By and large, these OTC plans are accessible for use related to other effective treatments. Because they can address multiple pathways that are involved in the formation of acne, combination regimens are better suited to address the numerous factors that are involved in the pathogenesis of acne as well as the variety of complexion issues that are associated with the condition. Combination regimens may yield better results, despite the fact that these agents are effective in treating disease. QoL scores and self-assessment of facial skin conditions both showed significant improvements from week 12 to baseline. The study participants did not experience any AEs related to the product.

The viability of prophylactic antitoxins and betadine skin readiness on cranial cutaneous *C. acnes*—A planned report.

Foundation

Cutibacterium acnes, previously known as *Propionibacterium acnes*, is progressively perceived as a reason for careful site disease and embed disappointment regardless of the utilization of prophylactic antimicrobials and germ-free careful arrangements. The point of this study was to explore whether *C. acnes* endures in the dermal layer of the skin after standard perioperative antitoxins and skin preparing with alcoholic betadine arrangement in successive patients going through a craniotomy.

At Flinders Medical Centre, a prospective observational single-center study was carried out. Grown-up patients going through a cranial neurosurgical intercession between October 2019 and Walk 2021 were qualified for consideration. Three swabs were taken from each patient after the standard preoperative antibiotic (cefazolin) was given: one preceding to preparing the skin with alcoholic betadine, one subsequent to preparing the skin, and a dermal swab once the skin was chiseled.

Results

73 patients were included. 61 patients in the "pre-prep" group had positive *C. acnes* cultures (83.6%), 12 patients in the "post-prep" group had positive cultures (16.4%), and 53 patients (72.6%) had positive cultures from dermal swabs. There was a significant reduction in positive skin cultures after surgical preparation was applied ($p = 0.00001$). After skin preparation, there was a nonsignificant decrease in the number of positive cultures in the dermal swabs ($p = 0.068$). The conclusion is that *C. acnes* continues to exist within the dermis of the scalp despite the standard prophylactic measures of using cefazolin and alcoholic betadine solution.

Patients treated with BPO in addition to tretinoin in the first and second reviews accomplished 21.6 and 16.2 mean fiery sore decreases from gauge versus 14.8 ($p < 0.001$) and 14.1 ($p = 0.018$) decreases in the vehicle arms, separately.

Treated patients furthermore detailed 29.7 and 24.2 mean decreases in nonfiery sores from benchmark in the two preliminaries versus 19.8 ($p < 0.001$) and 17.4 ($p < 0.001$) in the vehicle arms, separately.

In both studies, the combination therapy was tolerated well by the researchers, with application site pain (10.6%), dryness (4.9%), and exfoliation (4.1%) being the most frequently reported AEs.

They came to the conclusion that a fixed-dose regimen of encapsulated BPO and tretinoin was safe and effective for treating patients with moderate-to-severe acne.

The researchers wrote that treatment "reduced both inflammatory and noninflammatory lesions in subjects with moderate-to-severe acne" and "provided statistically significant improvements in IGA scores." The review met every essential endpoint and showed critical improvement over vehicle at 12 weeks, with no treatment-related serious unfriendly occasions.

PROJECTIVE PERSONIFICATION APPROACH TO THE EXPERIENCE OF PEOPLE WITH ACNE AND ACNE SCARRING

Significance

The relationship of skin breakout with close to home and social prosperity is not restricted to dynamic skin breakout on the grounds that skin breakout scarring can expand long after the end of dynamic injuries.

Objective

The objective of this study is to investigate the psychosocial weight of facial and truncal skin breakout [facial and truncal acne (FTA)] and skin breakout scars [acne scars (AS)] in an unconstrained way utilizing subjective exploration.

Participants, Setting, and Design

This qualitative study used local panels to find participants. In the form of letter completion, a personification exercise known as "Letter to My Disease" was developed for participants in two independent arms of an international qualitative study: FTA and AS.

Perceptions, psychosocial effects of FTA and AS, and coping behaviors were the main outcomes of the study.

Results

A sum of 60 members were enrolled for the FTA and AS study. 17 participants with FTA were female (57%), 21 (70%) were between the ages of 13 and 25 years, and 9 (30%) were between the ages of 26 and 40 years. 26 people (87%) had severe active acne, while 4 people (13%) had moderate active acne. 18 of the AS participants were women (60%), 9 (30%) were between the ages of 18 and 24 years, and 21 (70%) were between the ages of 25 and 45 years. 56 (FTA, 28; AS, 28) of these 60 participants completed the projective exercise "Letter to My Disease", and its analysis is the focus of this study. During the letter exercise, participants spontaneously expressed emotional and physical burden as well as the social stigma associated with their skin condition. The three main themes that emerged were the severity of the condition, attitudes, and beliefs, and connection to the personified condition.

Conclusions and Importance

Participants personified acne as an intruder and unwelcome companion that was responsible for their low self-esteem and emotional impairment, which was consistent with their skin condition. As a catalytic process and free-expression space, the joint analyses of letters (FTA and AS) highlight the struggle for self-acceptance and the ongoing burden of active acne, which begins in adolescence and continues into adulthood and beyond active lesions with AS.

ATROPHIC ACNE SCARS AND PATIENTS' SOCIAL FUNCTIONING AND EMOTIONAL WELL-BEING

Atrophic acne scars can have a substantial, negative affect on patients' QoL and social functioning, according to study findings published in the *Journal of the American Academy of Dermatology*.

The mixed-method study used qualitative interviews and a quantitative survey of patients in the United States, Canada, Brazil, France, Italy, and Germany from 2019 to 2020. Eligible participants were aged 18-55 years with mild-to-severe facial atrophic acne scars.

A total of 30 patients (5 from each country) participated in the 60-minute telephone semistructured interview—70% participants were aged 25-45 years, and 60% were women. Among the 723 patients (51.6% women) who participated in the quantitative survey, 12.7%, 71.8%, and 15.5% were aged 18-24, 25-45, and 46-55 years, respectively.

The average age at which the patients first developed atrophic acne scars was 19.1 years [standard error of the mean (SEM), 0.39], and the average duration of their scarring was 15.7 years (SEM, 0.35). Additionally, mild, moderate, and severe/very severe scarring affected 31.6%, 49.6%, and 18.8% of participants, respectively. In the qualitative interviews, reduced self-esteem and self-consciousness were recurrent themes expressed, along with ugliness/beauty. Self-esteem was the domain most affected by acne scars [3.57 on a Likert scale of 1 (no impact at all) to 5 (extreme impact)], followed by hygiene habits (3.43) and finances/expenses (3.03).

Among participants in the quantitative survey, 51.8% thought that they were unattractive owing to their acne scars and 25.7% felt "extremely" or "much less" attractive than others. Regarding their level of embarrassment/self-consciousness, among patients with severe acne, 20.1% responded "very much," 27.2% responded "a lot," and 34.5% responded "a little." Among those with mild acne, 6.2% responded "very much," 13.4% responded "a lot," and 48.5% responded "a little." In addition, 8.6% of those who took part in the quantitative survey believed that their work life had been affected "very much/extremely" and 15.9% believed that they had been unfairly dismissed from their jobs or turned down for jobs.

Among other findings, 32.9% of respondents to the quantitative survey said that their acne scars were the source of negative comments, 8.3% said that they were frequently the target of verbal and/or physical abuse because of their scars, and over 37% of respondents thought that their scars affected how others perceived them. Additionally, 19.7% of respondents reported being "very" or "extremely" bothered by their scars, 35.5% reported that their scars prevented them from participating in activities that they enjoy, and 43.2% reported that their scars had a negative impact on their relationships. Moreoever, respondents reported that they tried to hide their scars with clothes, hairstyles, or makeup.

Participants in the interview stated that the appearance of their scars, stigma, and daily life restrictions adversely affected their emotional well-being, with one participant responding, "It bothers me a lot and makes me sad."

Overall, 36.2% of the survey responders reported having no control over their scars, and 28.4% thought that nothing could be done to improve the appearance of their scars.

Potential study limitations include the lack of assessment of the survey's construct validity and reliability, and recruitment relied on self-reported scar severity.

"Acne scar management remains challenging, and scars may remain an indelible and permanent feature after acne," the researchers commented. "Therefore, effective therapies aimed at reducing the development of acne scarring are integral to prevent the associated debilitating psychosocial effects that may arise from acne scars."

EFFICACY OF ALPHA HYDROXY ACID COMBINED WITH INTENSE PULSED LIGHT IN THE TREATMENT OF ACNE VULGARIS: A META-ANALYSIS

Background

Patients with acne frequently receive multiple treatments at once. In any case, there has been no thorough audit of the viability of consolidating alpha hydroxy corrosive with intense pulsed light (IPL) for skin breakout vulgaris treatment.

The goal is to determine whether alpha hydroxy acids (AHAs) and IPL treatment for acne vulgaris is safe and effective.

In order to locate previous randomized controlled trials (RCTs) of AHA combined with IPL in the treatment of acne vulgaris, a comprehensive computer search of common biomedical databases, such as PubMed, Web of Science, the Cochrane Library, Embase, Wanfang, CNKI, SinoMed, and VIP, was carried out.

18 publications were included, and 1,435 common acne patients met the inclusion criteria. AHA and IPL were found to be more effective than the control group overall in the meta-analysis (OR 4.24; 95% CI 2.66–6.74; $p < 0.01$). There was a significant difference in total efficiency between AHA combined with IPL and AHA alone for acne vulgaris (OR 4.10; 95% CI 2.12–7.91; $p = 0.01$), and the combined efficacy of AHA and IPL was greater than that of IPL alone (OR 4.02; 95% CI 2.25–7.16; $p < 0.01$). Additionally, there was no difference in the incidence of adverse reactions between the AHA combined with IPL and control groups (OR 0.86; 95% CI 0.46–1.60; $p = 0.64$).

In conclusion, IPL-based AHA therapy performed better than other treatments.

CLINICAL AND METAGENOMIC PROFILING OF HORMONAL ACNE-PRONE SKIN IN VARIOUS POPULATIONS

Introduction

Acne is one of the most common skin problems with no known cause. It is frequently associated with women's menstrual cycles and possibly with the microbial profile and function. Despite its wide range of applications and effectiveness, it was slightly more expensive.

Our goal was to investigate the relationship between clinical skin parameters and microbial profiles and how hormonal fluctuations affect hormonal acne-prone skin in various populations.

Biophysical and topographical tools were used to evaluate skin features. For microbial profiling, we sequenced the microbiota of the facial skin and linked the results to the clinical parameters of the skin during the various menstrual cycles.

Results

We recognized contrasts between and inside hormonal stages in ladies of Chinese and Caucasian beginning. Changes were found in transepidermal water loss (TEWL), sebum level, hydration level, and pore volume. *Cutibacterium*, *Staphylococcus*, and *Streptococcus* were the most easily identified genera in both ethnic groups without any significant differences in the menstrual cycle. Interestingly, during the follicular phase, 11 bacterial metabolic pathways were downregulated in Chinese skin compared to Caucasian skin. Most of these pathways were related to skin redox balance, maybe showing a more vulnerable oxidative pressure reaction in Chinese versus Caucasian skin. The Chinese skin microbiome contained more *Novosphingobium* taxa, which have been shown to shield the skin from oxidative stress brought on by pollution.

Conclusions

Hence, this pilot concentrate on investigated a portion of the clinical and metagenomic changes in skin breakout inclined skin, and give direction to tailor-customized healthy skin systems during the period. Additionally, the skin redox status of acne-prone skin makes it easier to tailor individual skin care regimens.

NETWORK META-ANALYSIS IDENTIFIES MOST EFFECTIVE ACNE TREATMENTS

Topical acne treatment combinations, chemical peels, and photochemical therapy are the most effective treatments for mild-to-moderate acne, according to data from a systematic review and network meta-analysis (NMA) published in the *British Journal of Dermatology*.

A systematic review of RCTs of topical, oral, physical, and combined treatments for mild-to-moderate and moderate-to-severe acne vulgaris was carried out by the researchers, who also carried out separate analyses according to acne severity. They also conducted separate analyses for men and women in the case of treatment with hormonal contraceptives. Patients of all ages were included except for those with neonatal acne.

Investigators only included drug classes and interventions available in the UK, and a fixed class effects model was used across analyses. All control groups were included under a broader "placebo" control class. Using NMA techniques, investigators analyzed three endpoints: efficacy, treatment discontinuation for any reason (acceptability), and treatment discontinuation due to side effects (tolerability).

The NMA analysis included 173 publications on 179 RCTs, 112 of which dealt with mild-to-moderate acne and 67 with moderate-to-severe acne. Due to the small sample sizes of RCTs for mild-to-moderate acne, the results were biased-adjusted.

Topical retinoids, BPO, and their combination had a higher rate of discontinuation due to side effects than placebo for mild-to-moderate acne. Compared to a placebo, both physical and topical treatments (photochemical therapy and chemical peels) were effective. Compared to single topical treatments and placebo, combinations of clindamycin, BPO and a retinoid; BPO and a macrolide; clindamycin and a retinoid; and a microlide and an antifungal were more effective.

Topical retinoids alone or in combination with oral tetracycline for moderate-to-severe acne (bias-adjusted analysis), oral co-cyprindiol alone or in combination with oral tetracycline, and oral tetracycline alone had higher rates of discontinuation due to side effects than placebo. Oral isotretinoin, oral tetracyclines combined with topical treatments (azelaic acid, retinoid, or combination retinoid with BPO), and topical treatment combinations were the most effective treatments. In addition, photochemical and photodynamic treatments were more effective than placebo. Compared to combination treatments, monotherapies of oral tetracyclines or topical treatments had lower efficacy. There was no proof of an impact on treatment suspension under any condition by any treatment class contrasted and fake treatment at either skin breakout seriousness level, the examiners found. There was no evidence for the effectiveness of hormone-modifying agents; however, patients with polycystic ovary syndrome were excluded from the analysis.

The study was limited by the moderate-to-very-low quality of evidence from the RCTs included in the analysis.

Despite limited evidence, the study authors wrote that azelaic acid combined with oral tetracycline was considered "a good alternative for people with moderate-to-severe acne who have irritation to topical retinoids," and it also has a "possible side effect" which reduces the risk for hyperpigmentation in acne patients with darker skin.

Investigators conducted a systematic review of 173 RCTs of different treatments for mild-to-moderate and moderate-to-severe acne vulgaris and performed separate analyses by acne severity. Despite limited evidence, the study authors wrote that azelaic acid combined with oral tetracycline was considered "a good alternative for people with moderate-to-severe acne who have irritation to topical retinoids," and it also has a "possible side effect" which reduces the risk for hyperpigmentation in acne patients with darker skin.

A major limitation of the study was the low quality of evidence from the RCTs included in the analysis. Retinoids continue to be the best treatment for acne when used judiciously.

ORAL VITAMIN A FOR ACNE MANAGEMENT: A POSSIBLE SUBSTITUTE FOR ISOTRETINOIN

Background

Providers no longer have the ability to give their patients isotretinoin due to recent alterations to the iPLEDGE platform. When isotretinoin is not available, a potential alternative could be helpful. Vitamin A's application in the treatment of acne was the subject of research prior to the FDA's approval of isotretinoin, a vitamin A derivative.

Objective

The objective is to investigate whether vitamin A could be used in place of isotretinoin in situations where it is unavailable.

Methods

We led a survey of distributed writing from 1931 to 2021, in regard to the utilization of vitamin A in skin breakout treatment, utilizing PubMed and Google Researcher datasets. Nine examinations were chosen subsequent to looking into articles for pertinence to our point.

Results
Eight out of the nine examinations noted improvement in patients' skin breakout with vitamin A utilization. The doses used ranged from 36,000 to 500,000 I/U per day, with 100,000 I/U per day being the most prevalent. The majority of side effects were mucocutaneous.

Limitations
Many of the studies in our review were published >50 years ago, so they do not have the standard elements of clinical trials today.

Conclusions
Oral vitamin A might actually act as a substitute for isotretinoin in skin breakout administration for select patients. Be that as it may, because of its teratogenicity, potential for poisonousness, and long half-life, severe checking under the consideration of a clinical supplier is judicious. Since vitamin A is accessible without a remedy, severe checking cannot be guaranteed, and particularly cautious patient determination and schooling would be fundamental.

PATIENT-REPORTED OUTCOME MEASURES FOR HEALTH-RELATED QUALITY OF LIFE IN PATIENTS WITH ACNE VULGARIS: A SYSTEMATIC REVIEW OF MEASURE DEVELOPMENT AND MEASUREMENT PROPERTIES

Importance
There are a number of patient-reported outcome measures (PROMs) for acne patients' health-related quality of life (HRQoL). However, little is known about these PROMs' measurement properties and content validity.

Goal
The goal is to conduct a methodical analysis of PROMs for HRQoL in adults or adolescents with acne.

Data Sources
The eligible studies were retrieved from Embase (OVID) and PubMed.

Concentrate on Determination Full-text articles distributed in English or Spanish on improvement, pilot, or approval reads up for skin breakout unambiguous, dermatology-explicit, or conventional HRQoL PROMs were incorporated. Advancement concentrates on included unique improvement studies, regardless of whether not concentrated on in skin breakout patients per Agreement Based Guidelines for the Choice of Wellbeing Estimation Instruments (COSMIN) proposals. Over 50% of patients must have acne, or acne-specific subgroup analyses must be available, if a study included multiple diagnoses. Two independent reviewers assessed the abstract and full text.

Data Extraction and Synthesis
Two independent reviewers used the COSMIN checklist to evaluate the study's quality and extract and evaluate the data. The evidence's quality was graded according to a measurement property for each distinct PROM.

The remaining measurement properties (structural validity, internal consistency, cross-cultural validity, reliability, measurement error, criterion validity, construct validity, and responsiveness) as well as the PROM properties (target population, domains, recall period, and development language), PROM development and pilot studies, and content validity (relevance, comprehensiveness, and comprehensibility) are the primary outcomes and measures. Each measurement property of the included PROMs was assigned a quality of evidence. Based on the content validity and quality of the evidence of measurement properties, an overall recommendation level was established.

Results

We distinguished 54 skin inflammation PROM improvement or approval reads up for 10 skin breakout unambiguous PROMs, 6 dermatology-explicit PROMs, and 5 nonexclusive PROMs. Few PROMs had responsiveness studies. The CompAQ and Acne-Q are the only acne-specific PROMs with sufficient content validity evidence, and the Acne-Q and CompAQ can be recommended for use in acne clinical studies.

Relevance and Conclusions

There are currently two PROMs that can be used in acne clinical studies: the CompAQ and Acne-Q. All PROMs lacked evidence regarding content validity and other measurement properties; further exploration examining the nature of outstanding skin breakout unambiguous, dermatology-explicit, and nonexclusive HRQoL PROMs is expected to suggest their utilization.

ENDO-RADIOFREQUENCY SUBCISION FOR ACNE SCARS TREATMENT: A CASE SERIES STUDY

Background

Patients who suffer from acne scars experience significant psychosocial pain. Acne scars have been treated with a variety of interventions, each with varying degrees of efficacy and side effects. A multimodal strategy can accomplish improved results to working on the actual appearance of the patients that can altogether build the personal satisfaction. Subcision is a well-known treatment for rolling acne scars, but it needs to be improved in order to be more effective.

The study's objectives were to evaluate the safety and efficacy of Endo-Radiofrequency (Endo-RF) subcision for the treatment of acne scars.

Methods

Nine adult patients with atrophic acne scars were included in this study. One Endo-RF subcision is performed on each patient, and they are followed up on for 6 months. Biometric assessment with the Visioface 1000 D, the Mexameter and skin ultrasound imaging system, photographs taken after treatment, and the patient's level of satisfaction were used to evaluate outcome.

Results

The number of skin spots ($p < 0.05$) and fine and large pores ($p < 0.05$) decreased, indicating that patients had made significant progress from baseline. Additionally, the dermis and epidermis' density and thickness were significantly increased ($p < 0.05$).

Conclusions

The Endo-RF subcision technique is safe and effective for treating acne scars.

TAZAROTENE 0.045% LOTION FOR FEMALES WITH ACNE: ANALYSIS OF TWO ADULT AGE GROUPS

Background

Females matured ≥25 years might have skin inflammation with various etiology, show, weight, and treatment reaction than females of 18–24 years. This post hoc examination explored viability and well-being of tazarotene 0.045% salve in females ≥18 years or ≥25 years old.

Methods

Participants over the age of 9 years who had moderate-to-severe acne were randomly assigned, in two phase 3 double-blind studies, to receive either vehicle lotion or once-daily tazarotene 0.045% lotion for a period of 12 weeks. For females under the age of 18 years ($n = 744$) or under the age of 25 years ($n = 335$), pooled data were analyzed. Assessments included the Acne-QoL questionnaire, treatment-emergent adverse events (TEAEs), cutaneous safety and tolerability, and treatment success [a score of 0 (clear) or 1 (almost clear) or a two-grade reduction from baseline on the Evaluator's Global Severity Score].

Results

At week 12, women in both age groups treated with tazarotene had more significant decreases from the baseline than from the vehicle in provocative [18 years: 60.6% vs. 53.7%; ($p < 0.01$)]; ≥25 years: lesions that are not inflammatory (59.0% vs. 48.4% and 61.1% vs. 48.8%; $p > 0.05$) as well as inflammatory lesions (both $p = 0.01$). Paces of treatment achievement were more noteworthy with tazarotene versus vehicle; this distinction was critical for females ≥18 years. Skin breakout QoL upgrades were comparable across age gatherings and by and large more noteworthy with tazarotene than vehicle. The majority of TEAEs were mild to moderate in severity. No age-related patterns for security or decency were noticed.

Conclusions

Tazarotene 0.045% salve showed tantamount adequacy, improvement in personal satisfaction, and well-being in grown-up females matured ≥18 or ≥25 years with moderate-to-serious skin breakout. This cosmetically exquisite cream is a very much contemplated and significant treatment choice for all patients, especially grown-up females.

EFFICACY AND SAFETY OF TAZAROTENE LOTION 0.045% IN THE TREATMENT OF TRUNCAL ACNE VULGARIS

Background

In spite of the fact that truncal skin breakout is remembered to have the equivalent pathophysiology to facial skin inflammation, treatment reaction might vary in view of body region contribution. Prescribers have traditionally relied on oral treatments to treat truncal acne, possibly because oral treatments are more convenient than applying medication to the chest and back. The treatment of truncal acne may be best served by a lotion formulation. The FDA has approved tazarotene lotion (0.045%) for the treatment of acne vulgaris in adults over the age of 9 years. Arazlo lotion's efficacy and safety as a treatment for truncal acne were the goals of this pilot study.

Concentrate on Discoveries

The 12-week study was completed by 19 subjects ranging in age from 12 to 58 years. At each of the study follow-up visits, truncal IGA, the primary endpoint, decreased significantly. According to the truncal IGA score, 89% of subjects were clear or nearly clear at week 12. From the beginning to week 12, there were statistically significant decreases in the total, inflammatory, and noninflammatory lesion counts. Erythema, dryness, peeling, oiliness, pruritis, and burning were generally rated as trace or mild during treatment with tazarotene lotion 0.045%, and this treatment was well tolerated. Most subjects (64% or more) evaluated the cream as "Great" or "Fantastic" overall compared to their earlier medications.

Conclusions

Tazarotene salve 0.045% is demonstrated to be successful and all around endured for the administration of truncal skin breakout in this pilot study. Further examinations with fake treatment control and bigger populaces are justified.

ADVANCES IN TOPICAL MANAGEMENT OF ADOLESCENT FACIAL AND TRUNCAL ACNE: A PHASE 3 POOLED ANALYSIS OF SAFETY AND EFFICACY OF TRIFAROTENE 0.005% CREAM

Purpose

Acne vulgaris is extremely prevalent in young adults and adolescents. Acne assessment and treatment strategies that clinicians who treat these patients use on a daily basis are critical.

Methods

Post hoc examination of two huge scope stage 3 critical preliminaries of trifarotene 0.005% cream, zeroing in on adequacy, security, and bearableness in the subgroup of subjects matured 12–17, comprehensive.

Results

In patients with moderate acne between the ages of 12 and 17 years, trifarotene was effective and well tolerated on the trunk and face. Tolerability was good, and the rate of AEs was low enough to be considered acceptable.

Conclusions

Trifarotene monotherapy was related to great clinical viability, security, and bearableness. Patients appreciate the convenience of once-daily application, and the low concentration of trifarotene makes it suitable for use on large areas of skin like the trunk.

EPIDEMIOLOGY OF ACNE

Introduction

It is important to note that the prevalence of acne is increasing, and clinicians now see acne beginning in children as young as 8 or 9 years old. Although facial acne has received most of the attention in the medical literature, approximately 50% of patients with acne on their face also have lesions on their trunk (back or chest). Acne vulgaris is the most common skin condition among adolescents worldwide. This condition has been estimated to affect 85–90% of teenagers. It is important to note that the prevalence of acne is increasing. There have only been a few epidemiological studies of acne.

The natural course of acne is one of recurrence and remission. It is a chronic condition. Acne is frequently regarded as a skin condition that is relatively mild; nonetheless, negatively affecting personal satisfaction has been shown. Skin breakout has been related to unfortunate mental self-portrait, wretchedness, school truancy, tension, and even suicidality, a significant thought in the juvenile populace which as of now has a raised gamble for these emotional wellness issues. Likewise, enduring issues because of skin breakout can happen, including lesional hyperpigmentation and skin inflammation scarring. Misjudging the effect of skin inflammation on teenagers is a vital barricade to right-on-time and fruitful treatment. Further, prior treatment and effective administration might mean superior clinical results, lower risk for scarring, and a superior in general nature of life. Having a consideration methodology setup can assist with busying specialists offer fitting starting consideration for this practically omnipresent condition. For skin inflammation the executives suggest starting useful treatment at the earliest opportunity to limit the possible effect on life quality and long-haul sequelae.

Powerful skin breakout administration systems incorporate skin retinoids as a groundwork of treatment. Retinoids are viewed as the center gathering of skin breakout therapeutics because of various activities, including comedolytic and mitigating impacts, a deterrent impact by repressing development of skin inflammation forerunner sores (microcomedones), and an upkeep impact by normalizing epidermal turnover. What's more, skin retinoids have legitimate viability, security, and tolerability. Retinoids are accessible for use in more youthful patients, and in different details and fixations. The benefit of topical administration is improved local drug delivery to affected tissues with a low risk of systemic adverse effects.

LONG-TERM SAFETY AND EFFICACY OF CLASCOTERONE CREAM SHOWN IN ACNE TREATMENT

According to the findings of this extension study, clascoterone cream 1% demonstrated long-term efficacy and a favorable safety profile in patients with acne vulgaris who were older than 12 years old.

"Clascoterone cream 1% is a skin androgen receptor inhibitor endorsed for the treatment of skin inflammation vulgaris in patients matured (at least) 12 years of age," Lawrence F Eichenfield, MD, head of pediatric and adolescent dermatology at Rady Children's Hospital and teacher of dermatology and pediatrics and bad habit seat of the branch of dermatology at College of California, San Diego, partners wrote in a banner introduced at South Ocean side Conference.

Clascoterone cream 1% showed long-haul viability and an ideal security profile in patients matured more seasoned than 12 years with skin breakout vulgaris.

Patients who had completed one of the 12-week phase 3 clinical trials were included in the open-label, multicenter, long-term extension study. They applied clascoterone cream 1% to the face and to truncal skin inflammation two times every day for 9 extra months.

About 18.1% of patients in the subgroup of older patients experienced treatment-emergent AEs, the majority of which were mild and not thought to be related to the treatment.

Nasopharyngitis and upper respiratory parcel contamination were the most normally detailed treatment-emanant unfavorable occasions. "Among patients who completed the study without major protocol violation, the proportion achieving clear or almost clear skin of the face and trunk increased with duration of 1% clascoterone cream treatment and was highest for patients on-study for 12 months of treatment," the authors wrote.

ACNE SCARS IMPROVE WITH LASER PLUS TOPICAL TREATMENT

Use of an anhydrous gel with tripeptide and hexapeptides pre- and post-laser resurfacing significantly decreased postprocedural TEWL and erythema compared with a bland moisturizer, according to findings from a study published in *Clinical, Cosmetic and Investigational Dermatology*. The adjuvant therapy also increased improvement in acne scars and patient satisfaction.

Regenerating Skin Nectar with TriHex Technology (RSN; Alastin Skincare Inc.) was given to participants over the age of 18 years with grade 2 to 3 facial acne scars in the prospective, randomized study (or an uninteresting moisturizer (Cetaphil lotion; Galderma), which was used two times per day.

Participants attended seven study visits, including a screening and baseline visit 2 or more weeks prior to the first laser treatment, two visits for the laser treatment 1 month apart, and follow-up visits at day 4, 60 days after the last laser treatment. Assessments included TEWL, intensity of erythema, photography, Goodman and Baron qualitative scale, Global Aesthetic Improvement Scale, and patient satisfaction. A participant in each group had a 3-mm punch biopsy on the face before use of the products and 60 days after the second laser treatment. The study began in January 2020 and was completed in May 2021.

A total of five men and five women, 19–45 years of age, were included. Their mean age was 33.4 years, and four patients had skin type 1, two had type 2, three had type 3, and one had type 4.

Regarding TEWL, a statistically significant difference was found in lesional skin measurements at day 4 after both laser treatments. At day 4, after laser treatment 1, the RSN group had a mean change of 6.502 versus 21.59 in the control group ($p = 0.02$). At day 4 after laser treatment 2, a greater statistical difference of $p = 0.0001$ occurred, with an RSN group mean change of 2.858 versus 39.07 in the control group. For nonlesional skin, measurements for RSN participants were reduced before the first laser treatment (−5.098), compared with an increase in the control group of 2.061.

From day 4 after the laser procedure 1 to day 90 for both lesional and nonlesional skin, the erythema index consistently decreased in the RSN group compared to the control group. The RSN group had higher Goodman and Baron scores for acne scars than the control group. At day 30 after laser procedure 1, the RSN arm's mean improvement was −0.33, while the control group's improvement was −0.25. RSN participants had a mean improvement of −0.83 on day 90 after the second laser procedure, while control participants had a mean improvement of −0.40. At each visit following the initial laser procedure, participants in the RSN group rated their satisfaction with the improvement in acne scars as significantly higher than that of the control group, and this satisfaction was significantly higher at day 90.

The patient who underwent a biopsy and received the bland moisturizer had abnormally fragmented elastic fibers in the reticular dermis and lacked elastic fibers in the papillary dermis on day 0 of the study. On day 90, the properties of the elastin fibers in the reticular dermis began to change. On day 0 of the RSN participant's biopsy, elastic tissue stain revealed almost no elastic fibers in the superficial and deep dermis in the center of the specimen. On day 90, the papillary dermis contained relatively normal elastic fibers, and the reticular dermis contained additional fibers. On day 0, the RSN patient also had focally abnormally thin collagen bundles, and on day 90, normal-density collagen bundles slightly increased.

Suggested Readings

1. Sandoval AGW, Vaughn LT, Huang JT, Barbieri JS. Role of Tumor Necrosis Factor-α Inhibitors in the Treatment and Occurrence of Acne: A Systematic Review. JAMA Dermatol. 2023;159(5):504-9.
2. Adebamowo CA, Spiegelman D, Berkey CS, Danby FW, Rockett HH, Colditz GA, et al. Milk consumption and acne in adolescent girls. Dermatol Online J. 2006;12:1.
3. Adebamowo CA, Spiegelman D, Berkey CS, Danby FW, Rockett HH, Colditz GA, et al. Milk consumption and acne in teenaged boys. J Am Acad Dermatol. 2008;58:787-93.
4. Agak GW, Qin M, Nobe J, Kim MH, Krutzik SR, Tristan GR, et al. Propionibacterium acnes induces an IL-17 response in acne vulgaris that is regulated by vitamin A and vitamin D. J Invest Dermatol. 2014;134:366-73.
5. Akhavan A, Bershad S. Topical acne drugs: review of clinical properties, systemic exposure, and safety. Am J Clin Dermatol. 2003;4:473-92.
6. Alan S, Cenesizoglu E. Effects of hyperandrogenism and high body mass index on acne severity in women. Saudi Med J. 2014;35:886-9.
7. Alemzadeh R, Kichler J, Calhoun M. Spectrum of metabolic dysfunction in relationship with hyperandrogenemia in obese adolescent girls with polycystic ovary syndrome. Eur J Endocrinol. 2010;162:1093-9.
8. Alexis A, Heath CR, Halder RM. Folliculitis keloidalis nuchae and pseudofolliculitis barbae: are prevention and effective treatment within reach? Dermatol Clin. 2014;32:183-91.
9. Antoniou C, Dessinioti C, Stratigos AJ, Katsambas AD. Clinical and therapeutic approach to childhood acne: An update. Pediatr Dermatol. 2009;26:373-80.
10. Arowojolu AO, Gallo MF, Lopez LM, Grimes DA. Combined oral contraceptive pills for treatment of acne. Cochrane Database Syst Rev. 2012;(7):CD004425.
11. Asgharnia M, Mirblook F, Ahmad Soltani M. The Prevalence of Polycystic Ovary Syndrome (PCOS) in High School Students in Rasht in 2009 According to NIH Criteria. Int J Fertil Steril. 2011;4:156-9.
12. Ayhan M, Sancak B, Karaduman A, Arikan S, Sahin S. Colonization of neonate skin by Malassezia species: relationship with neonatal cephalic pustulosis. J Am Acad Dermatol. 2007;57:1012-8.
13. Bergman JN, Eichenfield LF. Neonatal acne and cephalic pustulosis: Is Malassezia the whole story? Arch Dermatol. 2002;138:255-7.
14. Bernier V, Weill FX, Hirigoyen V, Elleau C, Feyler A, Labrèze C, et al. Skin colonization by Malassezia species in neonates: A prospective study and relationship with neonatal cephalic pustulosis. Arch Dermatol. 2002;138:215-8.
15. Bettoli V, Zauli S, Virgili A. Is hormonal treatment still an option in acne today? Br J Dermatol. 2015;172 (Suppl 1):37-46.
16. Bhattacharya SM, Ghosh M. Insulin resistance and adolescent girls with polycystic ovary syndrome. J Pediatr Adolesc Gynecol. 2010;23:158-61.
17. Bree A, Siegfried E. Acne vulgaris in preadolescent children: recommendations for evaluation. Pediatr Dermatol. 2014;31:27-32.
18. Brodell LA, Hepper D, Lind A, Gru AA, Anadkat MJ. Histopathology of acneiform eruptions in patients treated with epidermal growth factor receptor inhibitors. J Cutan Pathol. 2013;40(10):865-70.
19. Brooke RC, Griffiths CE. Folliculitis decalvans. Clin Exp Dermatol. 2001;26:120-2.
20. Buhl T, Sulk M, Nowak P, Buddenkotte J, McDonald I, Aubert J, et al. Molecular and morphological characterization of inflammatory infiltrate in rosacea reveals activation of Th1/Th17 pathways. J Invest Dermatol. 2015;135:2198-208.
21. Cantatore-Francis JL, Glick SA. Childhood acne: Evaluation and management. Dermatol Ther. 2006;19:202-9.
22. O'Connor C, O'Grady C, Murphy M. Spotting fake news: a qualitative review of misinformation and conspiracy theories in acne vulgaris. Clin Exp Dermatol. 2022;47(9):1707-11.

23. Chen W, Obermayer-Pietsch B, Hong JB, Melnik BC, Yamasaki O, Dessinioti C, et al. Acne-associated syndromes: models for better understanding of acne pathogenesis. J Eur Acad Dermatol Venereol. 2011;25:637-46.
24. Chew EW, Bingham A, Burrows D. Incidence of acne vulgaris in patients with infantile acne. Clin Exp Dermatol. 1990;15:376-7.
25. Chicarilli ZN. Follicular occlusion triad: hidradenitis suppuritiva, acne conglobate and dissecting cellulitis of the scalp. Ann Plast Surg. 1987;18:230-7.
26. Choi JN. Chemotherapy induced iatrogenic injury of skin: new drugs and new concepts. Clin Dermatol. 2011;29:587-601.
27. Chronnell CMT, Ghali LR, Ali RS, Quinn AG, Holland DB, Bull JJ, et al. Human beta defensin-1 and -2 expression in human pilosebaceous units: upregulation in acne vulgaris lesions. J Invest Dermatol. 2001;117:1120-5.
28. Cretu S, Dascalu M, Salavastru CM. Acne care in health care providers during the COVID-19 pandemic: A national survey. Dermatol Ther. 2022;35(10):e15753.
29. Cunliffe WJ, Baron SE, Coulson IH. A clinical and therapeutic study of 29 patients with infantile acne. Br J Dermatol. 2001;145:463-6.
30. Davis SA, Sandoval LF, Gustafson CJ, Feldman SR, Cordoro KM. Treatment of preadolescent acne in the United States: an analysis of nationally representative data. Pediatr Dermatol. 2013;30:689-94.
31. Del Prete M, Mauriello MC, Faggiano A, Di Somma C, Monfrecola G, Fabbrocini G, et al. Insulin resistance and acne: a new risk factor for men? Endocrine. 2012;42:555-60.
32. Del Rosso J, Sugarman J, Gold M, Arekapdui K, Green L. A New Frontier in Acne Treatment: Encapsulated Benzoyl Peroxide and Tretinoin. SKIN J Cutan Med. 2022;6(2):s16.
33. Di Landro A, Cazzaniga S, Parazzini F, Ingordo V, Cusano F, Atzori L, et al; GISED Acne Study Group. Family history, body mass index, selected dietary factors, menstrual history, and risk of moderate to severe acne in adolescents and young adults. J Am Acad Dermatol. 2012;67:1129-35.
34. Draelos ZD, Carter E, Maloney JM, Elewski B, Poulin Y, Lynde C, et al; United States/Canada Dapsone Gel Study Group. Two randomized studies demonstrate the efficacy and safety of dapsone gel, 5% for the treatment of acne. J Am Acad Dermatol. 2007;56:439.e1-10.
35. Dréno B, Bettoli V, Ochsendorf F, Perez-Lopez M, Mobacken H, Degreef H, et al. An expert view on the treatment of acne with systemic antibiotics and/or oral isotretinoin in the light of the new European recommendations. Eur J Dermatol. 2006;15:565-71.
36. Dréno B, Blouin E, Moyse D, Bodokh I, Knol AC, Khammari A. Acne in pregnant women: a French survey. Acta Derm Venereol. 2014;94:82-3.
37. Dréno B, Fischer TC, Perosino E, Poli F, Viera MS, Rendon MI, et al. Expert opinion: efficacy of superficial chemical peels in active acne management: what can we learn from the literature today? Evidence-based recommendations. J Eur Acad Dermatol Venereol. 2011;25:695-704.
38. Eichenfield LF, Krakowski AC, Piggot C, Del Rosso J, Baldwin H, Friedlander SF, et al; American Acne and Rosacea Society. Evidence-based recommendations for the diagnosis and treatment of pediatric acne. Pediatrics. 2013;131(Suppl. 3):S163-86.
39. Esmat SM, Abdel Hay RM, Abu Zeid OM, Hosni HN. The efficacy of laser-assisted hair removal in the treatment of acne keloidalis nuchae; a pilot study. Eur J Dermatol. 2012;22:645-50.
40. Friedlander SF, Eichenfield LF, Fowler JF Jr, Fried RG, Levy ML, Webster GF. Acne epidemiology and pathophysiology. Semin Cutan Med Surg. 2010;29(2 Suppl 1):2-4.
41. Gemmeke A, Wollina U. Folliculitis decalvans of the scalp: response to triple therapy with isotretinoin, clindamycin, and prednisolone. Acta Dermatovenereol Alp Pannonica Adriat. 2006;15:184-6.
42. Gollnick HP, Bettoli V, Lambert J, Araviiskaia E, Binic I, Dessinioti C, et al. A consensus-based practical and daily guide for the treatment of acne patients. J Eur Acad Dermatol Venereol. 2016;30:1480-90.
43. Goulden V, Stables GI, Cunliffe WJ. Prevalence of facial acne in adults. J Am Acad Dermatol. 1999;41:577-80.
44. Gupta MA, Gupta AK. The psychological comorbidity in acne. Clin Dermatol. 2001;19:360-3.
45. Gürok NG. The correlation between ABO blood types and acne vulgaris severity. J Cosmet Dermatol. 2023;22(8):2318-23.
46. Hahn S, Bering van Halteren W, Roesler S, Schmidt M, Kimmig R, Tan S, et al. The combination of increased ovarian volume and follicle number is associated with more severe hyperandrogenism in German women with polycystic ovary syndrome. Exp Clin Endocrinol Diabetes. 2006;114:175-81.

Suggested Readings

47. Harper JC. Evaluating hyperandrogenism: a challenge in acne management. J Drugs Dermatol. 2008;7: 527-30.
48. Hayashi N, Akamatsu H, Kawashima M. Establishment of grading criteria for acne severity. J Dermatol. 2008;35(5):295-60.
49. Hebert A, Eichenfield L, Thiboutot D, Stein Gold L, Vassileva S, Mihaylova Y, et al. Efficacy and safety of 1% clascoterone cream in patients aged > 12 years with acne vulgaris. J Drugs Dermatol. 2023;22(2):174-81.
50. Hurtado-Nedelec M, Chollet-Martin S, Nicaise-Roland P, Grootenboer-Mignot S, Ruimy R, Meyer O, et al. Characterization of the immune response in the synovitis, acne, pustulosis, hyperostosis, osteitis (SAPHO) syndrome. Rheumatology (Oxford). 2008;47:1160-7.
51. Husein-ElAhmed H. Management of acne vulgaris with hormonal therapies in adult female patients. Dermatol Ther. 2015;28:166-72.
52. Imperato-McGinley J, Gautier T, Cai LQ, Yee B, Epstein J, Pochi P. The androgen control of sebum production. Studies of subjects with dihydrotestosterone deficiency and complete androgen insensitivity. J Clin Endocrinol Metab. 1993;76:524-8.
53. Ismail NH, Manaf ZA, Azizan NZ. High glycemic load diet, milk and ice cream consumption are related to acne vulgaris in Malaysian young adults: a case control study. BMC Dermatol. 2012;12:13.
54. Nowicki J, Mills M, Van Der Veken J, Pantelis I, Daniels S, Poonnoose S. The effectiveness of prophylactic antibiotics and betadine skin preparation on cranial cutaneous Cutibacterium acnes—A prospective study. J Clin Neurosci. 2022;100:33-6.
55. Jansen T, Burgdorf WH, Plewig G. Pathogenesis and treatment of acne in childhood. Pediatr Dermatol. 1997;14:17-21.
56. Jung JY, Yoon MY, Min SU, Hong JS, Choi YS, Suh DH. The influence of dietary patterns on acne vulgaris in Koreans. Eur J Dermatol. 2010;20:768-72.
57. Kamangar F, Shinkai K. Acne in the adult female patient: a practical approach. Int J Dermatol. 2012;51: 1162-11.
58. Kim J. Review of the innate immune response in acne vulgaris: activation of Toll-like receptor 2 in acne triggers inflammatory cytokine responses. Dermatology. 2005;211:193-8.
59. Kistowska M, Gehrke S, Jankovic D, Kerl K, Fettelschoss A, Feldmeyer L, et al. IL-1β drives inflammatory responses to Propionibacterium acnes in vitro and in vivo. J Invest Dermatol. 2014;134:677-85.
60. Kistowska M, Meier B, Proust T, Feldmeyer L, Cozzio A, Kuendig T, et al. Propionibacterium acnes promotes Th17 and Th17/Th1 responses in acne patients. J Invest Dermatol. 2015;135:110-8.
61. Goldberg JL, Dabade TS, Davis SA, Feldman SR, Krowchuk DP, Fleischer AB. Changing age of acne vulgaris visits: another sign of earlier puberty? Pediatr Dermatol. 2011;28:645-8.
62. Kurokawa I, Layton AM, Ogawa R. Updated treatment for acne: targeted therapy based on pathogenesis. Dermatol Ther (Heidelb). 2021;11(4):1129-39.
63. Kutlu Ö, Karadağ AS, Wollina U. Adult acne versus adolescent acne: A narrative review with a focus on epidemiology to treatment. An Bras Dermatol. 2023;98(1):75-83.
64. Lachiewicz AM, Wilkinson JM, Groben P, Ollila DW, Thomas NE. Muir-Torre syndrome. Am J Clin Dermatol. 2007;8:215-9.
65. Lacouture ME, Maitland ML, Segaert S, Setser A, Baran R, Fox LP, et al. A proposed EGFR inhibitor dermatologic adverse event-specific grading scale from the MASCC skin toxicity study group. Support Care Cancer. 2010;18:509-22.
66. Lacouture ME. Mechanisms of cutaneous toxicities to EGFR inhibitors. Nat Rev Cancer. 2006;6:803-12.
67. Lasek RJ, Chren MM. Acne vulgaris and the quality of life of adult dermatology patients. Arch Dermatol. 1998;134:454-8.
68. Eichenfield L, Kwong P, Lee S, Krowchuk D, Arekapudi K, Hebert A. Advances in Topical Management of Adolescent Facial and Truncal Acne: A Phase 3 Pooled Analysis of Safety and Efficacy of Trifarotene 0.005% Cream. J Drugs Dermatol. 2022;21(6):582-6.
69. Lee SE, Kim JM, Jeong SK, Choi EH, Zouboulis CC, Lee SH. Expression of protease-activated receptor-2 in SZ95 sebocytes and its role in sebaceous lipogenesis, inflammation, and innate immunity. J Invest Dermatol. 2015;135:2338.

70. Kircik L. Efficacy and Safety of Tazarotene Lotion, 0.045% in the Treatment of Truncal Acne Vulgaris. J Drugs Dermatol. 2022;21(7):713-6.
71. Li ZJ, Choi DK, Sohn KC, Seo MS, Lee HE, Lee Y, et al. Propionibacterium acnes activates the NLRP3 inflammasome in human sebocytes. J Invest Dermatol. 2014;134:2747-56.
72. Stein Gold L, Kircik L, Baldwin H, Callender V, Tanghetti E, Del Rosso J, et al. Tazarotene 0.045% Lotion for Females With Acne: Analysis of Two Adult Age Groups. J Drugs Dermatol. 2022;21(5):587-95.
73. Ljubojevic S, Pasic A, Lipozencic J, Skerlev M. Perifolliculitis capitis abscendens et suffodiens. J Eur Acad Dermatol Venereol. 2005;19:719-21.
74. Lolis MS, Bowe WP, Shalita AR. Acne and systemic disease. Med Clin North Am. 2009;93:1161-81.
75. Lucky AW, Biro FM, Huster GA, Morrison JA, Elder N. Acne vulgaris in early adolescent boys. Correlations with pubertal maturation and age. Arch Dermatol. 1991;127:210-6.
76. Lucky AW, Biro FM, Huster GA, Leach AD, Morrison JA, Ratterman J. Acne vulgaris in premenarchal girls. An early sign of puberty associated with rising levels of dehydroepiandrosterone. Arch Dermatol. 1994;130: 308-14.
77. Lucky AW. A review of infantile and pediatric acne. Dermatology. 1998;196:95-7.
78. Lucky AW. Hormonal correlates of acne and hirsutism. Am J Med. 1995;98:89S-94S.
79. Lucky AW. Quantitative documentation of a premenstrual flare of facial acne in adult women. Arch Dermatol. 2004;140:423-4.
80. Cook M, Perche P, Feldman S. Oral Vitamin A for Acne Management: A Possible Substitute for Isotretinoin. J Drugs Dermatol. 2022;21(6):683-6.
81. Mahé E, Morelon E, Lechaton S, Drappier JC, de Prost Y, Kreis H, et al. Acne in recipients of renal transplantation treated with sirolimus: clinical, microbiologic, histologic, therapeutic, and pathogenic aspects. J Am Acad Dermatol. 2006;55:139-42.
82. Mancini AJ, Baldwin HE, Eichenfield LF, Friedlander SF, Yan AC. Acne life cycle: the spectrum of pediatric disease. Semin Cutan Med Surg. 2011;30(3 Suppl):S2-5.
83. Mavranezouli I, Daly CH, Welton NJ, Deshpande S, Berg L, Bromham N, et al. A systematic review and network meta-analysis of topical pharmacological, oral pharmacological, physical and combined treatments for acne vulgaris. Br J Dermatol. 2022;187(5):639-49.
84. Miller IM, Echeverría B, Torrelo A, Jemec GB. Infantile acne treated with oral isotretinoin. Pediatr Dermatol. 2013;3:513-8.
85. Nilforoushzadeh MA, Heidari-Kharaji M, Fakhim T, Torkamaniha E, Nouri M, Rafiee S, et al. Endo-Radiofrequency subcision for acne scars treatment: A case series study. J Cosmet Dermatol. 2022;21(11):5651-6.
86. Monk B, Cunliffe WJ, Layton AM, Rhodes DJ. Acne induced by inhaled corticosteroids. Clin Exp Dermatol. 1993;18:148-50.
87. Mourelatos K, Eady EA, Cunliffe WJ, Clark SM, Cove JH. Temporal changes in sebum excretion and propionibacterial colonization in preadolescent children with and without acne. Br J Dermatol. 2007;156: 22-31.
88. Muto Y, Wang Z, Vanderberghe M, Two A, Gallo RL, Di Nardo A. Mast cells are key mediators of cathelicidin-initiated skin inflammation in rosacea. J Invest Dermatol. 2014;134:2728-36.
89. Nanney LB, Stoscheck CM, King LE Jr, Underwood RA, Holbrook KA. Immunolocalization of epidermal growth factor receptors in normal developing human skin. J Invest Dermatol. 1990;94:742-8.
90. Nast A, Dréno B, Bettoli V, Bukvic Mokos Z, Degitz K, Dressler C, et al. European evidence-based (S3) guideline for the treatment of acne—update 2016—short version. J Eur Acad Dermatol Venereol. 2016;30:1261-8.
91. Nast A, Dréno B, Bettoli V, Degitz K, Erdmann R, Finlay AY, et al. European evidence-based (S3) guidelines for the treatment of acne. J Eur Acad Dermatol Venereol. 2012;26(Suppl 1):1-29.
92. Niamba P, Weill FX, Sarlangue J, Labrèze C, Couprie B, Taïeh A. Is common neonatal cephalic pustulosis (neonatal acne) triggered by Malassezia sympodialis? Arch Dermatol. 1998;134:995-8.
93. Hrapovic N, Richard T, Messaraa C, Li X, Abbaspour A, Fabre S, et al. Clinical and metagenomic profiling of hormonal acne-prone skin in different populations. J Cosmet Dermatol. 2022;21(11):6233-42.
94. Oeff MK, Seltmann H, Hiroi N, Nastos A, Makrantonaki E, Bornstein SR, et al. Differential regulation of Toll-like receptor and CD14 pathways by retinoids and corticosteroids in human sebocytes. Dermatology. 2006;213:266.

Suggested Readings

95. Oh SW, Kim MY, Lee JS, Kim SC. Keratin 17 mutation in pachyonychia congenita type 2 patient with early onset steatocystoma multiplex and Hutchinson-like tooth deformity. J Dermatol. 2006;33:161-4.
96. Perez-Soler R, Saltz L. Cutaneous adverse effects with HER1/EGFR targeted agents: is there a silver lining? J Clin Oncol. 2005;23:5235-46.
97. Picardo M, Eichenfield LF, Tan J. Acne and Rosacea. Dermatol Ther (Heidelb). 2017;7(Suppl 1):43-52.
98. Tan J, Chavda R, Leclerc M, Dréno B. Projective Personification Approach to the Experience of People With Acne and Acne Scarring—Expressing the Unspoken. JAMA Dermatol. 2022;158(9):1005-12.
99. Pugashetti R, Shinkai K. Treatment of acne vulgaris in pregnant patients. Dermatol Ther. 2013;26:302-11.
100. Huang Q, Chen D, Pan S, Hu M, Wang P, Wang H, et al. Efficacy of alpha hydroxy acid combined with intense pulsed light in the treatment of acne vulgaris: A meta-analysis. J Cosmet Dermatol. 2022;21(11):5642-50.
101. Quinn M, Shinkai K, Pasch L, Kuzmich L, Cedars M, Huddleston H. Prevalence of androgenic alopecia in patients with polycystic ovary syndrome and characterization of associated clinical and biochemical features. Fertil Steril. 2014;101:1129-34.
102. Razavi Z, Moeini B, Shafiei Y, Bazmamoun H. Prevalence of anabolic steroid use and associated factors among body-builders in Hamadan, West Province of Iran. J Res Health Sci. 2014;14:163-6.
103. Rodriguez Baisi KE, Weaver AL, Shakshouk H, Tollefson MM. Acne incidence in preadolescents and association with increased body mass index: A population-based retrospective cohort study of 643 cases with age- and sex-matched community controls. Pediatr Dermatol. 2023;40(3):428-33.
104. Sand FL, Thomsen SF. Adalimumab for the treatment of refractory acne conglobata. JAMA Dermatol. 2013;149:1306-7.
105. Sardana K, Sharma RC, Sarkar R. Seasonal variation in acne vulgaris—myth or reality. J Dermatol. 2002;29(8):484-8.
106. Serna-Tamayo C, Janniger CK, Micali G, Schwartz RA. Neonatal and infantile acne vulgaris: an update. Cutis. 2014;94:13-6.
107. Smith RN, Braue A, Varigos GA, Mann NJ. The effect of a low glycemic load diet on acne vulgaris and the fatty acid composition of skin surface triglycerides. J Dermatol Sci. 2008;50:41-52.
108. Smolinski KN, Yan AC. Acne update: 2004. Curr Opin Pediatr. 2004;16:385-91.
109. Stoll S, Shalita AR, Webster GF, Kaplan R, Danesh S, Penstein A. The effect of the menstrual cycle on acne. J Am Acad Dermatol. 2001;45:957-60.
110. Sulk M, Seeliger S, Aubert J, Schwab VD, Cevikbas F, Rivier M, et al. Distribution and expression of non-neuronal transient receptor potential (TRPV) ion channels in rosacea. J Invest Dermatol. 2012;132:1253-62.
111. Tamaki C, Miyatake J, Yamagata T, Nozaki Y, Yu H, Sugiyama M, et al. Case of acne fulminans associated with hemophagocytosis. Nihon Naika Gakkai Zasshi. 2004;93:1632-3.
112. Tan J, Beissert S, Cook-Bolden F, Chavda R, Harper J, Hebert A, et al. Evaluation of psychological well-being and social impact of atrophic acne scarring: A multinational, mixed-methods study. JAAD Int. 2021;6:43-50.
113. Terzi E, Türsen B, Dursun P, Erdem T, Türsen Ü. The Relationship between ABO Blood Groups and Acne Vulgaris. Saudi J Med Med Sci. 2016;4(1):26-8.
114. Thiboutot D. Acne: hormonal concepts and therapy. Clin Dermatol. 2004;22:419-28.
115. Thiboutot DM, Craft N, Rissmann R, Gatlik E, Souquières M, Jones J, et al. Anti-IL-17A blockade did not significantly reduce inflammatory lesions in a placebo-controlled pilot study in adult patients with moderate to severe acne. J Dermatolog Treat. 2023;34(1):2138691.
116. Tosti A, Guerra L, Bettoli V. Solid facial edema as a complication of acne vulgaris in twins. J Am Acad Dermatol. 1987;17:843-4.
117. Uhara H, Kawachi S, Saida T. Solid facial edema in a patient with rosacea. J Dermatol. 2000;27:214-16.
118. Webster GF. Inflammatory acne represents hypersensitivity to Propionibacterium acnes. Dermatology. 1998;196(1):80-1.
119. Weinstein Velez M, Prezzano J, Bell M, Widgerow A. A single center, prospective, randomized, blinded study to evaluate the efficacy and safety of a topical tripeptide/hexapeptide anhydrous gel when used pre- and post- hybrid fractional laser for the treatment of acne scars. Clin Cosmet Investig Dermatol. 2022;15:2763-74.
120. Yamasaki K, Di Nardo A, Bardan A, Murakami M, Ohtake T, Coda A, et al. Increased serine protease activity and cathelicidin promotes skin inflammation in rosacea. Nat Med. 2007;13:975-80.

121. Yamasaki K, Kanada K, Macleod DT, Borkowski AW, Morizane S, Nakatsuji T, et al. TLR2 expression is increased in rosacea and stimulates enhanced serine protease production by keratinocytes. J Invest Dermatol. 2011;131:688-97.
122. Yamasaki K, Schauber J, Coda A, Lin H, Dorschner RA, Schechter NM, et al. Kallikrein-mediated proteolysis regulates the antimicrobial effects of cathelicidins in skin. FASEB J. 2006;20(12):2068-80.
123. Hopkins ZH, Thiboutot D, Homsi HA, Perez-Chada LM, Barbieri JS. Patient-Reported Outcome Measures for Health-Related Quality of Life in Patients With Acne Vulgaris: A Systematic Review of Measure Development and Measurement Properties. JAMA Dermatol. 2022;158(8):900-11.
124. Zaenglein AL, Pathy AL, Schlosser BJ, Alikhan A, Baldwin HE, Berson DS, et al. Guidelines of care for the management of acne vulgaris. J Am Acad Dermatol. 2016;74(5):945-73.e33.
125. Zouboulis CC, Bettoli V. Management of severe acne. Br J Dermatol. 2015;172(Suppl 1):27-36.
126. Zouboulis CC, Eady A, Philpott M, Goldsmith LA, Orfanos C, Cunliffe WC, et al. What is the pathogenesis of acne? Exp Dermatol. 2005;14:143-52.

Index

Page numbers followed by *b* refer to box, *f* refer to figure, *fc* refer to flowchart, and *t* refer to table.

A

ABO blood type 143
Abscess 74
Acanthosis nigricans 10, 57*f*, 61, 93*f*, 94*f*, 103
Acne 1, 5*f*-8*f*, 10, 12, 14, 26*f*, 28*f*, 34*f*, 36, 39*f*, 41*f*, 43*f*, 57*f*, 61, 81*f*, 90*f*, 96*f*, 99, 105, 106*f*, 108, 120*t*, 121*f*, 124*b*, 149, 154, 157
  acanthosis nigricans 101*f*
  adolescent 62, 62*t*
  adult-onset 21, 52, 61*b*, 62, 62*t*
  aestivalis 66, 112
  aggravator of 8*f*
  agminata 112
  antiandrogen therapy in 126*f*
  application in 134*t*
  boy with 31*f*
  causation of 20, 20*b*
  child with 45*b*
  childhood 39, 40*f*, 87*f*, 91, 109
  chronicity of 9*f*
  classical nodulocystic 32*f*
  classification of 2, 2*t*
  clinical manifestation of 52
  coal 64, 65
  coexist with 84*f*
  comedonal 61
  complications of 91, 97*fc*
  conditions in 10, 10*b*
  conglobata 35, 53*f*, 59*f*, 62, 72, 75, 111
  correlates, severity of 4*f*
  cosmetic 14, 55*f*
  cosmetica 65, 67
  cutibacterium 3, 6*f*, 11, 18, 20, 21, 35, 39*f*, 100, 108, 149, 153, 157
  cysts 31*f*
  detergent 65
  development of 11*fc*
  diagnosis of 99, 100
  diet in 131, 133
  differential diagnosis of 80
  drug 35*b*, 68, 70, 108
  early-onset 88*f*
  epidemiology of 162
  epidermal barrier impairments
    innate to 129
  eruption 60*f*
  etiology of 3*f*
  etiopathogenesis of 3, 11, 11*b*
  excoriée 55*f*, 67, 90*f*, 112
  female facial skin with 5*f*
  flare 123
  girl having 87*f*
  girl with 10*f*
  grade 37, 45, 106*f*
  granulomatous 68, 112
  histoclinical correlation of 21*f*
  hormonal 39, 80, 126, 128*fc*, 157
    therapy in 127*t*
  in adolescents, resistant 96*f*
  in boy 9*f*
  in smoker, severe 9*f*
  in teenager, mild 32*f*
  in women, early onset 149
  incidence 152
  indications for oral retinoid in 121*b*
  infantile 44, 91, 109
  inflammation in 20
  inflammatory 6*f*, 8*f*, 58*f*, 95*f*
    lesions of 48*f*
    papules of 81*f*
  keloidal scars in 93*f*
  keloidalis nuchae 59*f*, 75, 113
  late-onset 52*f*, 53*f*, 62*t*, 149
  lotion for females with 160
  major pathogenic factors in 3, 3*b*
  majority of 117
  management of 91, 126, 129, 158
  marking, papules of 43*f*
  mechanical 112
  mid-childhood 43*f*, 44, 45, 91
  mild 44*f*
    childhood 43*f*, 44*f*
  mild-to-moderate 33*f*, 153
  mimicking 83*f*, 84*f*
  moderate 33*f*, 44*f*
  moderate-to-severe 144, 152, 154
  natural course of 162
  neonatal 39, 109
  neoplastic conditions
    mimicking 86
  nodulocystic 93*f*
  noninflammatory 13
  occupational 63
  occurrence of 146
  oil 64, 65, 112
  oral isotretinoin in 122*b*
  papules of 43*f*, 84*f*
  pathogenesis 10, 17*f*
    of adult female 22
  pathogenic factor in 39*f*
  pathophysiology of 21, 21*b*
  pediatric 21, 22
    participants 144
  penile 77
  perpetuation of 10
  persistent 53*f*
    nodular lesions of 31*f*
  pitch 64, 112
    scars of 108*f*
  pityrosporum 121
  polymorphic inflammatory disease 30*f*
  pregnancy 79, 131
  premenstrual flare of 14
  prepubertal 22, 40*f*, 45
  primary lesions of 27*f*
  procedural management in 133
  psychological effects of 98
  pustules 82*f*
  radiation 66, 112
  role of genetics in 12, 12*b*

INDEX

rosacea 21, 23, 60f, 75
safely treats 150
scattered papules of 10f
sequelae of 91, 134t
severe 7f, 33f, 34f, 62, 101f
   active 155
severity of 7f, 37, 44f
side effects of topical treatment in 117
spectra of 21
steatocystoma with 81f, 82f
steroid 68, 70t
superficial ulcer in 93f
syndromes 70
systemic agents in 117
systemic drugs in 119fc
tarda 52
teenager with 101f
telltale evidence of 34f
temporal 31f, 42f
therapy-resistant 32f
topical agents in 113b
topical antimicrobials in 114b
topical medications in 117t
treatment of 106, 108fc, 109f, 110fc, 110t, 111fc, 113, 146, 157
tropical 65, 66, 112
truncal 29f, 89f, 102f, 161
type 39, 80
   of comedones in 36, 36b
unilateral 85f
user-friendly grading system for 38b
variants of 39, 61
varioliformis 75, 113
venenata 55f, 65
with facial edema 73
with hirsutism 94f
with insulin resistance 90f
with menstrual irregularity 94f
with polycystic ovary syndrome 88f
with psychological problems 67
Acne fulminans 21, 23, 35, 63, 103, 105, 111, 123
   etiology of 23
Acne lesion 82f, 83f
   adolescent with 82f
   type of 8f
Acne papule 54f, 57f, 93f, 96f
   excoriation of 58f
   milia mimicking 83f
Acne patient
   assessment of 99
   female 103b
   quality of life of 38t
Acne scar 92f, 154
   fillers for 142
   improve 163
   management 156
   punch techniques for 142
   treatment, endo-radiofrequency subcision for 160
Acne variants 52, 61b
   treatment of 109, 156
Acne vulgaris 1, 35, 39, 42f, 45, 46, 48f-51f, 64, 64t, 70, 70t, 87f, 91, 112, 143 159
   adolescent 49f
   early pustular lesion of 47f
   epidermal barrier dysfunctions in 129
   etiopathogenesis of 144
   grading in 46
   nodulocystic lesions 51f
   papulopustule of 49f
   signs in 91b
   with erythema 50f
   with facial pigmentation 51f
   with scars 50f
Acne-affected skin 130
Acneiform eruption 55f, 68, 77, 78b
   drugs inducing 16, 16b, 69b
Acneiform lesions 77, 78
   drug-induced 112
Acneiform nevi 79
Acne-prone skin 130
Actinomycin D 16, 78
Adalimumab 146
Adapalene 118, 132
Adrenal glands 22
Adrenal hyperplasia
   congenital 62, 104
   late-onset 53f
Adrenocorticotropic hormone 10, 22, 69
Affection, site of 46
Agent
   anti-inflammatory 115
   causative 65
   chemicals 24
   hormone-modifying 158
   hypoglycemic 132
   ingested 24
Alcohol 13
Alcoholic betadine solution 154
Allergic type 80
Alopecia 10, 105
   androgenetic 27f, 32f, 103
   patterned 61, 102f
Alpha hydroxy acid 135, 156
   efficacy of 156
Amineptine 16
Amoxicillin 118, 131
Androgen
   effect of 18f
   secreting tumor 62
Androgen-metabolizing enzymes 132
Androgen-secreting tumors 105
Angiogenic peptides 23
Ankylosing spondylitis 10
Anorexia 61
Anti-acne 112
   drugs, pregnancy category of systemic 131t
   topical 132t
   medications, side effects of topical 118t
Antibacterial agents, side effects of 120t
Antibiogram 100
Antibiotics 113
   topical 114
Antidepressants 69
Antimicrobial peptides 25
Antioxidants 133
APAAN syndrome 56f, 57f, 61, 70, 71, 94f
   with diabetes 94f
Apert's syndrome 12, 61, 70, 71
Arthralgia 72
Asthma 98
Asymmetric lesions 66
Atrophic acne 155, 160
   scars 155
Axilla mimicking hidradenitis suppurativa 82f
Azelaic acid 113, 116-118, 132, 148, 158
Azithromycin 118, 119, 131

B

Bacterial pustular eruption mimicking acne 81f
Bacterial pustules 82f
Benzoyl peroxide 109, 111, 113, 116-118, 132, 153
   face wash 107f
Beta hydroxy acids 135
Blocked pilosebaceous ducts 6f

INDEX

Blue-light therapy 135
Body dysmorphic disorder 67, 68
Body mass index 13, 128, 152
Body surface 79
Bone pain 63, 72
Breast tissue, lesions over 59*f*
Bulimia nervosa 61
Buserelin 16, 69

C

Cabergoline 16, 69
Calcium antagonist 16
Carbamazepine 16, 61, 69
Cathelicidin 20, 21
Causative organisms 20
Cefazolin 154
Cellular debris 27*f*
Cephalexin 118, 131
Cetaphil lotion 163
Cetuximab 16, 69
Cheilitis 107*f*, 122
Chemicals inducing chloracne 15, 15*b*
Chest pain 72
Chloracne 64, 64*t*, 65, 102, 103
  diagnosis of 37
  lesions 112
Chlorodiphenyl oxide 64
Cisplatin 16, 78
Clascoterone 148
  cream 146, 147
Cleansers 130
Clindamycin 114, 118, 132
  phosphate 144
Clofazimine 16, 61, 69
Clostridium 114
Combined oral contraceptive pills 117, 124, 124*b*, 128
Comedogenesis 4*f*, 5*f*
Comedogenic products 67
Comedonal acne, boy with 8*f*
Comedone 29*f*, 35, 36, 47*f*, 65
  absence of 68
  extraction 133, 134
  over back 29*f*
  papule pustule 27*f*
  types of 36
Complementary therapy 132
Comprehensive acne severity system 100*t*
Coronavirus disease 2019 (COVID-19) 148
Corticosteroids 126

Cosmetic
  chronic 14
  preparations 16
  role of 61
CRABPI genes 12
Craniofacial osteosclerosis 72
C-reactive protein 103
Crohn's disease 63
Cryotherapy 134
Cushing's syndrome 71, 104, 105
Cutaneous lesions 35
Cutibacterium acnes, role of 20
Cw6 gene 12
Cyclophosphamide 16, 78
Cyclosporine 16, 61
Cyproterone acetate 117, 126, 128
Cyst 35, 86
  aspiration of 135
  incision of 135
Cystic lesion 31*f*, 82*f*
  classical 31*f*
Cytotoxic drugs 78

D

Dactinomycin 61, 69
Daily activity 79
Daily work 79
Danazol 69
Dantrolene 16, 69
Dapsone 113*b*, 114*b*, 118*t*, 131, 132
  therapy 111
Darier's disease 84*f*
  papules of 84*f*
Dehydroepiandrosterone
  production of 22
  sulfate 22, 91
Demodex
  folliculorum 24
  species 24
Depression 77
Dermabrasion 136
Dermal matrix degeneration 24
Dermaroller 138
Dermatitis, signs of 130
Dermatology life quality index 99
Dermatosis papulosa nigra 81*f*
Diabetes 98
Diabetic mimicking acne 82*f*
Diabetic woman 53*f*
Disulfiram 16, 69
Dizygotic twins, monozygotic than 12
Dizziness 125

Doxycycline 118, 131
Dry skin 122
Ductal antigens 7*f*
Ductal hypercornification 3*f*
Ductal keratinocytes 4*f*
Dysmenorrhea 104

E

Ears 76
Eating disorder 68
Edema, areas of 79
Elevated testosterone 102*f*
Emotional disturbance 79
Encapsulated benzoyl peroxide cream 150
Endocrine
  abnormality 43*f*
  disorders 61, 62*t*
  profile, normal 94*f*
  tests 103
  work-up 104*b*
    indications for 103*b*
Enthesitis 72
Environmental factors
  influencing acne 12, 12*b*
Epidermal changes, medication-induced 130
Epidermal growth factor receptor 69, 112
  inhibitors 79*t*
Epidermis–superficial dermis 25
Epilepsy 98
Epistaxis 122
Erlotinib 16
Erythema 34*f*, 92*f*, 97, 148
  areas of 79
  intensity of 163
  nodosum 63, 111
Erythematotelangiectatic rosacea 76
Erythematotelangiectatic type 76, 86
Erythematous papules 47*f*
Erythromycin 114, 118, 131, 132
Ethinyl estradiol 128
Exanthem 123
Eyelid, milium near lower 42*f*

F

Face 65
Facial acne 52, 95*f*, 146, 154, 162
Facial edema 57*f*
Facial erythema 123
Facial palsy 85*f*

Facial skin inflammation vulgaris 147
Factors aggravating rosacea 23, 23b
Famotidine 16, 69
Fatal hepatotoxicity 125
Fatigue 125
Ferritin expression 24
Fluorouracil 16
Flutamide 125
Follicles, upper part of 5f
Follicle-stimulating hormone 96f, 101f
Follicular duct 6f, 19
Follicular epidermal hyperproliferation 17
Follicular occlusion tetrad 74, 75t
Folliculitis mimicking pustular acne 83f
Follitropin alfa 16, 69b
Fractional lasers 141

G

Gabapentin 16, 69
Galderma 163
Ganciclovir 16, 61, 69
Gastrointestinal symptoms 119
Gefitinib 16
Genetics 11
Germinative cells 20
Glucocorticoids 22
Glucose tolerance test 95f
  abnormal 94f, 95f
Glucose-6-phosphate dehydrogenase 111
Gnathophyma 76
Gonadotropin-releasing hormone agonists 128
Gram-negative folliculitis 66, 112
Granulomatous rosacea 77
Green-light therapy 135

H

Hair follicle 25
HAIR-AN syndrome 70, 71
Headache 122, 125
Healthy skin systems 157
Helicobacter pylori 24
Hematuria 122
Hidradenitis suppurativa 10, 58f, 59f, 72, 73, 75
  affecting gluteal region 58f
  stages of 74, 74t
Hirsutism 10, 41f, 96f, 103, 105, 123

Hirsutism acanthosis nigricans 102f
Hormonal contraceptives 124, 157
Hormonal therapy 107f, 124
Hormone 15, 16, 69
  profile 104, 105
  abnormal 95f
  altered 101f
Human epidermal cells 15
Human immunodeficiency virus 119
Human β-defensins 20
Hyperostosis 10, 12, 72
Hypertrophic scars 37, 97
Hyperuricemia 123
Hypervitaminosis A 121

I

Icepick scars 93f
Immune system 23, 123
Infection 79
Inflammation
  antibody-mediated 18
  depth of 25t
  hypothesis of 19
  pathophysiology of 19
Inflammatory bowel disease 151
Inflammatory lesions 36, 47f, 50f, 66, 100, 154, 161
Inflammatory nodular lesions 36
Infliximab 146
Innate immune system 21
Innate immunity 21
  abnormal 23
Insomnia 14
Insulin resistance 10, 90f
Insulin-like growth factor 140
Intracranial hypertension 120
Intralesional corticosteroids 134
Intralesional steroids 113
Isoniazid 16, 55f, 61, 69
Isopropyl myristate 5f
Isosorbide mononitrate 16, 69
Isotretinoin 118t
Isotretinoin
  drug 23
  substitute for 158
  treatment 122

K

Kahn's criteria, modified 73b
Keloid 36, 37
  lesions 113
  scar 54f

Keratotic papules 30f
Klebsiella 100

L

Lapatinib 16
Laser plus topical treatment 163
Lesions 65
  extensive 42f
  monomorphic 60f
  noninflamed 28f, 30f
  noninflammatory 36, 46, 61, 148, 154
  premenstrual 10f
  temporal 54f
  typical 74
Life-threatening 79
Lipid profiles, abnormal 102f
Lithium 16, 61, 69
Liver enzymes 103
Lupus erythematosus 120
Luteinizing hormone 96f, 101f, 104
Lymecycline 118, 120, 131
Lymphatic system 123

M

Macrophages 7f
Malassezia
  globosa 20
  sympodialis 20
Maternal hormones, effect of 17
Medroxyprogesterone 69
Meibomian glands 77
Menopausal symptoms 128
Menstrual cycle, phase of 14
Menstrual irregularity 95f
Menstruation 14
Mesalazine 16, 69
Metabolic syndrome 104
Methotrexate 16, 78
Metronidazole 114
Microbial organisms 24
Microbiologic tests 100
Microcomedone 4f, 41f
Microdermabrasion 136
Microneedle fractional radiofrequency 139
Microthermal zones 141
Milia, skin-colored papules of 83f
Minocycline 114, 118, 131
  induced pigmentation 92f
  therapy 92f
Moisturizers 130
Molluscum contagiosum mimicking papules 81f

INDEX

Mononuclear cells 100
Musculoskeletal problems 98
Myeloblasts 103
Myelocytes 103
Myocardial infarction 125

N

Nadifloxacin 114
Nail dystrophy 123
Nandrolone 69
Nasal crease, pseudoacne of 66
Nasal dryness 122
Nasopharyngitis 122
Necrotic skin 141
Neurocutaneous mechanisms 23
Neuroendocrine regulatory
   mechanism 19
Neurophysiology 20
Neutropenia 122
Nicotinamide, topical 116, 132
Nilvadipine 16, 61
Nodular lesions 32*f*
Nodules 47*f*, 65, 86
Nodulocystic lesions 49*f*, 54*f*
   deep 102
   healing with scar 32*f*
Nonclassical congenital adrenal
   hyperplasia 62, 104
Noninfective disease 6*f*
Noninflammatory papules 29*f*
Nonsteroidal anti-inflammatory
   drugs 109, 113, 132
Novosphingobium taxa 157
Nuclear retinoic acid 115

O

Obesity 96*f*
Occupation 14
Occupational acne, salient
   features of 65*t*
Ocular rosacea 76
O-hydroxybenzoic acid 115
Oily skin 26*f*
Oligomenorrhea 95*f*, 101*f*,
   102*f*, 105
   persistent 96*f*
Omega-3 fatty acid 13
Oral contraceptive pill 15, 111,
   124
Oral isotretinoin 117
   mechanism of action of 121*f*
Oral retinoids 95*f*, 120
   complications of 123*t*
Oral tetracyclines 117

Oral vitamin 158
Osteitis 10, 12
Osteolysis 72
Osteoma cutis 98, 113
Otophyma 76
Oxytetracycline 118, 131

P

PAC syndrome 70
Pain 79
Palmoplantar pustulosis 73
Panitumumab 16
PAPA syndrome 12, 61, 63, 70, 71,
   73, 113
PAPASH syndrome 70, 71
Papular lesions, developing 49*f*
Papule 35, 36, 46, 47*f*, 65, 86
   number of 79
   syringoma, skin-colored 83*f*
Papulopustular eruption 79, 112
   severity of 79*t*
Papulopustular rosacea 76
Para-aminobenzoic acid 115
Paronychia 123
PASH syndrome 71
Pentostatin 16, 69
Peroxide 37
Peroxisome proliferator-activated
   receptor 11, 18
Personal protective equipment 148
Phenobarbitone 16, 69
Phenytoin 16, 61, 69
Photoprotection 131
Photosensitive reaction 123
Phymatous rosacea 76
Pilonidal sinus 75
Pilosebaceous unit abnormalities
   24, 24*t*
Pimozide 16, 61, 69
Pityrosporum folliculitis 68
Plasma cells 100
Platelet 140
   derived growth factor 140
   rich plasma 140
Polychlorinated biphenyls 15
Polycystic ovarian
   disease 104
   syndrome 10, 33*f*, 35, 62, 71,
     88, 95*f*, 96*f*, 101*f*
Polycystic ovary 96*f*
Polymorphic lesions 47*f*
Pomade acne 64, 65
Post-acne scarring 134
Postinflammatory pigmentation
   135

Potassium iodine 16
Prednisolone 131
Predominantly pustules 30*f*
Pregnancy 14
Prepubertal girl 42*f*
Prerosacea 75
Proinflammatory cytokines,
   production of 39*f*
Prolactin levels, abnormal 101*f*
Promyelocytes 103
Propionibacterium acnes 153
Propylene glycol 6*f*
Proteinuria 122
Pruritus 79, 122
Pseudocysts 46, 65
Psoriasis 98
Psychocutaneous disorders 67
Psychological stress 35, 97
Punch excision and grafting 142
Punch floatation technique 142
Punch incision and elevation 142
Pustule 35, 46, 47*f*, 65, 86
   number of 79
Pustulosis 10, 12
Pyoderma gangrenosum 10, 12,
   61
Pyogenic arthritis 10, 12, 61
Pyogenic granuloma 63, 98, 113
Pyrazinamide 16, 61, 69

Q

Quality of life 98, 106, 144
   assessment of 26
   health-related 159
   inventory 99
Quinine 16

R

Radiation 15
Ramipril 16, 69
Reactions, severe 113
Reactive oxygen species 24*t*, 25
Red papules 148
Red-light therapy 135
Reduce inflammatory lesions 152
Refractory acne treatment 145
Resorcinol 113, 114, 132
Retinoic acid 37
   topical 106*f*
Retinoid 109, 113, 115, 120,
   148, 158
   mode of action of 121
   topical 111, 114, 117, 158
Retinol moisturizer 153

INDEX

Retroauricular papules 54f
Rheumatoid arthritis 77
Rhinophyma 76
Ribavirin 15
Ribonucleic acid 114
Risperidone 16, 61, 69
Ritonavir 16, 61, 69
Rosacea 24, 24b, 60f
   etiological factors of 24f
   fulminans 77
   granulosa 60f
   inflammatory 75
   pathogenesis of 24
   risk factors in 24, 24b
   solid facial edema of 98
   subtype of 24, 76b
   type 80
   vascular 75

S

SAHA syndrome 56f, 61, 70, 71, 96f, 125
Salicylic acid 113, 115, 132, 135, 148
Sandpaper comedones 27f, 28f, 36
SAPHO syndrome 12, 61, 70-72, 72t, 102, 103
   diagnosis of 73b
Scalp, dissecting cellulitis of 75
Scar 37, 74, 86, 134t, 136
   box 37
   deep irregular 53f
   disfiguring 51f
   formation, pathogenesis of 21, 25
   hormone profile, abnormal 95f
   moderate acne with 33f
   permanent 97
   pigmented 55f
   post acne, superficial 92f
   superficial 108f
   varioliform 93f
Seasonal variation 15
Sebaceous gland hyperplasia 20
Sebolamellar sheath, rupture of 6f
Seborrhea 6f, 7f, 10, 40f, 42f, 47f, 88f, 91, 94f, 96f, 101f, 107f
   marked 103
   premenstrual 8f
Sebum production, increased 17
Selumetinib 16
Senile comedones 85f

Sensitive skin 79, 80
Serratia 100
Sertraline 16, 61, 69
Sex hormone-binding globulin 124
Sinus 74
Sirolimus 16
Skin
   care 130
      role of 129
   caucasian 157
   disorder 153
   inflammation 162
      scarring 162
   lesions 63, 122
   sensitivity and cosmetic intolerance syndrome 79
   type 130
Smoking 13
Sodium
   fluoride 16
   sulfacetamide 113, 132
Solid facial edema 60f, 98, 113
Spironolactone 117, 125
Stanozolol 69
Staphylococcus 157
   aureus 100, 122
Steatocystoma, cystic lesions of 82f
Steatocytoma 82f
Steroid
   acne, diagnosis of 69
   rosacea 69
Stevens–Johnson syndrome 120, 140
Stratum corneum 129
Streptococcus 157
Stress 14
Subcision 137
Submarine comedones 28f
Sulfamethoxazole 118-120, 131
Sulfur 16, 69, 113, 132
   precipitate 118
   topical 115
Sunlight 15
Synovitis 10, 12, 72
Syringoma 84f
Systemic retinoids 107f

T

T cells 7f
Tacrolimus 16
Tazarotene 160-162
   lotion

      efficacy of 161
      safety of 161
Tenderness 79
Tetrachlorodibenzodioxin 112
Tetrachlorodibenzo-p-dioxin 14
Tetracycline 112, 118, 120, 131
Thiouracil 16, 69
Thiourea 16, 69
Thyroid
   diseases 77
   replacement 132
Tinea faciei 82f
Topiramate 16, 69
Toxic epidermal necrolysis 120
Trametinib 16
Trauma, severe self-induced 93f
Tretinoin 115, 118, 132
Triamcinolone acetonide 135
Triazoloquinoxalines 15
Trichloroacetic acid 133
Trichostasis spinulosa 84f
Trifarotene
   efficacy of 162
   monotherapy 162
Trimethoprim 118-120, 131
Troxidone 16, 69
Truncal acne 95f, 154, 162
   vulgaris, treatment of 161
Tuberculoderma 68
Tumor necrosis factor-alpha inhibitors, role of 146

U

Ultraviolet radiation 15
Upper respiratory parcel 163

V

Vascular endothelial growth factor 25
Virilizing syndrome 105
Visible follicular opening 27f
Vitamin
   B12 15, 16, 61, 69
   B6 15
Vulgaris treatment 156
V-zone acne with pustule 30f

X

XYY genotype 2

Z

Zinc 113, 116, 131, 132
   coceth sulfate 130
   topical 116

EU GSPR Authorised Reprsentative
Logos Europe, 9 rue Nicolas Poussin
1700, La Rochelle, France
Phone: +33 (0) 6 67 93 73 78
E-mail: contact@logoseurope.eu

www.ingramcontent.com/pod-product-compliance
Ingram Content Group UK Ltd.
Pitfield, Milton Keynes, MK11 3LW, UK
UKHW051138270226
468476UK00003B/26